Diagnosis and Management of Musculoskeletal Disorders

Diagnosis and Management of Musculoskeletal Disorders

Editor: Joel Reynolds

AMERICAN
MEDICAL PUBLISHERS
www.americanmedicalpublishers.com

AMERICAN
MEDICAL PUBLISHERS
www.americanmedicalpublishers.com

Cataloging-in-Publication Data

Diagnosis and management of musculoskeletal disorders / edited by Joel Reynolds.
p. cm.
Includes bibliographical references and index.
ISBN 978-1-63927-392-8
1. Musculoskeletal system--Diseases. 2. Orthopedics. 3. Bones--Diseases.
4. Joints--Diseases. I. Reynolds, Joel.
RC925 .H36 2021
616.74--dc23

American Medical Publishers,
41 Flatbush Avenue,
1st Floor, New York,
NY 11217, USA

ISBN 978-1-63927-392-8 (Hardback)

Contents

Preface

In my initial years as a student, I used to run to the library at every possible instance to grab a book and learn something new. Books were my primary source of knowledge and I would not have come such a long way without all that I learnt from them. Thus, when I was approached to edit this book; I became understandably nostalgic. It was an absolute honor to be considered worthy of guiding the current generation as well as those to come. I put all my knowledge and hard work into making this book most beneficial for its readers.

The human musculoskeletal system enables humans to move with the help of their skeletal and muscular systems. It consists of joints, ligaments, nerves, muscles, tendons and the structures that support limbs, back and neck. Any injury or pain in the human musculoskeletal system is known as a musculoskeletal disorder. It can be caused by an interaction of physical factors with ergonomic, occupational, psychological and social factors. Sudden exertion or continuous repetitive motion that exposes the musculoskeletal system to repeated force, vibration and uncomfortable postures can lead to these disorders. Different body parts such as upper and lower back, shoulders, necks, arms, hands, legs and feet are affected by the disorders of the musculoskeletal system. Some of the common musculoskeletal disorders are tendinitis, carpal tunnel syndrome, back pain, epicondylitis and tension neck syndrome. This book unravels the recent studies in the field of musculoskeletal disorders. It also elucidates some of the vital pieces of work conducted across the world, on various topics related this field. The book, with its detailed analyses and data, will prove immensely beneficial to professionals and students involved in this area at various levels.

I wish to thank my publisher for supporting me at every step. I would also like to thank all the authors who have contributed their researches in this book. I hope this book will be a valuable contribution to the progress of the field.

Editor

Risk factors for neck pain among forklift truck operators

U. Flodin[1*], B. Rolander[2,3], H. Löfgren[4], B. Krapi[1], F. Nyqvist[1] and C. Wåhlin[1,5]

Abstract

Background: No previous research has been performed into neck pain among forklift operators. This is a common complaint among these workers, who number around 150,000 in Sweden and six million in Europe. The aim of the study was to examine long-term exposure to unnatural neck positions among forklift operators as a risk factor for neck pain.

Methods: A retrospective cohort study was conducted of all eligible employees at a high-level warehouse. Forklift operators and office workers answered an 18-page questionnaire comprising questions about joint pain, work tasks, work postures and year of start for all items. By using person years in the exposed and less-exposed groups before start of neck pain we were able to calculate Incident Rate ratios for various exposures.

Results: Forty nine percent of the forklift operators reported having experienced neck pain compared to 30 % of office workers. Being a forklift operator was associated with an increased risk of neck pain (OR = 5.1, 95% CI 1.4–18.2). Holding the head in an unnatural position resulted in significantly increased risks for neck pain, irrespective of type of position. The risks for neck pain remained after taking other ergonomic exposures and psychosocial aspects into consideration.

Conclusions: This is the first published study showing that forklift operators have an increased risk of neck pain. The results are therefore of significance for improving work schedules, the adjustment of work tasks for these workers and the design of the vehicles.

Keywords: Forklift operators, Neck pain, Ergonomics, Work postures, Retrospective cohort study, Occupational medicine

Background

Risk factors for persistent neck pain in workers are described in a great number of papers. A Swedish review by the Swedish council on health technology assessment was published in 2012 [1]. It focused on the impact of work on the incidence of symptoms and disorders in the neck and shoulders and upper extremities. The review concluded that there is a lack of high quality research to support the association between long-term pronounced flexion, extension or rotation of the head and the development of neck and shoulder pain. This review only scrutinized cohort studies and randomized controlled trials. The cohort studies included in the review covered the general population of Denmark [2–4]; a number of industrial and service sectors [5]; office workers [6]; female nurses [7] and industrial forestry workers [8]. There are at least eight epidemiological studies of forklift operators. However, seven of them do not focus on neck pain [9] and only one addresses neck pain [10]. That study does not, however, evaluate the specific role of neck positions and does not distinguish forklift operators from drivers of earth-moving machines and buses in public transport.

The work of forklift truck operators in large, high-level warehouses involves extension of the neck when loading and unloading the forklift on shelves at high levels – up to 12 levels above the operators. Throughout the workday they repeatedly rotate their heads when reversing the forklift some hundred metres at a time. They also lean to the side to get a better view when loading and unloading their vehicle. Thus, these forklift truck operators are exposed to a variety of non-neutral head positions in their daily work.

* Correspondence: ulf.flodin@regionostergotland.se
[1]Occupational and Environmental Medicine, and Department of Clinical and Experimental Medicine, Linköping University, Östergötland, 581 85 Linköping, Sweden

Our clinic was given the opportunity to perform a retrospective cohort study on a large group of forklift operators at a large warehouse in southern Sweden. A literature review we performed found no other studies of forklift operators with a specific focus on neck pain. The present study gives us a greater understanding of the association between non-neutral head positions at work and neck pain among forklift operators. The aim of the study was to examine long-term exposure to unnatural neck positions among forklift operators as a risk factor for neck pain.

Methods

Study population

This is a retrospective cohort study. All permanently employed staff at a warehouse, which included forklift operators and administrative personnel, were invited to participate. The study was supported by the union and the human resource managers. Four hundred and twenty nine questionnaires were posted to all workers at their home addresses in May 2014. After three postal reminders, 194 subjects (45%) had replied to the questionnaire. The study was approved by the Regional Ethical Review Board at the University of Linköping, Sweden (2014 02 26 Dnr. 2013/418–31).

Exposure and risk factors

The workplace was first visited by two experienced ergonomists who documented, photographed and filmed the workplace. They were particularly interested in significantly extended, rotated and lateral flexed neck movements among forklift operators. Some of these were interviewed about what they perceived as awkward postures. This information formed the basis for the questions in the questionnaire. Three types of forklift truck are used at the warehouse: the low-lift order picker, the reach decker and the counterbalanced tilting mast. The low-lifting order picker is operated in a standing position; in the other two types of forklift truck the operator is seated. Most of the workers switch between the three. All of them require the operator to hold his/her head in unnatural positions. When reversing the truck the operator rotates the head at least 45 degrees; when loading the fork at high levels he/she holds the head a lateral flexed position, in combination with rotation and extension (backward bending).

The questionnaire

Exposure information for the employees was collected by means of an 18-page questionnaire containing 41 questions evaluating workplace conditions; demands and health, including job title; start and end of employment; type of forklift truck; work tasks and position of the neck while working. They were also asked about whether they had ever had neck pain; experience of neck pain in the previous seven days; onset and end of neck pain; shoulder pain and a work ability single-item question. Questions about pain and work ability have been used in previous studies [11, 12]. Only self-reported measures were used to classify workers with neck pain and/or shoulder pain for the main outcome. For this study, the definition of having neck pain is based on the question "Do you have or have you had pain, ache or discomfort in your neck?" with a yes/no answer. If yes, the informant gave the year of start and end of symptoms. The definition of having shoulder pain is based on the question "Do you have or have you had pain, ache or discomfort in your shoulders?" with a yes/no answer. If yes, the informant gave the year of start and end of symptoms. Of particular interest were neck positions used in daily work, including neck extension, rotation and lateral flexion and the years of the start and end of exposure to these unnatural positions. General self-reported health was obtained by the question: "In general, would you say your health is…?", with five anchor points ranging between excellent and poor [13]. The worker's work satisfaction was measured on a score graded from 0 to 10, where a higher score indicates greater satisfaction. Work-related stress in the previous week was measured on a score graded from 0 to 10, where a higher score indicates higher stress level. Freedom of work was asked by the question: "Do you have the freedom to plan how you do your work?", using a 4-item scale ranging from "strongly disagree" to "strongly agree". Co-worker support was also measured by a 4-item scale. The Borg CR10 scale was used to evaluate perceived physically strenuous work [14]. All data were collected in the second quarter of 2014 from the 194 subjects who answered the questionnaire.

Statistics

Table 1 shows the univariate analyses which were performed on the two cohorts to compare demographics, health and lifestyle, work tasks and psychosocial factors between exposed (forklift operators) and less exposed (office workers). T-tests for prevalence were used for the continuous variables and cross tabulated chi-square tests for the categorical variables. Frequencies were presented in counted numbers with percentages for categorical variables and standard deviation (SD) for continuous variables. Analyses were performed using SPSS, version 23 (IBM SPSS Inc., Armonk, NY). A probability value of 0.05 (5%) was considered statistically significant. A univariate logistic regression analysis was performed (Table 2) using affirmed neck pain as the dependent variable and various potential risk factors as independent variables, in order to calculate odds ratios for neck pain during current employment (OR). Since neck and shoulder pain commonly overlap, a third combined outcome variable for neck and shoulder pain was included in this analysis. To exclude neck pain with no

Table 1 Presentation of the study populations with health outcomes, work tasks and ergonomic and psychosocial conditions

Variable	Forklift operators (*n* = 150)	Mean	SD[a]	%[b]	Office workers (*n* = 44)	Mean	SD	%	*P* Value
Demographics									
Men	110			73	24			55	0.04
Women	40			27	18			41	0.04
Age (range:21–66)		40.4	9.60			37.3	9.42		0.70
Length of employment		9.8	4.41			7.3	5.25		< 0.01
Health and lifestyle									
Has experienced neck pain	74			49	13			30	0.02
Neck pain during the previous 7 days	42			28	4			9	0.48
Intensity of neck pain		5.04	2.47			5.0	2.00		0.90
Sick leave due to neck pain	26			17	0			0	< 0.01
Shoulder pain	95			63	17			39	< 0.01
Shoulder pain during the previous 7 days	53			35	4			9	0.03
Intensity of shoulder pain		5.28	2.52			4.36	2.29		0.14
Perceived good health	121			81	39			89	0.08
Ever smoked	84			56	30			68	0.15
Work tasks									
Has previously worked as forklift operator[c]	150			100	18			41	< 0.01
Low-lifting order picker	123			82	14			32	< 0.01
Counterbalanced tilting mast	129			86	15			34	< 0.01
Reach decker	100			67	11			25	< 0.01
Never sits at work	56			37	7			16	0.02
Sits at work part of the day	42			28	8			18	0.08
Sits at work 100%	52			35	29			66	< 0.01
Works in drafts or cold	69			46	5			11	< 0.01
Floor bumps when operating forklift	69			46	5			11	< 0.01
Neck extension	108			72	9			20	< 0.01
Neck lateral flexion	104			69	8			18	< 0.01
Neck rotation	124			83	12			27	< 0.01
Monotonous arm/ hand movements	119			79	19			43	< 0.01
Heavy lifting arms/ hands	112			75	13			30	< 0.01
Work involving hands above shoulder level	100			67	7			16	< 0.01
Psychosocial factors									
Satisfied with work		7.15	1.94			8.1	1.40		0.04
Co-worker support	135			90	43			98	< 0.01
Freedom of work	105			70	39			89	< 0.01
Stress due to high work pace		5.2	2.82			5.4	2.81		0.64
Physically strenuous work		13.6	2.63			8.8	2.34		< 0.01
Work ability now compared with personal best		7.1	1.98			8.6	1.43		< 0.01

Chi squared cross-tabulations (categorical variables) and t-tests (continuous variables) for comparisons between the groups
[a]Standard deviation
[b]Missing values not taken into consideration when calculating percentages
[c]Office workers may operate forklifts on rare occasions

Table 2 Unadjusted odds ratios[a] for ever having had neck pain, shoulder pain or combined after various exposures during current employment

	Neck pain $n = 71$		Shoulder pain $n = 95$		Combined $n = 106$	
Risk factors	OR	95% CI	OR	95% CI	OR	95% CI
Age years						
18–32	Reference level		Reference level		Reference level	
33–37	0.88	0.37–2.07	0.90	0.39–2.11	0.69	0.29–1.65
38–46	1.45	0.62–3.38	0.95	0.40–2.23	1.08	0.44–2.63
47–66	1.13	0.47–2.68	1.29	0.55–3.00	1.11	0.45–2.75
Female gender	1.00	0.52–1.94	1.07	0.56–2.05	1.13	0.57–2.24
Forklift operator	5.19	1.48–18.2	3.89	1.44–10.5	3.26	1.29–8.29
Extension	3.77	1.92–7.40	2.56	1.39–4.74	3.22	1.70–6.10
Rotation	3.94	1.82–8.54	3.22	1.64–6.32	3.09	1.56–6.09
Lateral flexion	3.30	1.71–6.36	2.65	1.43–4.91	2.86	1.51–5.40
Monotonous work hands arms	4.00	1.79–8.95	3.16	1.57–6.37	3.52	1.74–7.12
Heavy physical work	2.28	1.12–4.61	3.29	1.67–6.46	2.99	1.52–5.88
Work involving hands above shoulder level	2.91	1.53–5.55	3.33	1.79–6.20	3.78	1.97–7.24
Stress due to high work pace	2.62	1.29–5.30	1.56	0.82–2.97	2.03	1.05–3.92
Has previously smoked	1.62	0.70–3.74	2.88	1.16–7.18	2.36	0.90–6.23

[a]Odds ratios from univariate logistic regression analysis using perceived neck pain, shoulder pain and combined as dependent variable and potential risk factors as independent

possible connection to the studied exposure, 16 subjects whose pain onset occurred before present employment were removed from the analysis (Tables 2 and 3).

Taking person years into consideration, the risk from exposure was calculated in a multivariate Poisson regression model. The total length of employment was calculated for each individual, either ending in 2014 or up to the first year of perceived neck pain. The exposure time was calculated from the total amount of time spent with the neck in non-neutral postures. Minimum exposure time is one calendar year. The numbers of cases in the exposed and unexposed groups were calculated. The two groups were analyzed in a regression model in order to obtain incidence rate ratios (IRR) (Table 3). All analyses were adjusted for age and gender. Poisson and the binominal regression analyses were performed with the software STATA 12 (Statistical Software StataCorp LP, US). A probability value of 0.05 (5%) was considered statistically significant. Possible confounding factors were those variables shown in Table 2 to be risk factors for neck pain. Collinearity was tested in a nonparametric Spearman's rank correlation test for every item adjusted for in the multiple regression models. To avoid interference between correlating predictors, the multiple regression analysis was carried out in three steps adjusted for different categories of work-related exposure.

Results

The characteristics of the study populations, consisting of forklift operators and office workers, are presented in Table 1. Their occupational titles are those held at the time of the questionnaire. The study presents data concerning the demographics, illness, lifestyle, exposure and psychosocial factors of forklift operators and office workers. A total of 194 employees (of whom two did not state their gender) completed the questionnaire and participated in the analysis, i.e. 45% (see "study population" above). The average age of forklift operators was 40.4 years (SD 9.6, range: 21–66) and of office workers 37.3 years (SD 9.4, range 20–63). Average length of employment was 9.8 years (SD 4.4) for forklift operators and 7.3 years (SD 5.2) for office workers. Seventy-four forklift operators (49%) and 13 (30%) office workers replied that they had at some time in adult life experienced neck pain. Intensity of neck pain on a scale from 1 to 10 was similar in both groups (mean 5). Experience of neck pain during the seven days before answering the questionnaire was reported by 28% of the forklift operators and 9% of the office workers (n.s.). Ever having been on sick leave for neck pain was significantly more common among forklift operators (17%) than among office workers (0%) $p < 0.001$. For shoulder pain, see Table 1. Many office workers started as forklift operators before later switching to office work, which explains why 41% of the office workers reported that they had at some time operated a forklift truck. Working with the head in unnatural positions (extended, in lateral flexion and/or rotated) was significantly more common among forklift operators than among office workers. Thirty-five percent of the forklift operators and 66% of the office workers

Table 3 Incidence rate ratios for neck pain by years of exposure adjusted for age and gender, psychosocial aspects and hand/shoulder work

	A = age and gendSer		B = A+ Psychosocial aspects		C = A+ Hand/shoulder work	
Neck postures and exposure time	IRR[a]	95% CI[b]	IRR	95% CI	IRR	95% CI
Extension						
Non exposed	Reference level		Reference level		Reference level	
1–2 years	**3.09**	**1.08–8.86**	1.23	0.97–8.85	2.09	0.70–6.28
3–4 years	**5.34**	**2.42–11.78**	**4.63**	**2.00–10.72**	**3.56**	**1.52–8.36**
5–9 years	**2.01**	**1.00–4.03**	1.89	0.91–3.92	1.38	0.63–2.99
10- years	1.04	0.48–2.20	1.05	0.48–2.31	0.71	0.32–1.60
Rotation						
Non exposed	Reference level		Reference level		Reference level	
1–2 years	**7.10**	**2.63–19.14**	**5.86**	**2.08–16.50**	**6.24**	**1.97–19.79**
3–4 years	**5.70**	**2.47–13.27**	**5.00**	**2.09–11.99**	**4.76**	**1.67–13.65**
5–9 years	1.70	0.78–3.74	1.49	0.67–3.31	1.58	0.62–4.04
10- years	1.24	0.53–2.91	1.13	0.47–2.71	1.11	0.39–3.14
Lateral flexion						
Non exposed	Reference level		Reference level		Reference level	
1–2 years	**5.60**	**2.23–14.09**	**4.51**	**1.67–12.13**	**4.35**	**1.68–11.29**
3–4 years	**3.76**	**1.80–7.80**	**3.54**	**1.67–7.49**	**3.06**	**1.40–6.69**
5–9 years	1.55	0.79–3.05	1.37	0.68–2.77	1.30	0.64–2.66
10- years	0.90	0.41–1.94	0.84	0.37–1.89	0.72	0.31–1.64

Bold numbers are those statistically significant at 95% confidence level
Poisson multivariate regression model. Person years were calculated from years of employment and years of exposure up to the debut of perceived neck pain
[a]Incidence rate ratio
[b]95% Confidence interval. Column B; Psychosocial factors included: mental stress, lack of co-worker support and freedom to perform your work. Column C; Hand/shoulder work includes monotonous work with arms/hands, heavy lifting and work involving hands above shoulder level

reported sitting for 100% of the working day. Thirty-seven percent of the forklift operators and 16% of the office workers reported that they did not sit at all. Twenty-eight percent of forklift operators said that they sat for part of the day compared with 18% of office workers (Table 1).

Work satisfaction, on a 10 degree scale, was higher for office workers (8.1) than for forklift operators (7.15) ($p = 0.04$). Good co-worker support was reported by 90% of the forklift operators as compared with 98% of the office workers ($p < 0.001$). Eighty-nine percent of office workers reported that they were free to decide how to perform their work, as compared with 70% of forklift operators 70% ($p < 0.001$). There were no reported differences in perceived stressed from a high work pace. Forklift operators had a significantly higher physical workload than office workers, 13.6 versus 8.8 $p < 0.01$ on a 20-item scale. Current work ability compared to peak ability was significantly lower among forklift operators than in office workers: 7.1 versus 8.6 $p < 0.01$ on a 10-item scale.

Odds ratios (OR) for potential risk factors are presented in Table 2. Ever having worked as a forklift operator is associated with an increased risk of having neck pain (OR = 5.19; 95 CI 1.48–18.2. Holding the head in unnatural positions also resulted in an increased risk of neck pain; extended (OR = 3.77; 95% CI 1.92–7.4), rotated (OR = 3.9; 95% 1.8–8.5 CI) or laterally flexed (OR =3.3; 95% 1.7–6.4 CI). Monotonous hand and arm work, heavy manual work and manual work tasks above shoulder-level as well as mental stress were associated with neck pain. There was no significant association between age or gender and neck pain (Table 2). Similar results were obtained for shoulder pain (Table 2).

In an incident rate ratio (IRR) analysis of neck pain we looked at length of exposure to unnatural neck positions (Table 3), with person years up to the first year of neck pain or the end of the study period for the exposed group and the corresponding time for the unexposed subjects. The results reveal that 1–2 years of neck extension at work leads to a higher risk of neck pain than the corresponding length of employment for non-exposed workers (IRR = 3.09; 95% CI 1.08–8.9). Three to four years of neck extension further increased the risk of neck pain (IRR = 5.34; 95% CI 2.4–11.8). Of all the types of exposure in this model – extension, rotation and lateral flexion of the neck – the first four years of exposure are most strongly associated with increased risk of neck pain, when age and gender have been taken into account (Table 3, column A).When the psychosocial factors of mental stress, lack of co-worker support and freedom to perform work are taken into account in the Poisson regression, the IRR for neck pain from unnatural neck positions were somewhat weakened (Table 3, column B). When ergonomically strenuous hand/arm work are included in the Poisson regression, the IRR for neck pain from extension, 3–4 years, still presents an increased risk (IRR = 3.56; 95% CI 1.52–8.36) (for more details, see Table 3, column C). Exposure to rotation as a forklift operator for at least one year resulted in a significantly increased risk of neck pain; for rotation 1–2 years (IRR = 5.86; 95% CI 2.08–16.5).

Discussion

Even working as a forklift operator with one's head in unnatural positions for a couple of years resulted in a significantly increased risk of developing neck pain compared to those working with their heads in natural positions. In this study, the work title 'forklift operator' was used as a proxy for holding one's head in unnatural positions, while the title 'office worker' was used as a proxy for more neutral head positions. The use of work titles makes it possible to translate ergonomic neck exposures into occupational titles rather than angles of neck position. This also helps us to understand and improve the ergonomic situation of forklift operators. An increased risk of neck pain was observed after 1–2 years of exposure; this then gradually reduced after 5–9 years of exposure. The reduced incident risk ratios by increasing number of years can be explained by the fact that forklift operators who developed neck pain were eventually obliged to leave the workplace. Since this is a retrospective cohort study rather than a prospective one, we are not able to include those workers who left. We can, however, make the assumption that those who left were more likely to be suffering from neck or other localized pain. This would involve a bias towards the null. But despite this phenomenon, the risks from operating forklifts remain.

The workplace where the study was performed is a major international company which offers many opportunities for career development. This explains why so many office workers have previously worked as forklift operators. It would have been interesting to evaluate the harmful effects of the three types of forklift truck (low-lifting order picker, reach decker and counterbalanced tilting mast). However, the operators switched between vehicles in order to get a more varied working day, which means that we cannot distinguish the effects of the individual types of vehicle.

Other studies have analyzed the association between neck positions and neck pain. Van den Heuvel et al. [15] looked at neck extension and found an association with neck and shoulder symptoms (OR =2.4 significant) in a group of office workers. The odds ratio for neck extension among forklift operators in our study is 3.7 (Table 2). The result seems reasonable, even with higher risk estimates up to 5.34 (Column A, Table 3), since forklift operators are exposed to more strenuous neck positions than office workers.

Van den Heuvel et al. [15] also studied the effects of neck rotation on neck pain risk among office workers. Their group found a crude OR of 2.6, significant, at rotation over 45 degrees for 14–45% of working time, while Marcus et al. [16] found only a slightly elevated risk among computer users (HR 1.17, N.S.) and Ariens et al. [5] reported an RR of 1.4 (N.S.) in their mixed occupation cohort. Again, the neck pain risk we found from rotation in a group of forklift operators (OR 3.9, Table 2) seems reasonable given that forklift operators are more exposed to unnatural head positions than the two other cohorts studied. For lateral flexion we found an OR of 3.3 (Table 2). To the best of our knowledge, the only previous study to have evaluated the association between neck/shoulder pain and lateral neck flexion, by Marcus et al. [16], found a non-significant association. However, they chose a minimal tilt angle for their study (> 3 degrees). According to our workplace observations of the forklift operators, exposure to lateral flexion, rotation and extension was more pronounced in our study than in a study by Marcus et al. [16].

We have chosen office workers as the reference group. A review of neck pain among office workers by Paksaichol et al. [17] was based on seven prospective cohort studies. They found only female gender and previous neck pain to be strong risk factors for the onset of new episodes of neck pain. Our reference group of office workers had a higher proportion of women (41%) than the exposed group of forklift operators (27%). This is a possible negative confounder which may reduce the effects of the ergonomic exposure among the forklift operators. We have therefore adjusted for gender in Table 3. We have also adjusted for age since it is a common risk factor for pain. These adjustments could explain the higher risks observed in Table 3 than in Table 2, where there is no adjustment for age and gender.

Psychological factors associated with neck pain are also commonly discussed in the literature. In one review, McLean et al. [18] report high job demands and poor social work support among office workers as strong risk factors for neck pain. In a review of office workers by Deokhoon et al. [19], they found that low satisfaction with the workplace environment, low work task variation, keyboard position and self-perceived muscular tension, were risk factors for developing neck pain. In our study we included some of these psychosocial work exposures, but they did not greatly affect the risk of neck pain from unnatural neck positions (Table 3, Column B). Since previous studies have identified risk factors for neck pain to be work positions which involve holding the hands above shoulder level [2, 8]; heavy physical work [2, 4] and monotonous hand/arm work [4, 20], we included these ergonomic exposures in our Poisson regression. Here, the risks from the unnatural neck positions remained, albeit somewhat weaker (Table 3, Column C).

In our study we examined the effect of three unnatural positions: extension, lateral flexion and rotation. We did not focus on exposure to neck flexion, since our study group of forklift operators does not assume that position very frequently. Previous studies give considerable support to the contention that the effects of exposure to neck flexion are harmful [4, 5, 21, 22]. When comparing prevalence of ever having had neck pain in our material (49% of forklift operators and 30% of office workers, Table 1) with studies of workers in the general population, the annual prevalence of neck pain varies from 27% in Norway to 33% in the UK and 47% in Quebec, Canada [23]. The annual prevalence of neck pain varies between occupations. A recent Swedish study shows that neck pain is common among workers in public dentistry, with an annual prevalence of 60–67% [24]. Cote et al. [23] showed in their review that neck pain ranged from 17% among dentists to 72% among dental hygienists. For office workers, the one-year prevalence of neck pain varied from 17.7% among Norwegian administrative workers to 63% among Swedish secretaries. For blue-collar workers, the annual prevalence of neck pain among Swedish crane operators is 74% [23]. Working with the cervical spine in flexion for long periods of time may increase the risk of neck pain. In a study by Marcus et al. [16], people exposed to a head position which involves tilting the head at an angle greater than 3° were 50% more likely to develop neck/shoulder pain than people who were not exposed to this kind of head position. In conclusion, Cote P et al. [23] found that neck pain is an important cause of disability. Likewise they found that physical and psychosocial exposures at the workplace contribute to an increased risk of cervical pain. Another review by McLean et al. [18] evaluated the link between occupational exposures and neck pain. They found an association between neck pain and psycho-social factors apart from age and earlier neck injury. Most occupational risk factors were only of limited evidence. The one-week prevalence in our material was 28% among the forklift operators and 9% among the office workers. In Sweden generally, the one-week prevalence of neck pain varies from 7% of office workers to 53% of female plant workers in the laminate industry [23]. When comparing different prevalence rates found in the literature it is important to bear in mind that the questionnaires used in the various studies will have differed. Comparisons within studies will therefore be more accurate than those between studies.

Methodology

The strengths of this study are the long follow-up time (with a mean exposure time of 9.8 years for the forklift operators) and the fairly homogenous observed exposure situation. The exposure took place at two large warehouses belonging to one large company. A weakness of the study is the overall response rate of 45%. Our recruiting method was to invite all workers to participate and answer a questionnaire about experienced health and work environment. We invited every worker to participate independently of health status. We did not specifically approach those with neck pain. The study was supported both by the union and the human resource manager, who informed and encouraged all workers at their staff meetings to participate in the study. In the invitation the workers were guaranteed that their questionnaire answers would not be made available to anyone other than the research team. Three reminders were given. The response rate was 40% for the forklift operators and 60% for the office workers. The difference in response rates can probably be explained by the fact that it is likely to be easier for office workers than for forklift operators to answer a questionnaire. However, one can also imagine that those forklift operators who do not have neck pain might be less motivated to answer the questionnaire than their colleagues who do have symptoms. This would give falsely high risk estimates for unnatural neck positions. To correct for possible skewedness we have added the number of person years in the group of forklift operators who did not have neck pain by 50% as for simulating the same answer percentage in the forklift operators as in the office workers. By adding person years only in the non-symptomatic group we have constructed a worst-case biased scenario. This simulation gives an IRR for extension of the neck IRR = 2.7, 95% CI 1.1–6.4. Thus, the risks associated with unnatural neck positions remain. Another explanation for the low response frequency is the high percentage of immigrants with a poor knowledge of Swedish among the forklift operators. However, this would not bias the final results, since there is no reason to assume that the immigrant workers would have a higher or lower proportion of neck pain than their native Swedish colleagues.

We have conducted a retrospective cohort study with one exposed group, forklift operators, which we compare with a less exposed group, office workers. However, a certain degree of misclassification occurred since some office workers said that they had been exposed to unnatural neck positions. This is shown in Table 1, where we present a cross-sectional perspective. Thus, a non-differential misclassification has occurred, which would lower the prevalence rate ratios presented in Table 2. In Table 3, where we used person years as a measure of exposure to unnatural neck positions instead of occupational title, the misclassification is minimized.

Information about exposure was obtained by means of a questionnaire. We did not measure the angles of head rotation, extension or lateral flexion. We did, however, spend several days observing the subjects at work. We systematically recorded that the forklift operators held their heads in unnatural positions for most of their working hours, unlike the office workers, who spent most of their working time with natural head positions. In this study we have focused on the outcome variable neck pain. Our definition of neck pain is the answers of the respondents to the question "Do you have or have you had pain, ache or discomfort in your neck?" combined with a question about year of start and end of pain. This is a broad question which is intended to include workers with different degrees of pain intensity. We used the answers to this question to calculate the prevalence of ever having had neck/ or shoulder pain as a forklift operator or office worker in Table 1. Table 2 presents the odds ratios for prevalence for these two occupational groups.

Respondents give a more precise description of their pain in a question which asks about the intensity of pain in the previous seven days, on a scale from 0 = no pain up to 10 = pain as intense as pain can be. Mean pain intensity among forklift operators and office workers was similar, about 5 (Table 1). We have also reported risk indicators for neck pain and shoulder pain in Table 2. Because we asked about year of start and end of neck pain, we could calculate years of exposure before neck pain onset, the results of which are presented in Table 3. To avoid interference between correlating predictors, the multiple regression analysis was performed in three steps adjusted for different categories of work-related exposure.

There is an association between neck and shoulder pain because they share many of the same work-related risk factors. These include awkward postures, unnatural, static positions and mental stress due to high work pace. The forklift operators use both neck and shoulder muscles in their work. How muscle activation patterns and cervical range of motion are related to neck and shoulder pain could be studied further for this group of workers. No clinical or radiological examinations were performed so diagnosis using ICD-10 was not carried out. The diagnoses of the respondents were not elucidated. In the Swedish health care system, neck pain can be given a variety of classifications such as cervicalgia ICD code M 54.2; cervico-brachial syndrome ICD code M 53.1 (if pain radiates into the arms); and cervicocranial syndrome M53.0 (if the neck pain radiates up into the head). In some cases, a specific diagnosis can identified, such as herniated discs in the cervical spine ICD code M 50.1; spondylosis M47, or spinal stenosis M48. For a more precise analysis of the correlation between unnatural neck positions and specific diagnoses it would have been necessary to perform a thorough medical and radiological examination with Magnetic Resonance Imaging (MRI). Although this was not possible in our study, we nevertheless consider it valuable to try to establish the association between unnatural head positions and neck pain. Neck pain is a highly distressing condition. In our clinical experience, all advances in our understanding of how the risk of neck pain can be reduced are important, even if precise anatomical diagnoses are not available.

The sample size of our study is not very large. However, since the risk of neck pain from the exposure is high and the proportion of exposed subjects is also high, the number of subjects in this study is sufficient for us to be able to draw conclusions. Thus, the statistical significance tests resulted in the lower 95% confidence intervals exceeding the null for a large part of the associations. When working with a binary outcome, sample size is important for achieving sufficient statistical power. When one is addressing specific exposures, their proportion must also be taken into consideration: the exposed group should be at least 30% of the total number of participants in the analysis [25]. These are requirements are fulfilled in our study.

Practical implications

The present study is, to the best of our knowledge, the first ever published about the association between forklift operating and neck pain. The results are in line with other studies of unnatural neck positions at work. There are 150,000 forklift operators in Sweden according to the manufacturing industry and Statistics Sweden. In Europe there are some six million forklift operators and globally about 20 million. The numbers are calculated by multiplying the numbers of forklift trucks sold every year by eleven (i.e. the lifetime of a forklift truck) multiplied again by two (the number of operators using one truck during a work shift) [26]. According to our results, 49% of forklift operators suffer from periodic neck pain. Furthermore, 28% reported neck pain during the previous week. Neck pain is obviously a major problem for forklift operators; it impacts their personal life as well as society.

The designers of forklift vehicles are aware of the problem and are working on solutions. We hope that this study will encourage them to prioritize the development of better-designed and more ergonomic vehicles.

Even 1–2 years of forklift driving with the head in an unnatural position increases the risk of neck pain. The condition is handicapping and makes some kinds of work impossible to perform. Efforts should therefore be made to improve the working conditions of forklift operators; this includes physical and organizational factors as well as improving operator ergonomics. Since a forklift machine is used for about eleven years, it is worthwhile looking at how the machines already in use can be improved while we wait for new, ergonomically-superior forklift trucks to be available.

Conclusions

This is the first published study showing that forklift operators have an increased risk of neck pain. Even 1–2 years of forklift driving increases the risk of neck pain. Efforts should therefore be made to improve the working conditions of forklift operators. The results are of significance for improving work schedules and adjustment of work tasks for about 150,000 workers in Sweden and six million in Europe and, should also be of interest for those designing the vehicles.

Abbreviations

CI: Confidence interval; ICD: International Statistical Classification of Disease and Related Health Problems; IRR: Incident rate ratio; MRI: Magnetic resonance imaging; N.S: Non significant; OR: Odds ratio; SD: Standard deviation

Acknowledgements

The authors would like to thank Anna-Lena Hällsten for her excellent support and assistance with this project. We would also like to express our gratitude to all the participants in the study who completed the questionnaire.

Funding

This study was supported by grants from Medical Research Council of Southeast Sweden.

Authors' contributions

UF, CW and BR wrote part of the application for research funding, contributed to the creating of the questionnaire, was a member of the group creating contact with the enterprise in order to make this study possible. Also wrote part of the manuscript. FN worked with management of the data set, statistical analysis and wrote parts of the methodology section in the article. HL contributed to the application for research funding, to the discussions among the authors how to interpret the results and to the revision of the manuscript. BK has taken part in the planning process of the study and contributed to the questionnaire with observations from the workplace of the exposure situations, thereby improving the questionnaire. He has compiled relevant literature for the background and discussion part of our paper. All authors have read and approved the final manuscript.

Consent for publication

Not applicable.

Competing interests

The authors declare that they have no competing interests.

Author details

[1]Occupational and Environmental Medicine, and Department of Clinical and Experimental Medicine, Linköping University, Östergötland, 581 85 Linköping, Sweden. [2]Department of Behavioral Science and Social Work, School of Health Sciences, Jönköping University, Jönköping, Sweden. [3]Futurum, Academy for Health and Care, Region Jönköping County, Jönköping, Sweden. [4]Neuro-Orthopedic Center, Ryhov Hospital, Jönköping, Sweden. [5]Unit of Intervention and Implementation Research, Institute for Environmental Medicine, Karolinska Institutet, Stockholm, Sweden.

References

1. Arbetets betydesle för uppkomst av besvär och sjukdomar. Nacken och övre rörelseapparaten. En systematisk litteraturöversikt. Stockholm:Statens beredning för medicinsk utvärdering (SBU); 2012.
2. Andersen JH, Haahr JP, Frost P. Risk factors for more severe regional musculoskeletal symptoms: a two-year prospective study of a general working population. Arthritis Rheum. 2007;56(4):1355–64.
3. Andersen JH, Harhoff M, Grimstrup S, Vilstrup I, Lassen CF, Brandt LP, et al. Computer mouse use predicts acute pain but not prolonged or chronic pain in the neck and shoulder. Occup Environ Med. 2008;65(2):126–31.
4. Andersen JH, Kaergaard A, Mikkelsen S, Jensen UF, Frost P, Bonde JP, et al. Risk factors in the onset of neck/shoulder pain in a prospective study of workers in industrial and service companies. Occup Environ Med. 2003;60(9): 649–54.
5. Ariens GA, Bongers PM, Douwes M, Miedema MC, Hoogendoorn WE, van der Wal G, et al. Are neck flexion, neck rotation, and sitting at work risk factors for neck pain? Results of a prospective cohort study. Occup Environ Med. 2001;58(3):200–7.
6. Bergqvist U, Knave B, Voss M, Wibom R. A longitudinal study of VDT work and health. Int J Hum Comput Interact. 1992;4:197–219.
7. Smedley J, Inskip H, Trevelyan F, Buckle P, Cooper C, et al. Risk factors for incident neck and shoulder pain in hospital nurses. Occup Environ Med. 2003;60(11):864–9.
8. Viikari-Juntura E, Martikainen R, Luukkonen R, Mutanen P, Takala EP, Riihimaki H. Longitudinal study on work related and individual risk factors affecting radiating neck pain. Occup Environ Med. 2001;58(5):345–52.
9. Waters T, Genaidy A, Deddens J, Barriera-Viruet H. Lower back disorders among forklift operators: an emerging occupational health problem? Am J Ind Med. 2005;47(4):333–40.
10. Bovenzi M. A prospective cohort study of neck and shoulder pain in professional drivers. Ergonomics. 2015;58(7):1103–16.
11. Jonker D, Gustafsson E, Rolander B, Arvidsson I, Nordander C. Health surveillance under adverse ergonomics conditions–validity of a screening method adapted for the occupational health service. Ergonomics. 2015; 58(9):1519–28.
12. Roelen CA, van Rhenen W, Groothoff JW, van der Klink JJ, Twisk JW, Heymans MW. Work ability as prognostic risk marker of disability pension: single-item work ability score versus multi-item work ability index. Scand J Work Environ Health. 2014;40(4):428–31.
13. DeSalvo KB, Jones TM, Peabody J, McDonald J, Fihn S, Fan V, et al. Health care expenditure prediction with a single item, self-rated health measure. Med Care. 2009;47(4):440–7.
14. Borg G. Psychophysical scaling with applications in physical work and the perception of exertion. Scand J Work Environ Health. 1990;16 Suppl 1:55–8.
15. van den Heuvel SG, van der Beek AJ, Blatter BM, Bongers PM. Do work-related physical factors predict neck and upper limb symptoms in office workers? Int Arch Occup and Environ Health. 2006;79(7):585–92.
16. Marcus M, Gerr F, Monteilh C, Ortiz DJ, Gentry E, Cohen S, et al. A prospective study of computer users: II. Postural risk factors for musculoskeletal symptoms and disorders. Am J Ind Med. 2002;41(4):236–49.
17. Paksaichol A, Janwantanakul P, Purepong N, Pensri P, van der Beek AJ. Office workers' risk factors for the development of non-specific neck pain: a systematic review of prospective cohort studies. Occup Environ Med. 2012; 69(9):610–8.
18. McLean SM, May S, Klaber-Moffett J, Sharp DM, Gardiner E. Risk factors for the onset of non-specific neck pain: a systematic review. J Epidemiol Community Health. 2010;64(7):565–72.
19. Jun D, Zoe M, Johnston V, O'Leary S. Physical risk factors for developing non-specific neck pain in office workers: a systematic review and meta-analysis. Int Arch Occup Environ Health. 2017;90(5):373–410.
20. Jensen C. Development of neck and hand-wrist symptoms in relation to duration of computer use at work. Scand J Work Environ Health. 2003;29(3): 197–205.
21. Hamberg-van Reenen HH, Ariens GA, Blatter BM, van der Beek AJ, Twisk JW, van Mechelen W, et al. Is an imbalance between physical capacity and exposure to work-related physical factors associated with low-back, neck or shoulder pain? Scand J Work Environ Health. 2006;32(3):190–7.

22. Nordander C, Hansson GA, Ohlsson K, Arvidsson I, Balogh I, Stromberg U, et al. Exposure-response relationships for work-related neck and shoulder musculoskeletal disorders - analyses of pooled uniform data sets. Appl Ergons. 2016;55:70–84.
23. Cote P, van der Velde G, Cassidy JD, Carroll LJ, Hogg-Johnson S, Holm LW, et al. The burden and determinants of neck pain in workers: results of the bone and joint decade 2000-2010 task force on neck pain and its associated disorders. Spine. 2008;33(4 Suppl):S60–74.
24. Rolander B, Wahlin C, Johnston V, Wagman P, Lindmark U. Changes in division of labour and tasks within public dentistry: relationship to employees work demands, health and work ability. Acta Odontol Scand. 2016:1–9.
25. Hajian-Tilaki K. Sample size estimation in epidemiologic studies. Caspian J Intern Med. 2011;2(4):289–98.
26. Warmbold J. World ranking for industrial trucks 2014/2015. dhf Intralogistik. 2015.

2

Self-care of chronic musculoskeletal pain – experiences and attitudes of patients and health care providers

Irena Kovačević[1*], Višnja Majerić Kogler[2], Tihana Magdić Turković[3], Lidija Fumić Dunkić[3], Željko Ivanec[3] and Davorina Petek[4]

Abstract

Background: Self-care is often the first choice for people with chronic musculoskeletal pain. Self-care includes the use of non-prescription medications with no doctor's supervision, as well as the use of other modern and traditional treatment methods with no consultation of the health care provider. Self-care may have positive effects on the successful outcome of a multidisciplinary approach to treatment. The aim of this study was to investigate the experiences and attitudes of patients and health care providers to the self-care of chronic musculoskeletal pain.

Methods: Qualitative Phenomenological study, where the data were collected by the method of an audio-taped interview in 15 patients at the outpatient clinic for pain management and in 20 health care providers involved in the treatment of those patients. The interviews were transcribed verbatim and analyzed by principles of Interpretative Thematic Analysis.

Results: Topics identified in patients: a) positive aspects of self-care, b) a need for pain self-care, c) social aspects of pain self-care. Topics identified in health care providers: a) aspects of self-care, b) a need for self-care c) risks of self-care. Most of patients have positive attitude to self-care and this is the first step to pain management and to care for itself. The most frequent factors influencing decision about the self-care are heavy pain, unavailability of the doctor, long awaiting time for the therapy, or ineffectiveness of methods of conventional medicine. The health care providers believe that self-care of chronic musculoskeletal pain may be a patient's contribution to clinical treatment. However, good awareness of methods used is important in this context, to avoid adverse effects of self-care.

Conclusion: Patients understand the self-care of musculoskeletal pain as an individually adjusted treatment and believe in its effectiveness. Health care providers support self-care as an adjunction to clinical management only, and think that self-care of musculoskeletal pain acts as a placebo, with a short-lived effect on chronic musculoskeletal pain.

Keywords: Self-care, Chronic musculoskeletal pain, Attitudes, Patients, Health care providers, Qualitative study

Background

Due to its unique neurobiological ground and the influence on physical function, quality of life and medical outcome, chronic pain can be considered chronic disease [1]. The prevalence of pain varies depending on the age, life style and general health in the population [2]. The incidence of pain doubles around the age of sixty and has the tendency to further increase with each decade of life [3].

The chronic pain has been recognized as one that lasts longer than its normally expected resolution time [4] and an acute warning function of physiologic nociception is not present [5]. A pain is usually considered chronic if it lasts, or is present, for more than 3 to 6 months [6]. It has been estimated that chronic pain is present in approximately 20% of people globally [7–10] and accounts for 15% to 20% of all visits to the doctor's office [11, 12]. Persons with chronic pain generally suffer from multiple physical and also psychological consequences of pain [13, 14]. Chronic pain increases the healthcare costs and cause losses in working hours due to absence from workplace [15, 16].

* Correspondence: irena.kovacevic1@gmail.com
[1]University of Applied Health Sciences, Mlinarska 38, 10 000 Zagreb, Croatia

Negative experiences related to chronic pain can be considered the main life events, particularly among unemployed, but among employed too, because pain affects their working capacity [17]. Other emotional problems also occur, such as the feeling of futility and loss of control in everyday life or on working place [17]. People feel like victims, which is associated with the inability to accept its own situation regarding the pain [17]. Disorders of musculoskeletal system are the most common causes of chronic pain, leading to physical damage, limitations of working capacity, and unemployment in the long term [18]. According to the ICD 11, chronic musculoskeletal pain is defined as "persistent or recurrent pain that arises as part of a disease process directly affecting bone(s), joint(s), muscle(s), or related soft tissue(s)" [19]. For example, musculoskeletal disorders account for 53% of absences from working place in Norway and are the main reason for disability pensions [20]. Musculoskeletal pain thereby poses a huge economic burden [21].

It is known that the population of elderly people is rapidly growing worldwide [22]. Increasing age is often associated with complex health problems and is frequently combined with long-lasting musculoskeletal pain. The prevalence rate in communities of elderly people is even 60% [23, 24]. There is no significant difference in the prevalence of musculoskeletal pain between rural and urban populations. Social isolation is deemed to be more expressed in rural areas, which negatively impacts the perception of pain [25].

As reported by some authors, persons with chronic musculoskeletal pain are not satisfied with the effects of clinical treatment [26]. They believe that the health system, particularly doctors, does not take them seriously [26]. Doctors also believe that they are not able to do a lot for persons with chronic musculoskeletal pain and that the medical treatments have a little or no effect [26]. This is one of the main reasons why is self-care usually the first choice for the treatment of early disease symptoms [27]. "Self-care may be defined as the care taken by individuals towards their own health and well being, In practice it includes the actions people take to stay fit and maintain good physical and mental health; meet social and psychological needs; prevent illness or accidents; avoid unnecessary risks; care and self-medicate for minor ailments and long-term conditions; and maintain health and well being after an acute illness or discharge from hospital"[28].

The self-care implies the use of one or more medications not prescribed by a doctor, and procedures not supervised by the health service. It includes the use of herbal or pharmacological products, medications previously prescribed for similar cases, some medications from home pharmacy, or too short use of prescribed treatment [29]. It can also be defined as the use of medications as well as modern and traditional methods without consultations with the doctor (or other health care provider), or with no prescription and treatment supervision [30]. Considering various definitions and terms that describe the care about one's own health, such as self-management, self-medication and self-treatment, the term self-care seems to be the most appropriate for this report since it covers more aspects and more different methods of care about patient's own health investigated in this study.

Musculoskeletal pain is the most frequent reason for the use of complementary and alternative medicine (CAM) [31]. According to the investigation of Breivik H et al. [7] the most common self-care methods are the massage, physical therapy and acupuncture. In that study 38% of subjects reported that those methods were highly or very useful.

Asking for assistance of relatives as a strategy to cope with a pain can be useful, and stressful at the same time, because people who are in pain hardly accept the change of their role and asking for assistance [17]. The family is often a source of information and the transmission of traditional treatment methods and personal experiences from one generation to another [32]. Role of women in the family is the most important in this sense [33].

Self-care is related to increasing age [34, 35], which increases the risk of adverse events in self-care. The level of knowledge regarding methods and duration of treatment, and possible interaction of self-care with the use of already prescribed medications or the other form of treatment for another indication is lower in elderly population [36]. Younger generations, on the contrary, have better access to relevant information about self-care methods [34, 35].

Self-care of pain may have positive impact to pain alleviation and general disability, as well as to increase of psychological well-being such as lower level of stress, depression and anxiety [37].

Self-care studies are frequently carried out by the use of qualitative methods [38]. The aim of this study was to investigate experiences, needs and attitudes of patients regarding the self-care of chronic musculoskeletal pain, as a part of comprehensive care of chronic pain, ways to make decisions about the self-care, and expectations about the outcomes. We aimed to get an insight in the group of chronic pain patients that received the highest level of medical treatment of their chronic pain. At the same time, data regarding health care providers' attitudes about patient's self-care of musculoskeletal pain and its possible usefulness in relations to conventional medicine were collected.

In tis report, the first part of a larger mixed methods study aimed to test factors that are possibly associated with the good outcome of chronic pain treatment is presented. This part of the study explored the patient's activation and his role in improvement of his condition.

Methods

A qualitative, phenomenological approach was used, which allows understanding of certain phenomenon from the aspect of those who experienced it. It includes investigator's intuition and open-minded acceptance of all adapted experiences and standpoints.

Procedure

A series of a total of 35 semi-structured interviews, among them 15 with patients and 20 with health care providers, was carried out. Each subject was assigned an alias, to maintain the anonymity. By a method of audiotaped interview patients were asked about their understanding of the self-care phenomenon, their attitudes about self-care, and needs fulfilled in the self-care of chronic musculoskeletal pain (Table 1). The same method was used to ask health care providers about their attitudes regarding the patient's self-care of musculoskeletal pain (Table 2). Interviews were carried out until saturation was attained. The saturation was defined and attained when answers in the last interviews were repeated and no new codes appeared in the analytical process [39]. All of interviews were carried out at the Outpatient Clinic for Pain Management, Sisters of Charity Clinical Hospital Centre Zagreb, Croatia, during the scheduled follow up or treatment visit. Conversations were transcribed verbatim and processed by a thematic analysis.

Analysis

The thematic analysis was done according to Braun and Clarke [40] settings because it allows identification and analysis of topics within collected data and consequently the precise answer to study questions asked [40]. The aim of this qualitative analysis was to come to general conclusions or starting hypotheses for a quantitative study.

Following identification of key topics in line with the study questions and marking quotations containing terms relevant for the selected topic, the data were reduced based on the agreement between two independent investigators. Selected quotations were coded by an open codes which revealed characteristics derived from the text by an inductive method. Eventually a code list was formed. Based on code lists, related topics were grouped into categories/themes. Coding as a process developed relationships between main categories in line with the study questions and aim of the study.

In data interpretation the context of individual topics and codes, evident from the original text was respected. During the coding process, data from new interviews were continuously compared with data already analyzed. For the understanding and interpretation of phenomena studied, basic (raw) data were used eventually. Since the answers were coded by two independent investigators, the level of agreement for codes of each respective topic was determined by calculation of the agreement coefficient (Cohen's kappa coefficient).

Participants

Two subject groups were formed. Purposeful sampling method of participants of both groups was chosen according to the preselected criteria determined by the research question [41]. The participants were sought in the population of patients who received the highest level of medical pain management in the Outpatient Clinic for Pain Management so it was homogeneous in this characteristic, but we looked for the variety in patients' age, gender, education and location of living (rural/urban) (Table 3). We included the patients with experience of chronic pain of different duration, different intensity and location to capture a wide range of perspectives on self-care and gain a greater insight into phenomena of self- care in this population from all

Table 1 List of questions for the semi-structured interview with patients

Study questions	Asked questions
Self-care attitude	What do you thing about self-care and what is your attitude about pain self-care?
Self-care decision	In what cases you decide to practice pain self-care?
	Please describe what influenced your decision to practice pain self-care
	• regarding the length of the pain
	• regarding the site and intensity of your pain
Self-care experiences	What do you expect from self-care?
	How satisfied are you with the outcome/result of self-care?
Self-care methods	Please describe your experiences with different methods of pain self-care?
Self-care information source	In what way and from whom you got the information about pain self-care?
Family tradition in self-care	Please describe the impact of family tradition to your decision to practice pain self-care.

Table 2 List of questions for the semi-structured interview with health care providers

Study questions	Asked questions
Self-care attitude	What do you think about patient's self-care of pain and what is your attitude about this?
Self-care decision	In your opinion and experience, why patients decide to practice pain self-care?
Relation of self-care to clinical benefits in pain management	In what way is pain self-care related to successful outcome of medical management?

aspects. A group of patients comprised 15 subjects, (until saturation) who were visiting the pain clinic. Before the start of interview patients were asked whether they practice self-care. If the answer was yes, the interview proceeded. Therefore the inclusion criteria were patients aged > 18 who practice self-care, any level of education and any place of residence, any type of chronic musculoskeletal pain and any duration of pain (> 3 month) (Table 3) while the exclusion criteria were age < 18 years, non-musculoskeletal pain and acute pain.

The other group of 20 subjects (until saturation) comprised health care providers, experts for pain management or those experienced in management of patients in pain on primary care level. The subjects from health care provider group were nurses and doctors who differ in their age, gender, level of education, workplace, and professional experience (Table 4). Inclusion criteria for the health care provider sample were: specialist in anesthesiology, specialist in family medicine, nurse anesthetist, anesthesia technician, family medicine nurse, with variation in age, gender, level of education, workplace, and professional experience (Table 4). Although all health care workers see patients in pain, we limited our sample to the health care providers at two level of care that are most frequently involved in care of patients with chronic pain.

Inclusion criteria were selected based on the aim of the study (Tables 1 and 2) and available literature data.

Results

In total, 35 subjects entered the study: 15 patients from the Outpatient Clinic for Pain Management and 20 health care providers from the Department of Anesthesiology, Department of Surgery, and from general practice. Demographic characteristics of patient group are described in Table 3 and health care provider group in Table 4. The average age in patient group was 47 years. Most of them were employed, with prevailing secondary school education and the place of residence in a large urban area. The subjects from health care provider group were mostly nurses and technicians from the Department of Anesthesiology, Department of Surgery, Outpatient Clinic for Pain Management, and from general practice, as well as doctors – specialists or residents in anesthesiology. Their average length of service was 20 years.

From interviews, topics for each study groups were selected, representing their experiences in pain self-care.

Duration and site of chronic musculoskeletal pain

Mean duration of the pain was 10.26 years (0.4–30.0 yrs). The shortest period of pain was 4 months and the longest one was 30 years.

The most common site of pain was lumbosacral region, followed by the cervical part of spine, pelvis and legs. An average intensity of pain evaluated by the pain assessment scale (0 – no pain, 10 – the worst possible pain) was 8 (6–10).

Table 3 Demographic characteristics of patient group

Characteristic		*n* = 15
Age		47.13 years (29–72)
Gender	M	5
	F	10
Employment status	Employed	13
	Retired	2
Educational level	Secondary school	10
	University or college degree	3
	Master's or Ph.D. degree	2
Place of residence	Country	1
	Inhabited place with 5.000–50.000 inhabitants	3
	Town with > 50.000 inhabitants	11

Table 4 Demographic characteristics of health care provider group

Characteristic		$n = 20$
Age		40,9 years (24–66)
Gender	M	5
	F	15
Profession	Specialist in anesthesiology	5
	Family doctor	1
	Resident in anesthesiology	2
	Nurse/technician at the anesthesiology department	11
	Nurse/technician in family medicine	1
Professional experience	Years of service	
	< 5	3
	5–9	4
	10–20	5
	> 20	8

Methods of self-care

The most common methods of pain self-care were the use of herbal products (various sorts of tea), and local administration of creams, gels and compresses. In addition, patients reported the use of acupuncture, yoga, meditation, exercise and walking. Patients often combine different methods of pain self-care.

Themes, derived from the analysis

Three themes were recognized from analyzed interviews in each study group. Data were collected from the patient group revealed the following themes: positive aspects of self-care, need for self-care, and social aspects of self-care. Levels of agreement between two independent investigators for each theme were as follows:

1. Positive aspects of self-care, $\kappa = 0.89$
2. Need for pain self-care, $\kappa = 0.71$
3. Social aspects of self-care, $\kappa = 0.90$

Three themes recognized on the basis of data from the health care provider group were: positive aspects of self-care, need for self-care, and risks of self-care.

Levels of agreement for each topic were as follows:

1. Positive aspects of self-care, $\kappa = 0.87$
2. Need for pain self-care, $\kappa = 1.0$
3. Risks of self-care, $\kappa = 0.69$

After the first round of topic reading and recognizing, the topics were interpreted in the next round (Tables 5 and 6).

Positive aspects of self-care

Results of this study reveal that the self-care is associated with patient's activation where she/he does not simply wait for professional assistance but do something for himself, wishing to take the control over his/her pain. The self-care allows an individual treatment of pain because patients believe they know the best their bodies and their pain and are able on the best possible way assess what procedures are most appropriate for them. By self-care patients avoid a routine therapy which is the same for all of them. Patients tend to use healthy and natural treatment methods which are gentle and less aggressive than clinical ones, thus at the same time reducing the need for use of analgesics. The psychological effect of self-care is also emphasized. A power of belief that something is helpful may result in pain relief in the patient (at least in the short-term).

„Why not? I am always open to all options. That what one believe, will surely help her/him"", (P-13) (P – patient).

„Because I am somehow poisoned by all of those treatments, I avoid, really avoid... because I am full of chemistry, really. "(P-9).

„...I think that a human, a person can at most help itself..."(P-2).

The health care providers agree with patients that self-care has a positive psychological effect and contributes to better psychic condition. Such a patient is easier to treat clinically. They also see higher activation in better informed patients. Unlike patients, health care providers think that self-care also reduce the burden of health services, while patients do not recognize or mention that.

...those people put themselves a goal to take control over their pain as soon as possible, that they do not want to take a sick-leave, they wish to be vital, to have a quality of life, and in this respect the self-care makes sense." (HP-17) (HP – health care provider).

Table 5 Interpretation of patient topics

Positive aspects of self-care	Activation of patients (something that the patient can do for himself)
	Individuality of self-care:
	-desire to control the pain
	-healthy natural methods
	-integrated actions
	-psychological effect
	Easier to tolerate the pain
Need for pain self-care	Something should be done if the doctor is not visited
	Awkward and long-lasting pain
	Pain alleviating
	Improving functionality and quality of life
	Better effect of alternative and medicine combination
	Too much medication from conventional medicine
	Conventional methods exhausted
	Disappointment with conventional medicine
Social aspects of self-care	Information about self-care
	Tradition
	Experiences from others, sharing of experience
	Support from the environment

"I support this, anyone knows its limits and needs the best. "(ZR-19).

„The self-care of pain has its place in the pain management and can be practiced until visit to doctor's office, physicians are less burdened, and anything that is harmless can be tried." (HP-1).

Table 6 Interpretation of health care provider topics

Positive aspects of self-care	Activation of the patient:
	- Awareness
	- Care for her–/himself
	- Empowered patient
	Psychological effect
	Lower burden for health services
	Lower consumption of analgesics
Need for self-care	The first form of treatment
	Avoiding of doctors (self-care preferred)
	Unavailability of doctors
	In mild conditions
	In acute conditions
Risks of self-care	Adverse effects
	Short-lived effect
	Mistakes in self-care
	Late diagnosis of pain causes
	Masking of symptoms
	Exaggeration

Need for self-care

The patients consider self-care essential in cases when something has to be done, for example, when the pain is intense and long-lasting but they do not visit the doctor, or when methods of clinical medicine are exhausted and they are disappointed with the treatment results. On the other hand, self-care can be an adjunct to clinical treatment (which is insufficient). While clinical medicine look for causes of pain, the patient try to help itself thereby improving its functionality and quality of life. The health care providers think that self-care is the first step in the pain management, particularly in some milder and acute conditions. They also think that patients prefer self-care to avoid the doctor, but there are also cases where the doctor is unavailable, or patients have to wait a long time for the examination or treatment.

„Any self-care is welcome as long as it acts and I really think that all of us should take this way first, and then possibly, if this fails, go further or combine various treatment methods. "(P-14).

„When I simply exhausted all of options with my doctor, when even doctors did not know how to help me, then I had to go myself. (P-12).

„Well, because traditional, conventional medicine did not help me." (P-2).

„...because to reach the therapy is very difficult. I think, you should wait for the physiatrist minimally for two months and then another two months for the therapy. "(P-15).

„It is good to start with some self-care prior to visit any institution. "(HP-13).

Social aspects of self-care

Patients talk to the family, friends and colleagues about their pain, thereby share their opinions and experiences. In addition to the Internet and various popular journals, those options are important source of information about methods of self-care. Family tradition plays a great role in transmission of positive experiences about the use of certain self-care methods from one generation to another.

„All of this was through my family, meaning my parents, my mother. Well yes, I was told by my mom, she was told by my grandma, I think, or maybe my aunt." (P-13);

„...Any available information was transmitted to me, and I transmit it further to my children. "(P-8).

„Well, through my friend." (P-11).

„In the company where I am currently employed, a lot of people are dedicated to alternative treatment methods and they are really open to this so that experiences are frequently shared. "(P-14);

„Well, I do not know, most frequently, I am pretty often on the Internet and in this way I receive the alternative, really good tips are available, advices are healthy, all is natural.. "(P-9); „Through the Internet, through various media. "(P-11); „... Then I read in the newspaper... "(P-14).

Risks of self-care

While patients do not see anything disputable in self-care processes, health care providers still emphasize that self-care may have adverse effects. Aberrances may occur in self-care which may result in symptom masking of certain serious conditions and in the late diagnosis of pain causes. Uninformed patients may exaggerate in the use of various self-care methods, thereby jeopardize their own health.

„Masking of symptoms by certain medications, such as analgesics, may potentially be dangerous for the patient." (HP-6).

"I think no, because they may come too late, when the pain is too heavy and then it is more difficult to treat it. "(HP-11).

„Patients persuade themselves that they get better with those various products and medications they use, thereby extending the period of treatment."(ZR-10).

Discussion

The results or this study indicate that patients see themselves as individuals different from the others and therefore they expect individual treatment procedure. The same finding was reported by other authors too, because patients see the realization of their individuality and freedom of choice right in the self-care [42]. The holistic view on the health, ability to take the control over its own health, and the preference of natural treatment methods, as well as the concern about potential side effects of pharmaceutical products, are predictors of increased use of self-care [43–45]. The self-care is also encouraged by other factors, such as long waiting time for the examination and therapy. These findings are supported by the results of other studies. Patients are dissatisfied because they wait long for health services, are far from their physicians, and sometimes working hours of doctor's office do not suit them [46, 47]. Reasons for self-care lie also in patient's distrust of physicians, while, on the other hand, patients sometimes do not want to bother physicians, particularly if the cause of pain is already known [48]. The self-care is also a method of choice in cases where conventional medicine failed, or its methods have already been exhausted. The results of this study are in line with other reported ones. For example, Siapush et al. [49] demonstrated that dissatisfaction with the conventional medicine was caused by two factors. One factor was dissatisfaction with the outcome of medical treatment and the other one was dissatisfaction with the physician or another responsible health care provider.

While the attitude of subjects from a patient group to self-care was mostly positive, subjects from a health care provider group assumed that self-care can only be an adjunct to the treatment of pain. This finding is supported by other authors, such as Correa-Velez et al. [50] who emphasized that other methods were only an adjunct to conventional treatment methods, and were not contrary to them. Although self-care with medications is a practice in many developing countries, particularly by an urban and educated population [51], health care providers in our study assumed that self-care should be confined to alternative methods. Albeit the patient's awareness of its need to make an effort for itself seems to be plausible, they warned to risks of self-care and its potential impact to diagnosis delay. They thought that patients undoubtedly should be well informed about methods used in the self-care. Non-awareness and use of various products in combination with prescribed medications may lead to interactions and adverse effects of self-care, such as intoxication or treatment failure [52–56].

Therefore health care providers in our study emphasized that self-care may carry potential risk for patient's health and may mask symptoms of more serious diseases, with consequent prolongation of diagnosis. To take the responsibility for care of its health and to participate actively in the treatment process, patients still should possess certain proficiency and skills [57].

The family was in our study an important source of information about self-care of musculoskeletal pain, mostly when considering chronic musculoskeletal pain self-care that has been practiced in the family and transmitted from one generation to another. One of our results that should also be emphasized is a social aspect of self-care because people who suffer from similar difficulties talk to each other and share their experiences. Friends and colleagues from the workplace are therefore a common source of information about alternative self-care methods. However, when use of medications was considered, most of patients reported exclusively healthcare providers as sources of information, namely family doctors or anesthesiologist from the outpatient clinic for pain management. Similar conclusions were also drawn by other authors. According to results of Nagarajaiah et al. [36], important sources of information about self-care with medications are family members and relatives, followed by healthcare providers and pharmacists. A study carried out in Slovenia demonstrated that relatives and pharmacists were the most common sources of information and tips about self-care, and that self-care was more frequent among younger subjects and those with higher educational level [48, 58].

Our study demonstrated that the patients started with self-care by taking various sorts of tea and by a local administration of ointments, gels and compresses. Self-care methods using the tea, herbs and herbal products are well known [59]. The next methods of choice were acupuncture, chiropractic, yoga, meditation, exercise and walking. Other studies reported the acupuncture, chiropractic, message and yoga as most frequently used methods [37]. The psychological effect and power of belief that self-care will help have also their place in positive aspects of self-care, as confirmed by the similar studies [60]. The main results of our study emphasized the positive aspect of self-care, which was manifested in empowerment of the patient itself, where the self-care was understood as an individually adjusted procedure. Health care providers supported the self-care because it boosted the patient's care about itself, but assumed that those procedures can be only an adjunct to the clinical treatment.

Advantages and limitations of the study

The attitudes and experiences of patients and health care providers of various profiles were studied at the same time.

Limitation

The patient sample was purposeful and not representative so that results cannot be translated to the whole population. We also did not expand the profile of health workers that are included in the treatment of chronic musculoskeletal pain especially specialists of physical medicine and physiotherapists.

Conclusions

Self-care of musculoskeletal chronic pain is understood as an activity of empowered patient and should be used by health care providers to further include patient in his treatment and motivate him for self-help within the safety of official medicine. Health care providers support self-care of musculoskeletal pain as an adjunct to clinical treatment. They, however, assume that self-care acts as a placebo, with short-time effect to chronic musculoskeletal pain. Because of possible risk of self-care adverse effects (late diagnosis and true cause of pain establishment) patients should be well informed about the methods used. Patients understand self-care of musculoskeletal pain as an individually adjusted procedure and believe in its effectiveness. They lack individualized care from conventional medicine. Family tradition methods are commonly used in the self-care.

Abbreviations

CAM: complementary and alternative medicine; HP: health care provider; P: patient

Acknowledgements

We would like to express our gratefulness to all of *health* care providers and patients who were engaged in interviews. Special thanks to the health team from the Outpatient Clinic for Pain Management for their understanding and facilities that allowed completion of all interviews.

Funding

No funding was received.

Authors' contributions

I.K. and D.P. developed the study design. IK conducted interviews at the Outpatient Clinic for Pain Management, audio-taped interviews transcribed verbatim, and along with D.P. completed thematic analysis of contents and overview of results. V.M.K. participated in study design development. T.M.T, L.F.D. and Ž.I. were engaged in realization of interviews and enrollment of patients who met inclusion criteria for interviews. All of authors participated in development of final manuscript version and approved it.

Consent for publication

Not applicable.

Competing interests

The authors declare they have no competing interests.

Author details

[1]University of Applied Health Sciences, Mlinarska 38, 10 000 Zagreb, Croatia. [2]School of Medicine, University of Zagreb, Šalata 3, Zagreb, Croatia. [3]Sisters of Charity University Hospital Centre, Vinogradska cesta 29, Zagreb, Croatia. [4]Department of Family Medicine, Faculty of Medicine, University of Ljubljana, Poljanski nasip 58, 1000 Ljubljana, Slovenia.

References

1. Institute of Medicine. Relieving pain in America: A blueprint for transforming prevention, care, education, and research. Washington, DC: The National Academies Press; 2011. p. 3. https://www.nap.edu/read/13172/chapter/2#3. Accessed 12 Jan 2018.
2. Jakobsson U, Klevsgard R, Westergren A, Rahm Hallberg I. Old people in pain: a comparative study. J Pain Symptom Manag. 2003;26:625–36.
3. American Geriatric Society Panel on Chronic Pain in Older Persons. The management of persistent pain in older persons: AGS panel on persistent pain in older persons. J Am Geriatr Soc. 2002;50:S205–24.
4. Bonica JJ. The management of pain. Philadelphia: Lea & Febiger; 1953.
5. Treede RD. Entstehung der Schmerzchronifizierung. In: Baron R, Koppert W, Strumpf M, Willweber-Strumpf A, editors. Praktische Schmerztherapie. Heidelberg: Springer; 2011. p. 3–13.
6. Merskey H, Bogduk N. Classification of chronic pain. 2nd ed. Seattle: IASP Press; 1994.
7. Breivik H, Collett B, Ventafridda V, Cohen R, Gallacher D. Survey of chronic pain in Europe: prevalence, impact on daily life, and treatment. Eur J Pain. 2006;10:287–333.
8. Goldberg DS, Summer JM. Pain as a global public health priority. BMC Public Health. 2011;11:770.
9. Gureje O, von Korff M, Kola L, Demyttenaere K, He Y, Posada-Villa J, Lepine JP, Angermeyer MC, Levinson D, de Girolamo G, Iwata N, Karam A, Borges GLG, de Graaf R, Browne MO, Stein DJ, Haro JM, Bromet EJ, Kessler RC, Alonso J. The relation between multiple pains and mental disorders: results from the world mental health surveys. Pain. 2008;135:82–91.
10. Institute of Medicine. Relieving pain in America: a blueprint for transforming prevention, care, education, and research. Washington, DC: The National Academies Press; 2011. p. 55-63. https://www.nap.edu/read/13172/chapter/4. Accessed 10 Jan 2018.
11. Koleva D. Pain in primary care: an Italian survey. Eur J Pub Health. 2005;15:475–9.
12. Mantyselka P, Kumpusalo E, Ahonen R, Kumpusalo A, Kauhanen J, Viinamaki H, Halonen P, Takala J. Pain as a reason to visit the doctor: a study in Finnish primary health care. Pain. 2001;89:175–80.
13. Thomas SPA. Phenomenological study of chronic pain. West J Nurs Res. 2000;22:683–99.
14. Corbett M, Foster NE, Ong SE. Living with low back pain – stories of hope and despair. Soc Sci Med. 2007;65:1584–94.
15. van Leeuwen MT, Blyth FM, March LM, Nicholas MK, Cousins MJ. Chronic pain and reduced work effectiveness: the hidden cost to Australian employers. Eur J Pain. 2006;10:161–6.
16. Phillips CJ, Harper C. The economics associated with persistent pain. Curr Opin Support Palliat Care. 2011;5:127–30.
17. Andersen LN, Kohberg M, Gram Herborg L, Søgaard K, Roessler KK. "Here we're all in the same boat" – a qualitative study o group based rehabilitation for sick-listed citizens with chronic pain. Scand J Psychol. 2014; 55:333–42.
18. Sarahroodi S, Maleki-Jamshid A, Sawalha AF, Mikaili P, Safaeian L. Pattern of self-medication with analgesics among Iranian university students in Central Iran. J Family Community Med. 2012;19:125–9.
19. Treede RD, Rief W, Barke A, Aziz Q, Bennett MI, Rafael Benoliel R, Cohen M, et al. A classification of chronic pain for ICD-11. Pain. 2015;156:1003–7.
20. Brage S. Musculosketal health problems and sickness absence - an epidemiological study of concepts, determinants, and consequences (dissertation). Institute of General Practice and Community Medicine: University of Oslo; 1998.
21. World Health Organization. The burden of musculoskeletal conditions at the start of the new millennium. World Health Organ Tech Rep Ser. 2003;919:1–218.
22. Cavanaugh JC, Blanchard-Fields F. Adult development and aging. 6th ed. Boston: Wadsworth/Cengage. Learning. 2011;
23. Bergman S, Herrström P, Högström K, Petersson IF, Svensson B, Jacobsson LT. Chronic musculoskeletal pain, prevalence rates, and sociodemographic associations in a Swedish population study. J Rheumatol. 2001;28:1369–77.
24. Woo J, Leung J, Lau E. Prevalence and correlates of musculoskeletal pain in Chinese elderly and the impact on 4-year physical function and quality of life. Public Health. 2009;123:549–56.
25. Docking RE, Fleming J, Brayne C, et al. Epidemiology of back pain in older adults: prevalence and risk factors for back pain onset. Rheumatology (Oxford). 2011;50:1645–53.
26. Steena E, Hauglib L. From pain to self-awareness - a qualitative analysis of the significance of group participation for persons with chronic musculoskeletal pain. Patient Educ Couns. 2001;42:35–46.
27. Ruehlman LS, Karoly P, Enders CA. Randomized controlled evaluation of an online chronic pain self-management. Pain. 2012;153:319–30.
28. World Self-Medication Industry. Responsible self-care and self-medication: A worldwide review of consumer surveys. 2014. http://www.wsmi.org/wp-content/data/pdf/wsmibro3.pdf. Accessed 3 Mar 2018.
29. Karimy M, Heidarnia A, Ghofrani F. Factors influencing self-medication among elderly urban centers in Zarandieh based on health belief model. Arak Med Univ J. 2011;14:70–8.
30. Hughes CM, McElnay JC, Fleming GF. Benefits and risks of self medication. Drug Saf. 2001;24:1027–37.
31. Artus M, Croft P, Lewis M. The use of CAMand conventional treatments among primary care consulters with chronic musculoskeletal pain. BMC Fam Pract. 2007;8:26.
32. World Health Organization. Legal status of traditional medicine and complementary/alternative medicine: A worldwide review. 2001. http://apps.who.int/medicinedocs/pdf/h2943e/h2943e.pdf. Accessed 4 Mar 2018.
33. Klemenc-Ketis Z, Hladnik Z, Kersnik JA. Cross sectional study of sex differences in self-medication practices among university students in Slovenia. Coll Antropol. 2011;35:329–34.
34. Kelly JP, Kaufman DW, Kelley K, Rosenberg L, Anderson TE, Mitchell AA. Recent trends in use of herbal and other natural products. Arch Intern Med. 2005;165:281–6.
35. Kishiyama SS, Leahy MJ, Zitzelberger TA, Guariglia R, Zajdel DP, Calvert JF, et al. Patterns of dietary supplement usage in demographically diverse old people. Altern Ther Health Med. 2005;11:48–53.
36. Nagarajaiah BH, Kishore MS, Shashi Kumar NS, Panchakshari P. Prevalence and pattern of self-medication practices among population of three districts of South Karnataka. Natl J Physiol Pharm Pharmacol. 2016;6:296–300.
37. Jafari F, A K, Rahmani E. Prevalence of self–medication among the elderly in Kermanshah-Iran. Global J Health Sci. 2015;7:360–5.
38. Matthias MS, Miech EJ, Myers LJ, Sargent C, Bair MJ. An expanded view of self-management: patients' perceptions of education and support in an intervention for chronic musculoskeletal pain. Pain Med. 2012;13:1018–28.
39. Moser A, Korstjens I. Series: practical guidance to qualitative research. Part 3: sampling, data collection and analysis. Eur J Gen Pract. 2018;24:9–18.
40. Braun V, Clarke V. Using thematic analysis in psychology. Qual Res Psychol. 2006;3:77–101.
41. Korstjens I, Moser A. Series: practical guidance to qualitative research. Part 2: context, research questions and designs. Eur J Gen Pract. 2017; 23:274–9.
42. Žuškin E, Pucarin Cvetković J, Kanceljak Macan B, Vitale K, Janev Holcer N, Čivljak M. The Art of Treatment: Historical View (Umijeće liječenja: povijesni prikaz). Soc psihijat. 2013;41:156–63.
43. Bucker B, Groenewold M, Schoefer Y, Schafer T. The use of complementary alternative medicine (CAM) in 1001 German adults: results of a population based telephone study. Gesundheitswesen. 2008;70:29–36.
44. Menniti-Ippolito F, Gargiulo L, Bologna E, Forcella E, Raschetti R. Use of unconventional medicine in Italy: a nation-wide survey. Eur J Clin Pharmacol. 2002;58:61–4.
45. Siahpush M. Postmodern attitudes about health: a population-based exploratory study. Complement Ther Med. 1999:164–9.
46. Babić-Banaszak A, Kovačić L, Mastilica M, Babić S, Ivanković D, Budak A. The Croatian health survey – patient's satisfaction with medical service in primary health care in Croatia. Coll Antropol. 2001;25:449–58.
47. Cvitanović H, Jančić E, Knežević E, Kuljanac I. Satisfaction of patients with healthcare quality in outpatients dermatology clinic Karlovac. Croatia Medicina Fluminensis. 2011;47:82–90.
48. Klemenc-Ketis Z, Mitrovic D. Patients' use of and attitudes towards self-medication in rural and remote Slovenian family medicine practices: a cross-sectional multicentre study. Rural Remote Health. 2017;17:3893. https://doi.org/10.22605/RRH3893

49. Siahpush M. Why do people favour alternative medicine? Aust N Z J Public Health. 1999;23:266–71.
50. Correa-Velez I, Clavarino A, Eastwood H. Surviving, relieving, repairing, and boosting up: reasons for using complementary/alternative medicine among patients with advanced cancer: a thematic analysis. J Paliat Med. 2005;8:953–61.
51. Sanghani S, Zaveri HG, Patel VJ. Self medication: prevalence and pattern in urban community. J pharmacovigilance. Drug Saf. 2008;5:95–8.
52. Blumenthal M, Busse WR, Goldberg A, Gruenwald J, Hall T, Riggins CW, et al. The complete German commission E monographs: therapeutic guide to herbal medicines. Austin: American Botanical Council; 1998.
53. Fugh-Berman A, Ernst E. Herb–drug interactions: review and assessment of report reliability. Brit J Clin Pharmacol. 2001;52:587–95.
54. Hurren KM, Lewis CL. Interaction between warfarin and bee pollen. Am J Helth Syst Pharm. 2010;67:2034–7.
55. Asadaq SNM, Inamdar MN, Asad M. Pharmacodynamic interaction with propranolol in ischemia-reperfusion induced myocardial damage. Pak J Pharm Sci. 2010;23:42–7.
56. Izzo AA, Di Carlo G, Borrelli F, Ernst E. Cardiovascular pharmacotherapy and herbal medicine: the risk of drug interaction. Int J Cardiol. 2006;98:1–14.
57. Newman S, Steed L, Mulligan K. Self-management interventions for chronic illness. Lancet. 2004;364:1523–37.
58. Klemenc-Ketiš Z, Kersnik J. The effect of demographic characteristics on self-medication patterns: a cross-sectional nationwide study from Slovenia. Coll Antropol. 2011;35:1237–42.
59. Goldman P. Herbal medicines today and the roots of modern pharmacology. Ann Intern Med. 2001;135:594–600.
60. Čižmešija T, Bergman-Markovac B. Use of complementary and alternative medicine in patients in primary health care. (Upotreba komplementarne i alternativne medicine kod pacijenata u primarnoj zdravstvenoj zaštiti). Acta Med Croatica. 2008;62:15–22.

3

Perioperative complications after surgical treatment in degenerative adult de novo scoliosis

Maciej J. K. Simon[1,2,3], Henry F. H. Halm[3] and Markus Quante[3*]

Abstract

Background: Degenerative adult de novo (DAD) scoliosis appears characteristically in the sixth or seventh decade with symptoms of severe back pain and radiculopathy or spinal claudication. The aim of this study was to enhance the knowledge of perioperative complications and detect possible risk factors in this selective DAD scoliosis surgery.

Methods: This retrospective study included only patients with DAD scoliosis undergone correction spondylodesis with previous failure of conservative treatment. Excluded were patients with other types of scoliosis and previous fusion surgeries. Patient epidemiological data, medical comorbidities and treatments were included. Intraoperative data and perioperative complications were documented. Analyses regarding early, late and no complications were undertaken.

Results: A total of 92 patients with a mean age of 67.29 ± 7.93 years and clinical follow-up visits of minimum 12 months were included. On average, 5.26 ± 2.24 segments were fused. Early complications (e.g. wound healing defects, paresis, screw loosing) occurred in 23 patients and often required a re-operation. Cardiac arrhythmias, pacemaker and coumarin derivative therapies were associated with increased perioperative complications. The transforaminal lumbar interbody fusion technique was associated with early complications. Adjacent segment failure occurred in 36% and was the major late complication. Twenty patients did not have any complications in the minimum follow-up.

Conclusions: This study analysed a selective DAD scoliosis collective and its' surgical treatment outcomes. It identified numerous perioperative complications (adjacent segment failure, postoperative paresis and epidural hematoma) and multiple possible predisposing risk factors (e.g. operative techniques and anti-coagulation therapies). This here gained information raises awareness in preoperative patient selection and preparation. Further studies in DAD scoliosis and a risk-adjusted patient selection/preparation are needed to improve treatment quality and outcomes.

Keywords: Correction spondylodesis, Degenerative adult de novo scoliosis, Perioperative complications

Background

Degenerative adult de novo (DAD) scoliosis is becoming increasingly a clinically important matter [1, 2]. Most of the patients are in the sixth to seventh decade or older and suffer from severe back pain that is mostly combined with signs of spinal or foraminal stenosis. These patients have no previous history of scoliosis and develop a spinal deformity first in late adulthood [3]. The aetiology of scoliosis can be primarily degenerative, secondary to previous surgery or due to metabolic changes – in particular, osteopenia or osteoporosis – and excludes idiopathic scoliosis [1]. The prevalence varies enormously in studies and reaches levels of up to 68% in a healthy adult population [4]. The natural history of DAD scoliosis shows a progression of degenerative changes to an increasingly worse stage, leading to further deformity [1, 5, 6]. Patients can develop severe impairments, but surgery should be considered only if sufficient conservative treatment has failed and

* Correspondence: mquante@schoen-kliniken.de
[3]Spinal Surgery Center, Schön Klink Neustadt, Am Kiebitzberg 10, 23730 Neustadt in Holstein, Germany

the patient is severely impaired regarding the activities of daily living.

Adult deformity surgery is technically difficult, has a high risk of complications and incompletely satisfactory outcomes [5, 7, 8]. Several intraoperative, perioperative and late-onset complications are common [9, 10]. Previous studies have identified certain surgical complications, but they contain a very heterogeneous patient collective ranging from adult idiopathic scoliosis, degenerative scoliosis, acquired, adult and iatrogenic kyphosis, and neuromuscular scoliosis, up to post-traumatic spinal deformities [10–13]. Further studies have the same problem regarding a clear risk assessment and outcome for a DAD scoliosis only collective [9, 14]. Despite previous reports, there is still a lack of information on DAD scoliosis-specific complications due to the mixture of scoliosis types in these studies. However, there seems to be a tendency towards an increased number of early complications for the group of DAD scoliosis cases.

DAD scoliosis surgery is an elective surgery and should consequently have a limited spectrum for complications. Therefore, this study premise is to collect and analyse intraoperative, perioperative and follow-up complication data of surgically treated patients exclusively with DAD scoliosis. As the next step, general and specific complications, as well as their possible risk factors for complications, were identified in this patient group in order to create a more disease surgical-specific risk pattern.

Methods

Diagnosis – Degenerative adult de novo (DAD) scoliosis

DAD scoliosis is a scoliosis form that develops in late adulthood. The degenerative deformation develops in the facet joints with dystrophic formation in the arthritis process or due to disc degeneration leading to frontal deviations or malrotations causing an curvature of the spine [1]. This process is mostly located in the thoracolumbar or lumbar spine [3, 15]. This form needs to be differentiated from the progressive idiopathic scoliosis. In the latter form the deformation was already present in childhood or adolescent life and progresses with increased age due to bony or degenerative changes [16, 17]. Furthermore, a distinct differentiation from secondary degenerative scoliosis with possible causes likes leg length discrepancies or vertebral fractures due to significant traumatic or metabolic changes is also fundamental [18, 19].

Identification and classification of scoliosis types is part of the clinical routine. However, classification of DAD scoliosis required a comprehensive medical history work-up with extended communication of referral and/or previous doctors of the patient, evaluation and comparison of past spinal radiographs or other type of spinal images to exclude any other origin of scoliosis (Fig. 1).

Exclusion criteria included diagnosis of any type of scoliosis of other origins (e.g. idiopathic, neuromuscular, congenital), which were excluded with an extended past medical history analysis, or previous radiologic images or fusion operations.

Study design

This retrospective study identified patients with DAD scoliosis, who underwent surgical procedures in the period from January 2007 until December 2009 with a minimum follow-up time of 12 months. During this time period, 622 deformity surgeries were performed at the authors' institution. Most of these cases were idiopathic nature ($n = 412$) followed by degenerative ($n = 92$), neuromuscular diseases ($n = 68$), congenital and other aetiology ($n = 33$ and 17). The internal registry of the spine surgery unit documents for quality management purposes precisely all surgical procedures (including type, technique, length, etc.) after each operation and data from the routine follow-up examinations. It was established to analyse complications and perform risk analysis/stratification for each patient according to the SPINE TANGO documentation system [20]. Inclusion criteria were the diagnosis of "DAD scoliosis" with a Cobb angle of at least 10° [21], persisting symptoms, failure of conservative treatment, and the procedure of a "correction spondylodesis".

The general symptoms were lumbago, spinal claudication and/or radicular pain. Prior to surgery, the patients had received conservative treatments (rest and avoidance of lifting heavy objects, adaption of lifestyle and antiphlogistic drugs, bracing, epidural and local facet joint injections and exercise) for a minimum of 3 to 6 months at our institution, excluding previous treatment time with the referral doctor. Only if conservative treatment failed, surgery was considered and performed after patient informed consent, including data collection, analysis and for scientific research purposes including publication followed by internal review board approval for analysis.

An ex-post analysis of prospective parameters was conducted for patients who had undergone primary correction spondylodesis in the authors' scoliosis centre for DAD scoliosis. All procedures performed in studies involving human participants were in accordance with the ethical standards of the institutional research committee and with the 1964 Helsinki declaration and its later amendments or comparable ethical standards.

Patient data

The patients' epidemiological data (gender, age and body mass index (BMI)), their therapies and medical comorbidities (obesity, osteoporosis, nicotine use, diabetes, chronic obstructive pulmonary disease (COPD), hypertension,

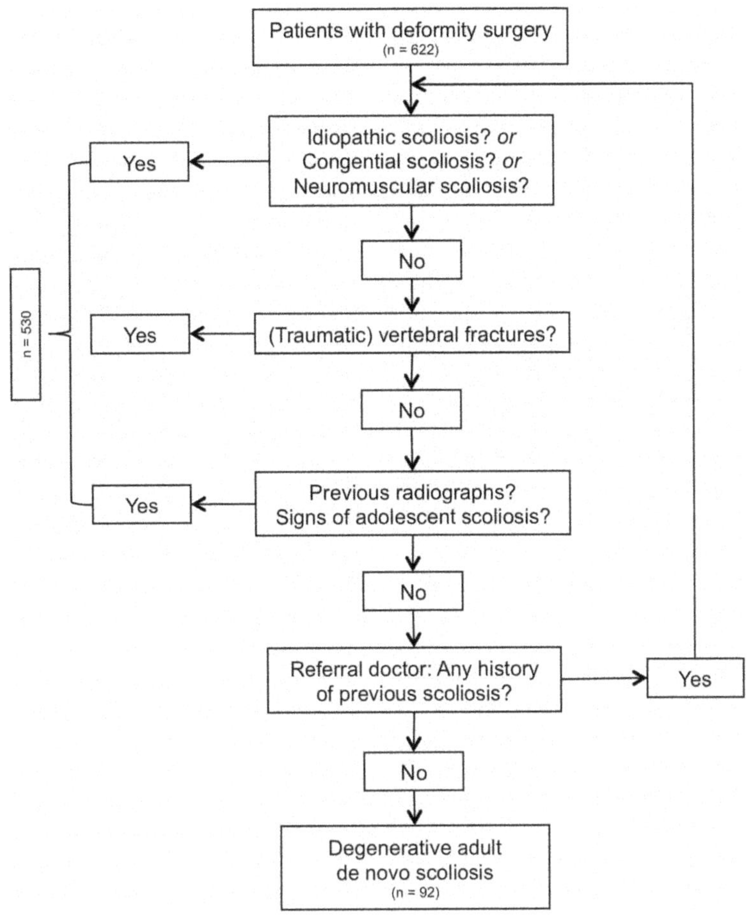

Fig. 1 The flow chart demonstrates patients with deformity surgery ($n = 622$) from 2007 until 2009 and the exclusion process of any type of scoliosis other than of degenerative adult de novo (DAD) scoliosis ($n = 92$). An extensive patient history was undertaken. If doubts arose, previous radiographic imaging was examined. Additionally, referral doctor and/or family physician were contacted to exclude other causes for scoliosis. Exclusion occurred when idiopathic ($n = 412$), neuromuscular ($n = 68$), congenital ($n = 33$) or vertebral fractures ($n = 17$) were answered with a "Yes" or radiographic images showed idiopathic or any scoliosis deformation other than DAD scoliosis

cardiac arrhythmias (CA), or pacemaker (PM) therapy) and anticoagulation therapies (such as acetylsalicylic acid or coumarin derivatives), neurological diseases (rheumatoid arthritis (RA) or steroid therapy), and whether they had previously had a non-instrumented spinal operation were preoperatively documented using a standardised procedure. The ASA (American Society of Anesthesiologists) physical status classification system was used to assess the fitness of each case before surgery.

This series represents all patients who underwent surgical treatment for DAD scoliosis between January 2007 and December 2009. None died before the minimum follow-up of 1 year, and none were lost to follow-up before that time. The mean follow-up time was 16.58 ± 13.89 months (range 12–36 months). Intraoperative data, as well as common surgical and specific spinal surgical postoperative information were analysed. Previous studies in adult deformity surgery identified several complications, however the postoperative time periods vary enormously (few days up to 12 weeks postoperatively) leading to different complication arrangements [9, 14, 22]. Due to the fact that the aim of this study was not only to include general surgical complications like wound healing, but also early problems related to the DAD scoliosis surgery (e.g. adjacent fractures, screw cut-outs), which tend to appear not immediately or are only recognized after a short observatory time and after regain of proper mobilization, the complication analysis led to the identification and classification of perioperative/early complications (≤ 30 days) and complications occurring >30 days after surgery.

Intraoperative and postoperative measurements

Operation times and the number of segments fused were recorded. The operative approach (dorsal only or dorsoventral) and additional techniques, such as a vertebroplasty, cement augmentation of the screws, transforaminal or anterior lumbar interbody fusion (TLIF or ALIF), were documented and had to be individually adapted for each patient. The estimated blood loss (EBL) was recorded by the cell salvage technician based on direct analysis of the suction loss and the use of surgical sponges. Additional confirmation was performed by the anaesthesiology service. The amount of erythrocyte concentrate (red blood cell (RBC) packs), fresh frozen plasma (FFP) packs and continuous autotransfusion system (CATS) blood used was documented.

Postoperative data was divided into two sections (early (≤ 30 days) and late (> 30 days including routine follow-up examinations). This data was further divided into common surgical (e.g. wound healing defects, infections) and specific spinal spinal (e.g. epidural hematoma, dural leak) complications. Radiological controls in form of a radiograph were undertaken during the postoperative stay and in the follow-ups. If the x-rays suggested a questionable screw/rod-placement or any other doubtable lesion, or if any neurological or other unexpected symptoms occurred, a computer-tomography or MRI was executed to identify the possible cause. Re-operations were accounted for.

Statistical analysis

Tables 1, 2, 3 and 4 report the summary statistics for all outcomes as well the summary statistics for all complications by group. Continuous variables are presented as mean ± SD, while categorical variables are presented as absolute numbers and percentages. Further, a subgroup analysis with respect to complications and all outcomes was conducted. Patients were divided into three groups, namely having experienced early (2), late (3) or no complications (4) at all. Columns 2, 3 and 4 of Tables 1, 2, 3 and 4 report the means of these subgroups and the p-values of their respective differences are reported in the three right-hand columns (5–7) of Tables 1, 2, 3 and 4. The p-values report the level of significance resulting from a t-test comparing the means of the subgroups. A p-value of ≤0.05

Table 1 Patient epidemiological data, medical disorders and treatments

		1		2		3		4		5	6	7
		Total		Early complications (< 30 d)		Late complications (> 30 d)		No complications		*p-value* $^{(3-2)}$	*p-value* $^{(4-2)}$	*p-value* $^{(4-3)}$
		n = 92	%	*n* = 23	%	*n* = 49	%	*n* = 20	%			
	Age (years)	67.2 ± 7.9		69.1 ± 8.3		67.2 ± 7.4		65.3 ± 8.5		0.34	0.14	0.35
	BMI (kg/m^2)	26.6 ± 3.4		27.0 ± 3.2		26.8 ± 3.2		25.9 ± 4.1		0.90	0.38	0.33
Gender	Male	28	30.4	7	30.4	13	26.5	8	40.0	0.73	0.52	0.28
	Female	64	69.6	16	69.5	36	73.5	12	60.0	0.73	0.52	0.28
ASA class	1	1	1.0	0	0.0	0	0.0	1	5.0	–	0.29	0.12
	2	62	67.3	13	56.5	35	71.4	14	70.0	0.22	0.37	0.91
	3	29	31.5	10	43.4	14	28.5	5	25.0	0.22	0.21	0.77
	4	0	0.0	0	0.0	0	0.0	0	0.0	–	–	–
	Obesity	20	21.7	4	17.3	11	22.4	5	25.0	0.63	0.55	0.82
	Smoker	26	31.7	6	30.0	12	28.5	8	40.0	0.91	0.52	0.38
	Type 1 Diabetes	8	8.9	4	8.6	4	8.6	0	0.0	0.29	0.05	0.18
	Type 2 Diabetes	11	11.5	5	12.7	6	12.7	0	0.0	0.26	< 0.05	0.10
	COPD	15	16.4	6	26.0	7	14.5	2	10.0	0.25	0.18	0.62
	Osteoporosis	23	25.0	6	26.0	14	28.5	3	15.0	0.83	0.38	0.24
	Neurological Disease	4	4.3	0	0.0	4	8.1	0	0.0	0.16	–	0.19
	Hypertension	34	36.9	11	47.8	16	32.6	7	35.0	0.22	0.41	0.85
	PM	5	5.4	3	13.0	2	4.0	0	0.0	0.17	0.10	0.37
	CA	19	22.6	9	40.9	9	21.4	1	5.0	0.10	< 0.05	0.10
	RA	7	7.6	2	8.6	4	8.1	1	5.0	0.94	0.64	0.65
	Cortisone	6	6.5	2	4.0	2	4.0	2	10.0	0.43	0.89	0.35
	ASS	7	7.6	1	10.2	5	10.2	1	5.0	0.41	0.92	0.49
	Coumarin derivative	8	8.6	4	17.3	2	4.0	2	10.0	0.06	0.50	0.35

Abbreviations: BMI body mass index, *ASA class* American Society of Anesthesiologists, *COPD* chronic obstructive pulmonary disease, *PM* pacemaker, *CA* cardiac arrhythmias, *RA* rheumatoid arthritis, *ASS* acetylsalicylic acid, coumarin derivative – phenprocoumon. Statistical analyses regarding *p*-values were performed between the three columns/groups, i.e. early complications (2), late complications (3) and no complications (4); see superscripted numbers (significance at $p < 0.05$ or at $p < 0.01$)

Table 2 Intraoperative data

	1		2		3		4		5	6	7
	Total		Early complications (< 30 d)		Late complications (> 30 d)		No complications		*p-value* $^{(3-2)}$	*p-value* $^{(4-2)}$	*p-value* $^{(4-3)}$
	n = 92	%	*n* = 23	%	*n* = 49	%	*n* = 20	%			
Previous Spine operations -Total	27	29.3	8	34.7	15	30.6	4	20.0	0.73	0.29	0.38
Nucelotomies	8	8.6	2	8.7	4	8.2	2	10.0	0.94	0.89	0.81
Spinal canal decompressions	19	20.6	6	26	11	22.4	2	10.0	0.74	0.18	0.24
Fused segments	5.2 ± 2.2		4.8 ± 1.9		5.6 ± 2.5		4.7 ± 1.6		0.16	0.89	0.14
Dorsoventral approach	35	38	8	34.7	23	46.9	4	20.0	0.34	0.29	< 0.05
Pedicle Screw augmentation	16	17.3	6	26	6	12.2	4	20.0	0.15	0.65	0.41
Vertebroplasty	17	18.4	6	26	7	14.3	4	20.0	0.23	0.65	0.56
ALIF	39	42.3	7	30.4	27	55.1	5	25.0	0.18	0.70	0.13
TLIF	54	58.6	17	73.9	26	53	11	55.0	0.11	0.25	0.89
Operation time (min)	341.1 ± 87.6		347.1 ± 102.7		361.1 ± 77.9		296.9 ± 78.9		0.57	0.10	< 0.01
Intraoperative blood loss (ml)	1567.3 ± 1098.4		1884.0 ± 1444.4		1602.7 ± 1065.3		1178.0 ± 580.3		0.39	0.05	0.10
CATS blood (ml)	344.9 ± 355.6		577.4 ± 522.7		353.5 ± 326.7		313.2 ± 235.8		0.97	0.72	0.62
Perioperative											
RBC	3.3 ± 5.5		5.6 ± 7.2		3.2 ± 5.3		0.9 ± 1.1		0.12	< 0.05	0.06
FFP	2.5 ± 4.7		4.4 ± 6.6		2.2 ± 4.2		1.1 ± 1.5		0.10	< 0.05	0.24

Abbreviations: ALIF and TLIF anterior and transforaminal lumbar interbody fusion, *RBC* red blood cell packs, *FFP* fresh frozen plasma units, *CATS-blood* continuous autotransfusion system blood. Statistical analyses regarding *p*-values were performed between the three columns/groups, i.e. early complications (2), late complications (3) and no complications (4); see superscripted numbers (significance at $p < 0.05$ or at $p < 0.01$)

Table 3 Postoperative complications and re-operations

	1		2		3		4		5	6	7
	Total		Early complications (< 30 d)		Late complications (> 30 d)		No complications		*p-value* $^{(3-2)}$	*p-value* $^{(4-2)}$	*p-value* $^{(4-3)}$
	n = 92	%	*n* = 23	%	*n* = 49	%	*n* = 20	%			
Wound healing defects	17	18.4	12	52.1	5	10.2	0	0	< 0.01	< 0.01	0.14
Wound dehiscence, delayed healing	10	10.9	6	26	4	8.2	0	0	< 0.05	< 0.05	0.18
Superficial infection	7	7.6	6	26	1	2.0	0	0	< 0.01	< 0.05	0.53
Operation due to wound healing defects	13	14.1	11	47.8	2	4.1	0	0	< 0.01	< 0.01	0.37
Postoperative Paresis	13	14.1	6	26	7	14.3	0	0	0.23	< 0.05	0.08
Epidural hematoma	6	6.5	5	21.7	1	2.0	0	0	< 0.01	< 0.05	0.53
Re-Operation	6	6.5	5	21.7	1	2.0	0	0	< 0.01	< 0.05	0.53
Dural leak	7	8.7	1	5.2	6	14.6	0	0	0.30	0.31	0.07
Re-Operation	1	1.2	1	5.2	0	0	0	0	0.14	0.31	–
Adjacent segment failure Total (n)	33	35.8	12	52.1	21	42.9	0	0	0.47	< 0.01	< 0.01
Adjacent segment failure during hospital stay	8	8.7	8	34.8	0	0	0	0	< 0.01	< 0.01	–
Re-Operation	8	8.7	8	34.8	0	0	0	0	< 0.01	< 0.01	–
Adjacent segment failure later on	25	27.2	4	17.4	21	42.8	0	0	< 0.01	< 0.01	< 0.01
After how many months	9.3 ± 6.3		6.7 ± 8.0		9.85 ± 6.1		0		0.19	< 0.01	< 0.01
Re-Operation	22	23.9	3	13.0	19	38.7	0	0	< 0.01	< 0.05	< 0.01

Statistical analyses regarding *p*-values were performed between the three columns/groups, i.e. early complications (2), late complications (3) and no complications (4); see superscripted numbers (significance at $p < 0.05$ or at $p < 0.01$)

Table 4 Early adjacent segment failure (ASF) complications requiring surgical treatment are listed below. (Sex: F = female, M = male)

Case	Sex, Age (years)	Previous operations	Fusion length	ASF	Cause and further treatment
1	M, 62	Yes	2	Yes	Patient had persitant back pain postoperatively and paresthesia in the lower extremity. MRI showed an adjacent vertebral fracture leading to an elongation of the initial fusion of up to 4 segments and second explorative operation due to persistant paresthesia. No specific cause was identifed for this. Sensation returned to normal in the further course.
2	F, 67	No	6	Yes	Early adjacent failure was caused by an osteoporotic cut out of the upper uncemented pedicle screws. This led to an elongation of the fusion by two segements with cement-augmentation.
3	F, 74	No	5	Yes	After the inital dorsoventral fusion, an osteoporotic adjacent segment failure in the upper instrumented vertebra caused the need of a fusion extension of one more segment with pedicle screw cement augmention. Thereafter, the patient developed a wound dehiscence. This led to a further operation for wound debridement and closure.
4	M, 65	No	6	Yes	This adjacent segment failure included a pedicle fracture causing a transient paresis of the hip flexion requiring immediate screw removal and nerve exploration. There was no nerve root damage. The fusion was elongated by 2 levels. The muscle regained full function in the follow-ups.
5	F, 72	No	4	Yes	This patient had a screw misplacement as idenfied by the CT-scan. The screw was causing irritation of the nerve root and had a cut out through upper vertebral plate. This complex cause of adjacent segment failure and spinal nerve compression lead to an early revision and elongation by one segment.
6	M, 85	No	5	Yes	This patient showed during the primary operation a poor bone quality (osteoporosis) with the need to use cement augmentation of the upper instrumented vertebra. During the early mobilisation process, the patient suffered an adjacent vertebral fracture with progression needing a revision with elongation of 2 more segments with careful cement augmentation.
7	F, 67	No	6	Yes	Due to osteoporotic bone, the upper pedicle screws were cement augmented. However, the poor bone quality caused an osteoporotic fracture with nerve irritation needing a revision surgery with elongation of the fusion by 2 segments. Unfortunately thereafter, a wound healing defect caused a further superfical wound revision.
8	F, 83	No	3	Yes	Due to a collapse of the upper vertebral plate during the mobilisation process, a surgical revision with elongation of 1 segment with cement augmentation was necessary.

shows that the mean outcomes were significantly different from one another for two groups. Column 5 in Tables 1, 2, 3 and 4 reports the difference in outcomes between patients with early and late complications, column 6 between no complications and early complications, and column 7 between no and late complications.

Results

From a total of 622 deformity surgeries in the years of 2007 until 2009, 92 patients with a DAD scoliosis were identified and included in this retrospective analysis. After failure of conservative treatment, these patients had a primary correction spondylodesis. The average follow-up time was 16.58 ± 13.89 months (minimum 12, maximum 31 months). The mean age was 67.29 ± 7.93 years. Sixty-four patients were female (69.6%) and 28 patients were male (30.4%). The overall BMI was 26.69 ± 3.48 kg/m^2 and 20.7% of patients were obese (BMI > 30 kg/m^2). The physical status of the patients was within the first three ASA classes (Table 1). More than a quarter (28.3%) of the patients smoked tobacco. Nineteen patients had diabetes mellitus (8 type 1 and 11 type 2). A quarter of the entire patient group had properly diagnosed osteoporosis (T-score: ≥ −2.5). Arterial hypertension was a medical comorbidity in 34 patients (37.0%) and 19 patients (20.7%) had a CA.

Twenty-seven patients (29.3%) had a previous non-instrumented spinal operation (an open spinal nucleotomy or spinal canal decompression in 8 (8.7%) and 19 (20.7%) patients, respectively). The average number of segments fused was 5.26 ± 2.24. All cases had fusion operations in segments T12-S1 (only 21.7% had fusions extended beyond these levels – total range from T4 until S1 with iliac screws)) with an average operation time of 341.19 ± 87.66 min (Table 2). Dorsoventral spondylodesis was performed in 35 cases (38.0%), whereas TLIF was undertaken in 54 patients (58.7%). Intraoperative estimated blood loss was 1567.33 ± 1098.42 ml and the CATS blood generation averaged at 344.94 ± 355.63 ml, which led to the use of 3.30 ± 5.55 RBC and 2.55 ± 4.73 FFP units.

Common surgical complications

In total, 17 wound healing defects were registered. Seven of these were superficial infections (Table 3). There was no correlation to diabetes mellitus or smoking. Nine postoperative electrolyte disturbances were quickly corrected and the eight urinary tract infections were uncomplicated and treated rapidly without further consequences (Table 4). There were no cases of thrombosis, pulmonary embolism or cerebrovascular insult (stroke). Two of the 92 patients died. One death within 30 days was due to postoperative disseminated intravascular coagulopathy in combination with systemic inflammatory response syndrome. The other death was due to an acute myocardial infarction several months after the operation (Table 4). The average hospital stay was 21.92 ± 10.05 days.

Specific spinal surgical complications

Postoperative weakness/paresis occurred in 13 patients. The muscle weakness was never below stage 3 (fair function) on the Janda muscle function scale (approximately 50% strength, movement against gravity). Nine patients had muscle function of stage 4 (strength reduced, but contraction can still move the joint against reduced resistance) and four patients showed reduced muscle strength of stage 3 at hospital discharge. However, in the follow-up visits all patients had returned to full muscle strength. Epidural haematoma occurred six times and in all six cases required a re-operation. Adjacent segment failure was the major complication, which happened in a total of 33 patients. In most cases ($n = 25$), it occurred several months after initial instrumentation (9.3 ± 6.3 months) and required in 22 patients another operation.

Another frequent complication was sciatic pain, which was observed in 22 patients (23.9%). Structural diagnostics were performed in each of the cases to identify a mechanical problem (6 epidural hematomas, 1 misplacement of pedicle screws, 1 adjacent segment failure). If it was due to a mechanical cause, it was surgically repaired. If no structural cause was identified, the pain resolved itself or an intensive pain-therapy regimen had to be started (14 patients) (Table 4).

Assessment of cases with early, late or no complications

Twenty-three patients had an early complication (≤ 30 days) following the spinal surgery. A late complication (> 30 days) occurred in a total of 49 patients. There were no significant predisposing biometric values identified regarding patient age, gender or BMI. There was no significant influence of illnesses or disorders detected regarding overall complications, but early complications tended to have a higher correlation with CA, PM and coumarin derivate therapies (Table 1).

The perioperative data show no significant differences in instrumentation length for both groups (4.82 ± 1.92 instrumented segments (early) versus 5.61 ± 2.51 (late complications)), either in the number of previous spinal surgeries or in the operating time (Table 2). A striking but non-statistically significant difference was seen in the percentage of TLIFs undertaken in the early complication group compared with the late complication group (73.9% versus 53.0%). However, the number of segments fused in these TLIF cases did not differ between these two groups. The majority of complications related to TLIF were of neurological nature. Most of these cases were classified as an early complication (6 cases of postoperative paresis, 10 cases of sciatic pain). All of these complications were transient. The postoperative paresis usually diminished within the hospital stay, whereas the sciatic pain was often prolonged but also temporary as seen in the follow-ups. Furthermore, the number of RBC and FFP units used was significantly higher in cases with early complications (Table 2).

A major late complication was adjacent segment failure (Table 3). In total, 25 cases of adjacent segment failure were observed in the follow-up visits. Twenty-two patients required surgical therapy with prolongation of the previous instrumented segments. Eight patients had an adjacent segment failure during their hospital stay (≤ 30 days) (Table 4). The causes were implant failure, screw loosening or fractured vertebral endplate, and led in all cases to a surgical revision. Sciatic pain occurred more often within 30 days postoperatively. However, intensive pain therapy was only necessary in five cases. In-hospital stay times differed significantly between the cases with early (31.65 ± 12.60 days) and late (20.16 ± 6.82 days) complications.

In comparison, a total of 20 patients did not have any complications early after the operation or later during the follow-up time of 15.80 ± 13.83 months (Table 5). These patients were slightly younger (65.3 ± 8.5 years) compared with the average age (67.29 ± 7.93 years) and had a slightly lower average BMI than the overall collective and the two complication groups (Table 1). An average of 4.75 ± 1.68 segments were fused (Table 2). Operation times were the shortest (296.90 ± 78.95 min) in comparison with the average operation time. Additionally, the estimated blood loss was the lowest at 1178 ± 580.33 ml, and thus these patients required the least amount of RBC and FFP units (Table 2).

Discussion

In the aging society, patient numbers with DAD scoliosis and required surgical treatments is increasing. Specific information regarding this entity is sparse and therefore assessment of surgical complications and outcomes trying to identify risk factors is essential. The current study with a DAD scoliosis only collective demonstrates that adjacent segment failure is the main complication (35.8%). DAD scoliosis surgery bears an increased risk

Table 5 Postoperative complications with conservative treatment, in-hospital stay and follow-up times

	1		2		3		4		5	6	7
	Total		Early complications (< 30 d)		Late complications (> 30 d)		No complications		*p-value* $^{(3-2)}$	*p-value* $^{(4-2)}$	*p-value* $^{(4-3)}$
	n = 92	%	*n* = 23	%	*n* = 49	%	*n* = 20	%			
Electrolyte disturbances	9	9.8	2	0.09	7	0.14	0	0.00	0.51	0.19	0.08
UTI	8	8.7	3	0.15	5	0.13	0	0.00	0.79	0.07	0.10
Sciatic pain	22	23.9	12	0.52	10	0.20	0	0.00	< 0.05	< 0.01	< 0.05
Hypoesthesia	3	3.3	1	0.04	2	0.04	0	0.00	0.96	0.36	0.37
Intensive pain-therapy	14	15.2	5	0.22	9	0.18	0	0.00	0.74	< 0.05	< 0.05
Thrombosis	0	0.0	0	0.00	0	0.00	0	0.00	–	–	–
Pulmonary embolism	0	0.0	0	0.00	0	0.00	0	0.00	–	–	–
Stroke	0	0.0	0	0.00	0	0.00	0	0.00	–	–	–
Death	2	2.2	1	0.04	1	0.02	0	0.00	0.58	0.36	0.53
Hospital Stay (d)	21.9 ± 10.0		31.6 ± 12.6		20.1 ± 6.8		15.0 ± 3.2		< 0.01	< 0.01	< 0.01
Follow-up time (months)	16.4 ± 13.8		14.1 ± 10.9		17.6 ± 15.2		15.8 ± 13.8		0.32	0.67	0.63

Abbreviations: UTI urinary tract infection. Duration of in-hospital stay is registered in days (d) and clinical follow-up visits are documented in months. Statistical analyses regarding *p*-values were performed between the three columns/groups, i.e. early complications (2), late complications (3) and no complications (4); see superscripted numbers (significance at $p < 0.05$ or at $p < 0.01$)

for various sorts of complications within 30 days after surgery as identified in 23 patients. In the further follow-up, 49 patients were documented to have a sort of late complication.

Early complications were typically wound healing dysfunctions, early adjacent segment failure, postoperative paresis or increased blood loss. Predisposing factors for these latter cases were CA, a PM or coumarin derivative therapy. In general, increased age and other co-factors (e.g. cigarette smoking, obesity or osteoporosis) are plausible contributing factors for complications following scoliosis surgery, as previously described [23]; the current results show that these can now be specifically attributed to DAD scoliosis patients as well. Factors such as CA, including PM therapy and coumarin derivative medication, were increased in patients with early complications. Generally, anticoagulation therapy management in spinal surgery is not simple [24, 25]. Poor anticoagulation management can be a cause of epidural or intraspinal haematomas, thromboembolisms or bleeding complications. However, the rate of occurrence of thromboembolisms in degenerative spinal surgeries (2.3%) is much lower than that for deformity or trauma surgery at 5.3% and 6.0%, respectively [26]. No thromboembolisms or pulmonary embolisms occurred in the current study. Postoperative haematomas may occur, but do not seem to be particularly predisposed by anticoagulative medication, as seen in the present study and a study by Cheng et al. [24].

Operative techniques, such as a TLIF, can be a risk factor for early complications, as during this process the spinal nerves are stressed, which may result in postoperative pain, sensory dysfunction or motor disabilities [27]. This is temporary in most cases, but can persist if nerves have been damaged [28]. With regard to the present results, TLIF did not seem to be a cause of major neurological complications, but should be recognised as a possible cause of minor neurological complications (transient paresis or hypoesthesia). The present results show that postoperative weakness or sensory dysfunctions resolved, in most cases, within three to 6 months after the operation. But, TLIF-technique increased operation times and blood loss, possibly leading to further postoperative complications. TLIF is not the only operation technique that may increase complication risks. Ventral surgery with support of the anterior column (ALIF) can enhance the posterior fusion stability and reconstruction of lumbar lordosis significantly [29], but the anterior approach is acquainted with an increased numbers of vascular injuries [12, 30]. However, the development of posterior fusion with TLIF techniques improved and now shows equally good results regarding fusion. But, posterior lumbar interbody fusion (PLIF) and TLIF are less effective than anterior methods in reconstructing lumbar lordosis. [31]. The selection of an operation procedure depends on the scoliosis length and severity, previous surgeries and/or bone quality and other possible confounders [32]. Therefore, each technique (e.g. ALIF) needs to be individually described to the patient carefully and explicitly explained regarding possible complications.

In contrast to our results, diabetes mellitus is regarded as a major complication factor in spinal fusion operations [33]. No significant correlation was identified in this analysed group. The results of whether insulin-dependent diabetes mellitus (IDDM) or non-insulin-dependent diabetes mellitus (NIDDM) is the more important risk factor are not completely constant but show a tendency towards IDDM [33, 34]. Cho and colleagues have shown that NIDDM was not a significant risk factor for perioperative complications or additional surgeries in spinal deformity surgery [35]. The reason for this discrepancy with diabetes being a risk factor in the literature and in the present study might be surgical invasiveness. This means that diabetes may be an influencing factor when the surgery is minor, such as in decompression operations or fusion surgeries of up to two levels, but is not of importance when fusion operations of three or more segments are performed [33–35].

The main problem in terms of early and late complications in the present study was adjacent segment failure with a total of 33 cases. Similarly, Etebar and Cahill identified in their collective that 18 of 125 patients had an adjacent segment failure problem after spinal instrumentation [36]. A majority of these were postmenopausal women. Only 22% were cigarette smokers. Most frequently, adjacent segment failure was not limited to the next segment alone. In the present study, a fair amount of patients who had adjacent segment degeneration were cigarette smoking (35.48%) or had osteoporosis (32.25%), however no significant correlation could be established. There are of course other factors that influence adjacent segment failure such as rigidity in adult spine deformities or the incorrect selection of fusion levels. These possible confounding factors were carefully considered before and during the surgery to optimize the outcome, maintain mobility/flexibility and avoidance of proximal or distal segment failure, as previous studies have analysed [37–39]. Even performance of an osteotomy confers a large risk of possible complications, but the outcome can improve significantly with such a procedure [38]. In this study of DAD scoliosis patients, 90 cases had at least three segments fused. This is often inevitable since this scoliosis type, with its degenerative nature and curvature length, make it prone to adjacent segment failure. In particular, early adjacent segment failure is of major interest, since the main reason was screw loosening or a fractured vertebral endplate, thus highlighting that the specific entity of DAD scoliosis is susceptible to early adjacent segment failure. Causes for adjacent segment failure other than misalignments in the sagittal or frontal plane are typically of a degenerative nature, based on metabolic changes which are specifically increased in this particular group of DAD scoliosis and make the adjacent segment less resilient. However, there have been no specific studies that showed a correlation between sagittal alignment and adjacent segment failure. In the current study, patients were not classified regarding their spinal balance. In future studies, the interaction between sagittal alignment and adjacent segment failure must be studied.

This study specifically focused on DAD scoliosis surgically treated patients in a retrospective manner; therefore, it has its limitations and requires careful interpretation of the results. First of all, the amount of patients included in this study is not great, but the limiting factor here was the exclusive investigation of DAD scoliosis as the sole scoliosis type, with the additional factor of no previous fusion surgeries. This might limit the case number, but leads to a clearer assessment and irreplaceable information for DAD scoliosis patients. Secondly, the follow-up times vary widely, but patients without complications and proper spinal fusion were only clinically monitored postoperatively for 1 year and thereafter should come in if problems occurred. This is not a long time to monitor patient outcomes, however, the main aspect of this retrospective study focused on perioperative and “early onset” complications, which are related to the surgical intervention. Nevertheless, patients have continuous and regular check-ups at the authors' department, but the long-term course of the patients was not part of this study focus. Furthermore, this patient collective consists of relatively morbid and elder people that have a great tendency of rapid health situation changes. Consequently after 1 or 2 years, one monitors many phenomena/changes of aging and general degeneration that are not the direct consequences of the spondylodesis operation. Once again, the aim of this current study was to primarily identify surgical related complications of this special collective of DAD scoliosis cases and therefore focused on the time period early after surgery. Third, the patients in this study were not subdivided according to the specific surgical approach undertaken, with each technique having a different set of complications. This current study was rather set up to monitor general complications and their occurrences. Establishing specific risk correlations should not be done due to the heterogeneous surgical techniques used. But, to achieve the best possible outcome, we had to individually adapt the surgical techniques for each patient. Penultimate, sagittal alignment was always part of the preoperative assessment and good sagittal balance was part of the surgical aim. However, at the times of surgery it was not in the main focus, therefore we cannot draw further conclucions. This needs to be the focus of newer studies. Lastly, the small sample size prevented us from drawing conclusive evidence from the statistical mean comparisons. Only a few subgroup outcomes differed from one another, possibly due to the lack of statistical power; we may have failed to reject the null hypothesis, when we should have rejected it. Furthermore, the small sample size did not permit us to conduct in depth statistical analysis such as regression analyses. The lack of random assignment and of a control group did not permit us to interpret our results as causal.

Conclusions

In summary, this study demonstrates that complications in DAD scoliosis surgery are not uncommon, as 25% of the patients required surgical revision within 30 days. The research exclusively limited to this very selective patient cohort is of major interest due to aging society and increased case numbers, and highlights that this elective operation has an increased risk profile. Assessing the risk factors (such as cardiac arrhythmias with anticoagulative therapies, various operative techniques e.g. TLIF, sagittal balance) can help in planning surgical strategies, estimating risk ratios and improving outcomes. Further studies with DAD scoliosis cohorts and long-term follow-ups are required to improve the risk profiles for these patients.

Abbreviations

ALIF: Anterior lumbar interbody fusion; ASA: American Society of Anesthesiologists; ASF: Adjacent segment failure; ASS: Acetylsalicylic acid; BMI: Body mass index; CA: Cardiac arrhythmias; CATS: Continuous autotransfusion system; COPD: Chronic obstructive pulmonary disease; d: Day(s); DAD: Degenerative adult de novo; EBL: Estimated blood loss; F: Female; FFP: Fresh frozen plasma; IDDM: Insulin dependent diabetes mellitus; M: Male; NIDDM: Non-insulin dependent diabetes mellitus; PLIF: Posterior lumbar interbody fusion; PM: Pacemaker; RA: Rheumatoid arthritis; RBC: Red blood cell; SD: Standard deviation; TLIF: Transforaminal lumbar interbody fusion; UTI: Urinary tract infusion

Acknowledgements

The authors thank Kristin Sorsch for her help with data acquisition and Lisa K Simon for her help with the statistical analysis.

Funding

No funding was obtained for this study.

Authors' contributions

MJKS: study concept design, data acquisition, data analysis, manuscript writing, final approval. HFHH: study concept design, data analysis, manuscript revising, final approval. MQ: study concept design, data analysis, manuscript writing and revising, final approval.

Consent for publication

Not applicable.

Competing interests

The authors declare that they have no competing interests.

Author details

[1]Department of Orthopedics, University Medical Center Hamburg-Eppendorf, Martinistrasse 52, 20246 Hamburg, Germany. [2]Department of Osteology and Biomechanics, University Medical Center Hamburg-Eppendorf, Martinistrasse 52, 20246 Hamburg, Germany. [3]Spinal Surgery Center, Schön Klink Neustadt, Am Kiebitzberg 10, 23730 Neustadt in Holstein, Germany.

References

1. Aebi M. The adult scoliosis. Eur Spine J. 2005;14:925–48.
2. Schwab F, Dubey A, Pagala M, Gamez L, Farcy JP. Adult scoliosis: a health assessment analysis by SF-36. Spine (Phila Pa 1976). 2003;28:602–6.
3. Grubb SA, Lipscomb HJ, Coonrad RW. Degenerative adult onset scoliosis. Spine. 1988;13:241–5.
4. Schwab F, Dubey A, Gamez L, El Fegoun AB, Hwang K, Pagala M, Farcy JP. Adult scoliosis: prevalence, SF-36, and nutritional parameters in an elderly volunteer population. Spine (Phila Pa 1976). 2005;30:1082–5.
5. Quante M, Richter A, Thomsen B, Koszegvary M, Halm H. Surgical management of adult scoliosis. The challenge of osteoporosis and adjacent level degeneration. Orthopade. 2009;38:159–69.
6. Kebaish KM. Degenerative (de novo) adult scoliosis. Semin Spine Surg. 2009; 21:7–15.
7. Schwab FJ, Lafage V, Farcy JP, Bridwell KH, Glassman S, Shainline MR. Predicting outcome and complications in the surgical treatment of adult scoliosis. Spine (Phila Pa 1976). 2008;33:2243–7.
8. Baron EM, Albert TJ. Medical complications of surgical treatment of adult spinal deformity and how to avoid them. Spine. 2006;31:S106–18.
9. Cho SK, Bridwell KH, Lenke LG, Yi JS, Pahys JM, Zebala LP, Kang MM, Cho W, Baldus CR. Major complications in revision adult deformity surgery: risk factors and clinical outcomes with 2- to 7-year follow-up. Spine (Phila Pa 1976). 2012;37:489–500.
10. Lapp MA, Bridwell KH, Lenke LG, Daniel Riew K, Linville DA, Eck KR, Ungacta FF. Long-term complications in adult spinal deformity patients having combined surgery a comparison of primary to revision patients. Spine. 2001; 26:973–83.
11. Yadla S, Maltenfort MG, Ratliff JK, Harrop JS. Adult scoliosis surgery outcomes: a systematic review. Neurosurg Focus. 2010;28:E3.
12. Glassman SD, Hamill CL, Bridwell KH, Schwab FJ, Dimar JR, Lowe TG. The impact of perioperative complications on clinical outcome in adult deformity surgery. Spine (Phila Pa 1976). 2007;32:2764–70.
13. Linville DA, Bridwell KH, Lenke LG, Vedantam R, Leicht P. Complications in the adult spinal deformity patient having combined surgery. Does revision increase the risk? Spine. 1999;24:355–63.
14. DeWald CJ, Stanley T. Instrumentation-related complications of multilevel fusions for adult spinal deformity patients over age 65: surgical considerations and treatment options in patients with poor bone quality. Spine (Phila Pa 1976). 2006;31:S144–51.
15. Ponseti I. The pathogenesis of adult scoliosis. Edinburgh: E & Livingstone; 1968.
16. Ascani E, Bartolozzi P, Logroscino CA, Marchetti PG, Ponte A, Savini R, Travaglini F, Binazzi R, Di Silvestre M. Natural history of untreated idiopathic scoliosis after skeletal maturity. Spine (Phila Pa 1976). 1986;11:784–9.
17. Rinella A, Bridwell K, Kim Y, Rudzki J, Edwards C, Roh M, Lenke L, Berra A. Late complications of adult idiopathic scoliosis primary fusions to L4 and above: the effect of age and distal fusion level. Spine (Phila Pa 1976). 2004; 29:318–25.
18. Bradford DS, Tay BK, Adult HSS. Scoliosis: surgical indications, operative management, complications, and outcomes. Spine (Phila Pa 1976). 1999;24: 2617–29.
19. Grubb SA, Lipscomb HJ. Diagnostic findings in painful adult scoliosis. Spine (Phila Pa 1976). 1992;17:518–27.
20. Aebi M, Grob DSSE. Spine Tango: a European spine registry promoted by the spine Society of Europe (SSE). Eur. Spine J. 2004;13:661–2.
21. Van Goethem J, Van Campenhout A, van den Hauwe L, Parizel PM. Scoliosis. Neuroimaging Clin N Am. 2007;17:105–15.
22. Emami A, Deviren V, Berven S, Smith JA, SS H, Bradford DS. Outcome and complications of long fusions to the sacrum in adult spine deformity: luque-galveston, combined iliac and sacral screws, and sacral fixation. Spine (Phila Pa 1976). 2002;27:776–86.
23. Tang H, Zhu J, Ji F, Wang S, Xie Y, Fei H. Risk factors for postoperative complication after spinal fusion and instrumentation in degenerative lumbar scoliosis patients. J Orthop Surg Res. 2014;9:15.

24. Cheng JS, Arnold PM, Anderson PA, Fischer D, Dettori JR. Anticoagulation risk in spine surgery. Spine. 2010;35:S117–24.
25. Quante M, Zamani R, Simon MJ, Klasen J, Bullmann V. Thromboprophylaxis and platelet aggregation inhibitors in spinal surgery: perioperative management. Orthopade. 2014;43:833–40.
26. Glotzbecker MP, Bono CM, Wood KB, Harris MB. Thromboembolic disease in spinal surgery: a systematic review. Spine. 2009;34:291–303.
27. Tormenti MJ, Maserati MB, Bonfield CM, Okonkwo DO, Kanter AS. Complications and radiographic correction in adult scoliosis following combined transpsoas extreme lateral interbody fusion and posterior pedicle screw instrumentation. Neurosurg Focus. 2010;28:E7.
28. Kim KT, Lee SH, Suk KS, Lee JH, Jeong BO. Outcome of pedicle subtraction osteotomies for fixed sagittal imbalance of multiple etiologies: a retrospective review of 140 patients. Spine (Phila Pa 1976). 2012;37:1667–75.
29. Hsieh PC, Koski TR, O'Shaughnessy BA, Sugrue P, Salehi S, Ondra S, Liu JC. Anterior lumbar interbody fusion in comparison with transforaminal lumbar interbody fusion: implications for the restoration of foraminal height, local disc angle, lumbar lordosis, and sagittal balance. J Neurosurg Spine. 2007;7: 379–86.
30. Daubs MD, Lenke LG, Cheh G, Stobbs G, Bridwell KH. Adult spinal deformity surgery: complications and outcomes in patients over age 60. Spine (Phila Pa 1976). 2007;32:2238–44.
31. Crandall DG, Revella J. Transforaminal lumbar interbody fusion versus anterior lumbar interbody fusion as an adjunct to posterior instrumented correction of degenerative lumbar scoliosis: three year clinical and radiographic outcomes. Spine (Phila Pa 1976). 2009;34:2126–33.
32. Cho KJ, Kim YT, Shin SH, Suk SI. Surgical treatment of adult degenerative scoliosis. Asian. Spine J. 2014;8:371–81.
33. Glassman SD, Alegre G, Carreon L, Dimar JR, Johnson JR. Perioperative complications of lumbar instrumentation and fusion in patients with diabetes mellitus. Spine J. 2003;3:496–501.
34. Deyo RA, Hickam D, Duckart JP, Piedra M. Complications after surgery for lumbar stenosis in a veteran population. Spine. 2013;38:1695–702.
35. Cho W, Lenke LG, Bridwell KH, Dorward IG, Shoda N, Baldus CR, Cho SK, Kang MM, Zebala LP, Pahys JM, Koester LA. Comparison of spinal deformity surgery in patients with non-insulin-dependent diabetes mellitus (NIDDM) versus controls. Spine. 2012;37:E978–84.
36. Etebar S, Cahill DW. Risk factors for adjacent-segment failure following lumbar fixation with rigid instrumentation for degenerative instability. J Neurosurg. 1999;90:163–9.
37. Voos K, Boachie-Adjei O, Rawlins BA. Multiple vertebral osteotomies in the treatment of rigid adult spine deformities. Spine. 2001;26:526–33.
38. Berjano P, Aebi M. Pedicle subtraction osteotomies (PSO) in the lumbar spine for sagittal deformities. Eur. Spine J. 2015;24(Suppl 1):S49–57.
39. Trobisch PD, Ducoffe AR, Lonner BS, Errico TJ. Choosing fusion levels in adolescent idiopathic scoliosis. J Am Acad Orthop Surg. 2013;21:519–28.

4

Subtle elbow instability associated with lateral epicondylitis

Sang Ho Kwak[1], Seung-Jun Lee[1*], Hee Seok Jeong[2], Min Uk Do[1] and Kuen Tak Suh[1]

Abstract

Background: In lateral epicondylitis, even in the absence of apparent instability, subtle instability can be found under anesthesia. We wanted to ascertain the following: (1) how many elbows surgically treated with lateral epicondylitis showed subtle instability during examination under anesthesia (EUA), (2) how effective magnetic resonance imaging (MRI) was in predicting subtle instability, and (3) if any difference existed in preoperative clinical data between elbows with and without subtle instability during EUA.

Methods: One hundred and twenty-two elbows (117 patients) diagnosed with intractable lateral epicondylitis underwent surgical treatment. No elbow showed apparent instability with conventional physical examination. Under general anesthesia, the elbows were examined for subtle instability via fluoroscopy and divided into unstable and stable groups. Potential prognostic factors and functional scores were assessed retrospectively. The MRIs were reviewed again by two radiologists.

Results: Seventeen elbows (unstable group, 13.9%) had subtle instability in EUA, while 105 elbows (stable group, 86.1%) did not. Lateral collateral ligament (LCL) complex injury was noted in the MRIs of 28 elbows. Fifteen elbows showed subtle instability among 28 elbows with abnormal MRI (positive predictive value, 53.6%), while 81 elbows did not show subtle instability among 82 elbows with normal MRI (negative predictive value, 98.7%). The preoperative visual analog scale score was higher in the unstable group than in the stable group ($p < 0.001$), and a history of multiple corticosteroid injections (≥3) was related to subtle instability in EUA ($p = 0.042$). Other factors showed no significant differences between both groups.

Conclusions: Subtle instability resulting from LCL complex injury was noted in elbows with lateral epicondylitis. This could be visualized with fluoroscopic EUA, and preoperative MRI could be used to exclude subtle instability. Surgeons should consider checking for subtle instability, especially when patients have a history of multiple corticosteroid injections (≥3) or severe pain and MRI indicates instability.

Keywords: Lateral, Epicondylitis, Tendinosis, Ligament, Instability, Elbow

Background

Lateral epicondylitis is usually diagnosed based on clinical history and physical examination. Excluding conditions that can mimic lateral epicondylitis is very important because symptoms cannot be fully relieved if such lesions are neglected. For a differential diagnosis, multiple modalities including simple radiography, ultrasonography, magnetic resonance imaging (MRI), and electrodiagnosis can be used.

* Correspondence: Ninanojune@naver.com
[1]Department of Orthopaedic Surgery, Pusan National University Yangsan Hospital, Pusan National University School of Medicine, 20, Geumo-ro, Mulgeum-eup, Yangsan-si, Gyeongsangnam-do, Republic of Korea

Associated ligament injuries in lateral epicondylitis were reported using MRI or via conventional physical examination. MRI can be used for differentiating other pathologic conditions such as plica, elbow arthritis, and osteochondral defect. In addition, concomitant ligament injuries involving the medial collateral ligament (MCL), lateral collateral ligament (LCL), and lateral ulnar collateral ligament (LUCL) have also been observed in MRI-diagnosed lateral epicondylitis [1, 2]. Associated ligament injuries can induce elbow instability eventually, and posterolateral rotatory instabilities after trauma, corticosteroid injection, and iatrogenic injury during debridement for lateral epicondylitis have been reported [3, 4]. In these reports, most of the patients showed apparent symptoms including instability via conventional physical examination, feeling of "pop," or prominent swelling of the elbow joint [3, 4]. However, Kalainov revealed that one patient showed unspecific physical examination and the posterolateral instability was detected only during general anesthesia [5]. Morrey et al. described lax LCL and LUCL found in fluoroscopy under local anesthesia or arthroscopic examination as subtle instability, which the authors reported as causes of refractory lateral epicondylitis [4]. Thus, even though conventional physical examination may not reveal associated ligament injuries, subtle instability can be found under specific examination with anesthesia. However, reports of subtle instability found in primary surgery for lateral epicondylitis are very rare, and except for one case [5], only one study reported about subtle instability under anesthesia and suggested a treatment algorithm [6].

In this study, we examined elbow instability in fluoroscopy during examination under anesthesia (EUA) and aimed to report the elbows that needed primary surgical interventions for lateral epicondylitis: (1) how many elbows had subtle instability, (2) how closely the EUA findings matched the MRI and operative findings in elbows with subtle instability, and (3) whether any differences existed regarding preoperative clinical data between elbows with and without subtle instability.

Methods

This was a retrospective case series study. After approval by our institutional board review (IRB number 05–2017-028), 173 consecutive elbows (168 patients) with lateral epicondylitis treated surgically between March 2011 to December 2016 were enrolled in this study. Definitive criteria for lateral epicondylitis included 1) pain at the elbow during the preceding 30 days and 2) pain at the lateral humeral epicondyle region and pain provoked by resisted extension of the wrist with the elbow extended [7]. All patients were treated with a combination of four conservative methods including NSAID administration, counterforce bracing, isometric exercise, and extensor muscle stretching. Injections including corticosteroid, autologous blood, or botulinum toxin were not given in our protocol. The surgical indication was intractable pain (visual analog scale [VAS] ≥ 4) after conservative treatment for at least 6 months. Simple radiographs were taken at initial diagnosis, and after deciding to treat with surgery, MRIs were performed. Elbows with previous trauma, including elbow dislocation and fracture ($n = 17$); deformities, including cubitus varus and valgus ($n = 11$); synovial plica and osteochondral defect on MRI ($n = 5$); and previous surgery for lateral epicondylitis ($n = 7$) were excluded. The mediolateral stress, posterolateral rotatory drawer, push-up, and tabletop tests were conducted again by two orthopedic specialists (KSH, LSJ) before surgery. If at least one examiner found any instability in these examinations, the patients ($n = 8$) were considered to have instability during conventional physical examination and excluded. None of the patients showed generalized ligament laxity (Beighton score < 4) [8]. Patients detected with synovial plicae intraoperatively ($n = 3$) were also excluded. Finally, 122 elbows (117 patients) were included in this study.

Identifying instability during EUA

The patients were placed in the supine position under general anesthesia. For valgus instability, the arm was positioned with the elbow in 30° flexion, humerus in full internal rotation, and forearm in pronation. Then, the manual valgus stress test was performed, and an anteroposterior (AP) image of the elbow was acquired using a fluoroscopic image intensifier [9]. A widening of more than 1 mm at the ulnohumeral joint was considered as subtle valgus instability [9]. For varus instability, the arm was positioned with the elbow in 15° flexion, humerus in full external rotation, and forearm in supination. Then, manual varus stress test was performed, and an AP fluoroscopic image was acquired. Since a previous study reported that the radiocapitellar joint is 0.47 mm more redundant compared with the ulnohumeral joint [10], a widening of over 1.5 mm at the radiocapitellar joint was considered as subtle varus instability (Fig. 1). In addition, a posterolateral pivot shift test was performed with the elbow in 90° flexion and forearm in supination [11]. If the longitudinal axis of the radius does not pass through the center of the capitellum, it was considered as a posterolateral instability [9]. Thereafter, a lateral image of the elbow was acquired to identify subtle posterolateral instability (Fig. 2a-c) [5]. If subtle instability was found, the contralateral asymptomatic elbow was examined to exclude underlying normal laxity of elbow joint.

Surgical exploration of ligament status

During surgery, intraarticular pathology was checked via arthrotomy, and 3 patients with synovial plicae were excluded. For patients without subtle instability, we performed open release of lateral epicondylitis. The LCL complex was not explored to minimize damage to the extensor tendon. For patients with subtle instability, additional exploration for unstable ligament was performed. For varus or posterolateral instability, the proximal LCL complex was explored by elevating the common extensor origin, and the distal LCL complex was explored by elevating the anconeus and extensor carpi ulnaris. For valgus instability, the MCL was explored via an additional medial longitudinal incision.

Preoperative clinical data and MRI evaluation

Demographic data that were considered as potential prognostic factors such as patient age, gender, duration of education, and involvement of the dominant hand were assessed retrospectively. Other potential prognostic factors

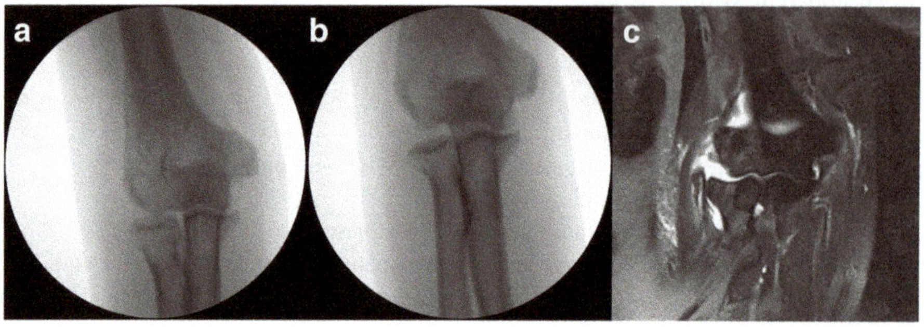

Fig. 1 a Intraoperative fluoroscopy image of a 53-year-old woman (patient #1). **b** Widening of the radiocapitellar joint was identified 2.3 mm in the varus stress view. **c** T2-weighted coronal magnetic resonance image showed rupture of the lateral collateral ligament and tear of the extensor tendon origin

such as duration of symptoms, smoking, body mass index (BMI), and history of multiple corticosteroid injections (≥3) were also assessed [7, 12–15]. Preoperatively, VAS score, Mayo Elbow Performance Score (MEPS), and Quick Disabilities of the Arm, Shoulder, and Hand (Quick DASH) score were assessed by an experienced orthopedic surgeon who did not attend the surgery. To identify ligament lesions in MRI, two radiologic specialists (TYM, HSJ), who had no knowledge of the intraoperative findings, reviewed the MRIs again.

Statistical analysis

Data were presented as mean ± standard deviation (SD). Categorical variables were analyzed using Fisher's exact test, and continuous variables were analyzed using the Mann-Whitney test. Statistical significance was defined as a P-value< 0.05. Data were analyzed with SPSS for Windows version 18.0 (SPSS, Chicago, Illinois, USA).

Results

Of the 122 elbows (117 patients), 17 elbows (16 patients) with subtle instability were assigned to the unstable group during EUA. One hundred and five elbows (101 patients) without instability were assigned to the stable group. All 17 elbows in the unstable group showed varus instability (radiocapitellar joint widening; range, 2.5~ 4.1 mm), and two showed additional posterolateral instability. No elbow in the unstable group showed valgus

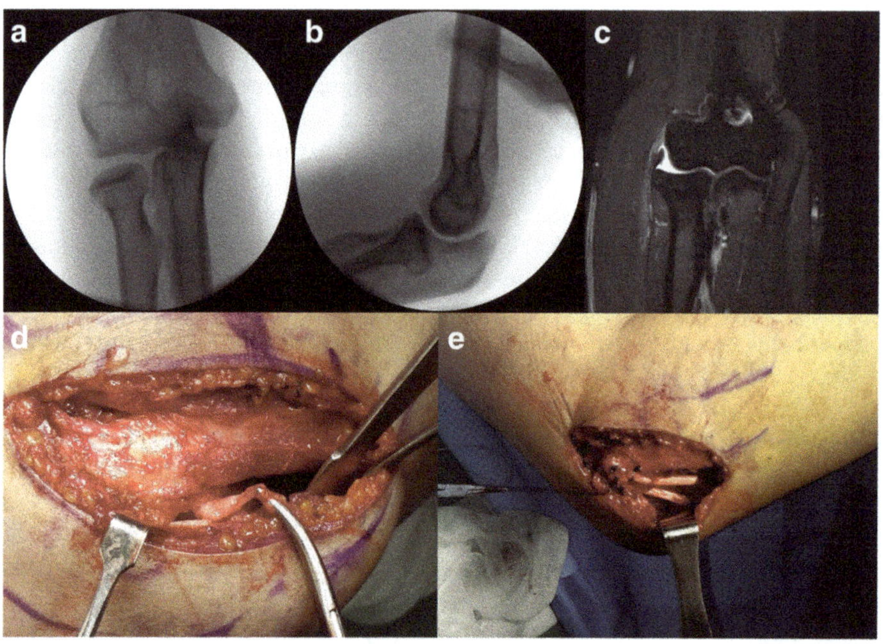

Fig. 2 a The 2.1 mm widening of the radiocapitellar joint was identified in the varus stress view of a 38-year-old man (patient #5). **b** The radial head was shifted posteriorly in the posterolateral pivot shift test. **c** T2-weighted coronal magnetic resonance image showed rupture of the lateral collateral ligament. **d** Intraoperatively, the definite lateral and lateral ulnar collateral ligaments were not found, except for thin fibrous tissue. **e** The lateral ulnar collateral ligament was reconstructed with a tibialis anterior allograft

instability under EUA (ulnohumeral joint widening; range, 0.13~ 0.66 mm). Except for 1 patient in the unstable group (patient 2), there was no patient who showed subtle instability on the contralateral asymptomatic elbow. In 105 elbows without subtle instability, the radiocapitellar and ulnohumeral joint widening was measured, ranging from 0.45 to 1.32 mm and 0.15 to 0. 75 mm, respectively.

One elbow in the unstable group and 11 elbows in the stable group did not undergo MRI for economic reason. Among 16 elbows which underwent MRI in the unstable group, 4 LCL + LUCL injuries, 6 LUCL injuries, and 5 LCL injuries were found. In 1 patient (patient 8), there was no notable ligament tear except for signal change on MRI taken preoperatively. In the stable group, 94 elbows underwent MRI, and 8 LCL and 5 LUCL injuries were noted on MRI. A combined LCL + LUCL injury was not identified. In both groups, no MCL injury was noted with MRI. Of all 28 elbows with LCL complex injuries on MRI, 15 showed subtle instability with EUA. Intraoperatively, in the unstable group, LCL complex abnormalities were confirmed at surgery in all cases; no functioning LCL and LUCL structure except the annular ligament was considered as a deficient LCL complex ($n = 8$) and remained a functioning structure despite that the defect or attenuation was considered as a partial loss of the LCL complex ($n = 9$) (Fig. 3). Capsules were not torn but attenuated in all patients (Table 1).

Duration of symptoms, gender, age, dominant hand involvement, occupation, educational periods, smoking, BMI, preoperative MEPS, and preoperative Quick DASH score were not different between both groups. The multiple corticosteroid injection rate (≥3) and preoperative VAS score were higher in the unstable group than in the stable group (Table 2).

Discussion

An elbow with significant instability can be detected via conventional physical examinations. However, it is difficult to demonstrate chronic ligament injury of subtle instability alone in the awake patient because of muscular restraints. Thus, EUA with muscle relaxation should be performed in these patients [16, 17]. On EUA, pathologic gapping of the lateral joint in the AP stress view or posterior translation of the radial head in the lateral stress view may provide evidence of lateral elbow instabilities and was applied in the current study [16]. Previously, EUA was not usually performed in lateral epicondylitis, and only arthroscopic EUA was reported [6]. In this study of 40 patients, 13 patients with dehiscence between 3 and 6 mm showed slight instability, and 2 patients with dehiscence over 6 mm showed severe instability. Arthroscopic examination had some potential advantages because there was no need for radiation and it was easy to perform anytime during the surgery. However, this procedure had a disadvantage in that surgeons could identify dehiscence on varus or valgus stress tests alone and obtain little information about posterolateral instability. Moreover, joint distension with saline can influence the tension of the capsule and ligament, causing some difficulties in analyzing the stability. Fluoroscopic EUA poses a risk of radiation exposure, and it might be difficult to note minor instability. However, it is possible to distinguish posterolateral instability from simple coronal instability, and it is easy to perform without any special technique. Moreover, it can provide more intuitive images of instability. Considering these advantages and disadvantages, the surgeon must decide which method to choose in identifying instability in EUA.

While few reports have been published about combined instability in EUA, there are several reports about associated ligament injuries with lateral epicondylitis identified via MRI. Potter et al. reported that 4 of 20 patients had associated radial collateral ligament injuries with MRI and those lesions were confirmed during surgery [17]. More recent studies have reported a positive correlation between the severity of common extensor tendon injury and that of LUCL injury [1, 2]. Moreover, in a study comparing 9 patients and 9 asymptomatic volunteers, MRI was reported to be effective in determining ligament abnormality in patients with subtle elbow

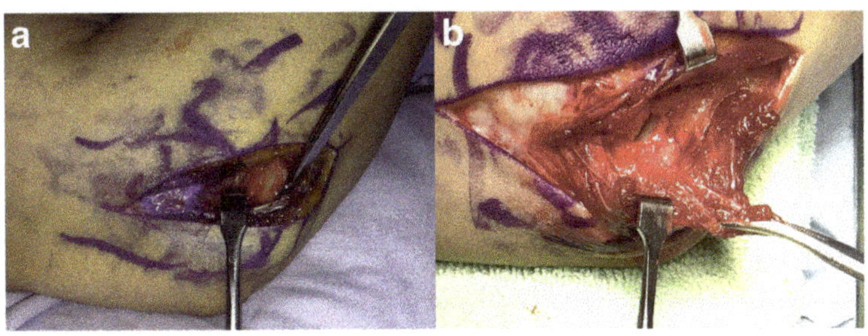

Fig. 3 a Example of a deficient LCL complex: no visible functioning LCL complex was found. **b** Example of partial defect of the LCL complex: there was a defect in the LCL complex, but a functional LCL complex partially remained

Table 1 Patient demographics, findings in MRI and EUA, and complication in unstable group

Patient	Gender	Age (decade)	Handedness	Duration of symptom	Multiple Injection history	Instability under EUA	MRI	Intraoperative findings of LCL complex
1	F	6th	Rt(D)	7	+	Var	LCL, LUCL	Deficient
2	F	6th	Rt(D)	24	+	Var	LUCL	Deficient
			Lt(ND)	24	+	Var	LUCL	Partial defect
3	M	6th	Rt(D)	36	+	Var,	LCL	Deficient
4	M	5th	Rt(D)	6	–	Var, Posterolat	LCL, LUCL	Partial defect
5	M	4th	Rt(D)	24	+	Var, Posterolat	LUCL	Deficient
6	F	6th	Rt(D)	12	+	Var	LUCL	Partial defect
7	F	7th	Lt(ND)	12	+	Var	LUCL	Deficient
8	M	5th	Rt(D)	10	+	Var	intact	Partial defect
9	F	5th	Lt(ND)	14	+	Var	LCL	Partial defect
10	F	5th	Lt(ND)	12	+	Var	LUCL	Deficient
11	F	6th	Rt(D)	60	+	Var	LCL	Deficient
12	M	5th	Rt(D)	10	+	Var	LCL	Partial defect
13	F	5th	Rt(D)	12	+	Var	Not taken	Partial defect
14	M	6th	Lt(ND)	14	+	Var	LCL	Partial defect
15	M	5th	Rt(D)	12	+	Var	LCL, LUCL	Partial defect
16	M	4th	Rt(D)	12	+	Var, Posterolat	LCL, LUCL	Deficient

EUA Examination under anesthesia, *MRI* Magnetic resonance image, *LCL* Lateral collateral ligament, *LUCL* Lateral ulnar collateral ligament

instability [18]. Thus, when suspected, it would be helpful to perform an MRI of the elbow. However, in elbows with lateral epicondylitis, MRI was not completely correlated with EUA and operative findings. In our study, 15 of the 28 abnormal elbow MRIs showed subtle instability (positive predictive value, 53.6%), while 81 of the 82 normal MRIs did not show subtle instability (negative predictive value, 98.7%). Considering the relatively low positive and high negative predictive value, we think MRI alone is not recommended in determining the surgical procedure, and EUA should be performed when there are ligament abnormalities in MRI.

It is clear that an unstable elbow with significant instability should be stabilized because detrimental

Table 2 Comparison of preoperative clinical data. Continuous variables were presented as mean (standard deviation)

	Unstable Group	Stable Group	*P*-value
Gender(M/F)	8/9	45/60	0.473
Age (year)	48.9 (6.61)	50.5 (7.47)	0.392
Dominant/Nondominant	12/5	65/40	0.344
Manual worker(+/−)	9/8	46/59	0.329
Duration (month)	17.7 (13.3)	14.5 (10.3)	0.321
Eductaion (year)	12.6 (2.18)	11.9 (2.37)	0.275
Multiple corticosteroid injection(> 3)(+/−)	16/1	76/29	0.042*
Smoking(+/−)	7/10	29/75	0.195.
BMI	23.6 (2.16)	24.3 (3.21)	0.373
Pre VAS	7.29 (0.99)	5.48 (1.20)	< 0.001*
Pre MEPS	59.1 (5.37)	61.8 (5.93)	0.061
Pre Quick DASH	56.4 (6.49)	54.6 (7.06)	0.333

VAS Visual analogue scale, *MEPS* Mayo Elbow Performance index Score, *Quick DASH* Quick Disabilities of the Arm, Shoulder and Hand Score
*$P < 0.05$

articular contact in the elbow joint usually leads to irreversible cartilage injury [19]. However, whether subtle instability during EUA should be surgically treated is controversial. Aoki et al. reported that a patient with mild lateral instability had a good outcome even with conventional debridement [20]. Coleman et al. reported that synovial fistulae developed in 2 patients postoperatively [21]. One patient with an irreparable defect in the elbow capsule during surgery had to undergo an anconeus flap operation, and the other was managed conservatively. There was no mention about instability in these 2 patients. However, Kalainov et al. reported that 3 patients with large fistulae with instability had to undergo LUCL reconstruction [5]. Moreover, several authors have recommended surgical correction for instability, which was only identified in EUA [16, 18]. We believe that such instabilities, identified during EUA, should preferably be corrected; however, evidence supporting this proposition is still lacking. It might also be unclear which procedure should be selected for subtle instability. Ligament repair, including imbrication or tensioning, could be an option [22]; however, ligamentous tissue often showed poor quality in cases of chronic posterolateral instability, and ligament reconstruction might provide more consistent results [18, 23, 24]. In our study, 13 patients underwent ligament reconstruction because ligament repair was not feasible. Thus, if surgeons decide to address subtle instability, they should prepare for ligament reconstruction as well as repair.

We investigated preoperative factors that were known to affect the prognosis of lateral epicondylitis, to determine which of the preoperative clinical data was different between the two groups. In conservative treatments, demographic factors including age and gender were reported to have no significant relationship with the prognosis of lateral epicondylitis, while the effect of site involvement was unclear. Manual work, high strain at work, long duration of symptoms, multiple musculoskeletal complaints, and low socioeconomic status were reported as poor prognostic factors at 12 months of treatment [7, 12, 14]. After surgical treatments, high baseline pain, sudden onset of symptoms, long duration, morbid obesity, smoking, a history of multiple corticosteroid injections (≥3), and young age were reported as potential risk factors for poor surgical outcome [13, 15]. The effect of gender on outcome was considered controversial [13, 25]. Some authors even mentioned previous corticosteroid injection as a cause of ligament tear [5, 26], and a history of multiple corticosteroid injections (≥3) was reported as the most significant risk factor for surgical treatment failure [17]. Among those factors, our results suggest that a high level of pain and history of multiple corticosteroid injections (≥3) are preoperative characteristics of lateral epicondylitis with subtle instability. However, patient's recollection of how many injections they received was inaccurate in our study, so we could not perform analysis based on the exact number of injections. Moreover, since the VAS score did not indicate the absolute value of pain, it was difficult to provide cut-off values for pain level predictive of subtle instability.

The present study revealed that some patients (13.9% of the patients that underwent surgery for chronic lateral epicondylitis) showed varus or posterolateral subtle instability during fluoroscopic EUA. To our knowledge, our study is the first to report the predictive value of MRI for subtle instability. Nevertheless, our study had several limitations. First, the number of patients in the unstable group was relatively small because subtle instability in EUA is uncommon in lateral epicondylitis. Therefore, results such as risk ratio could not be presented. Second, the force applied during the stress test was not identical. Thus, it was impossible to analyze the joint widening quantitatively. Third, exploration of the LCL complex was not performed in the stable group. Thus, the relationship between the structural status of ligaments and MRI findings was not revealed in this study. Further study should include a larger number of patients and the same force for stress test to overcome these limitations.

Conclusion

Subtle instability resulting from chronic LCL complex injury was noted in elbows with lateral epicondylitis. This is difficult to detect in conventional physical examination but can be easily visualized in fluoroscopic EUA. Preoperative MRIs can be used to exclude subtle instability with its high negative predictive value. The unstable group tended to have higher VAS scores than the stable group, and a history of multiple corticosteroid injections (≥3) was an indication of subtle instability. Although it was unclear whether surgical treatment of the LCL complex should be performed, surgeons should consider checking for subtle instability, especially when patients have a history of multiple corticosteroid injections (≥3) or severe pain and MRI indicates instability.

Abbreviations

BMI: Body mass index; ECRB: Extensor carpi radialis brevis; EUA: Examination under anesthesia; LCL: Lateral collateral ligament; LUCL: Lateral ulnar collateral ligament; MEPS: Mayo Elbow Performance Score; MRI: Magnetic resonance imaging; Quick DASH: Quick Disabilities of the Arm, Shoulder, and Hand; SD: Standard deviation; VAS: Visual analogue scale

Acknowledgements

We thank Tae Yong Moon for his help with the radiographic review.

Authors' contributions

SK, SL, and KS have contributed to the conception of the study, acquisition of data, or analysis of data. HJ contributed to the analysis of image data. MD, SK, and SL were involved in drafting the manuscript and revising it critically. All authors have read and approved the final version of the manuscript.

Competing interests

The authors declare that they have no competing interests.

Author details

[1]Department of Orthopaedic Surgery, Pusan National University Yangsan Hospital, Pusan National University School of Medicine, 20, Geumo-ro, Mulgeum-eup, Yangsan-si, Gyeongsangnam-do, Republic of Korea. [2]Department of Radiology, Pusan National University Yangsan Hospital, Pusan National University School of Medicine, 20, Geumo-ro, Mulgeum-eup, Yangsan-si, Gyeongsangnam-do, Republic of Korea.

References

1. Bredella M, Tirman P, Fritz R, Feller J, Wischer T, Genant H. MR imaging findings of lateral ulnar collateral ligament abnormalities in patients with lateral epicondylitis. AJR Am J Roentgenol. 1999;173(5):1379–82.
2. Qi L, Zhu Z-F, Li F, Wang R-F. MR imaging of patients with lateral epicondylitis of the elbow: is the common extensor tendon an isolated lesion? PLoS One. 2013;8(11):e79498.
3. Dzugan SS, Savoie FH, Field LD, O'Brien MJ, You Z. Acute radial ulno-humeral ligament injury in patients with chronic lateral epicondylitis: an observational report. J Shoulder Elb Surg. 2012;21(12):1651–5.
4. Morrey BF. Reoperation for failed surgical treatment of refractory lateral epicondylitis. J Shoulder Elb Surg. 1992;1(1):47–55.
5. Kalainov DM, Cohen MS. Posterolateral rotatory instability of the elbow in association with lateral epicondylitis. J Bone Joint Surg Am. 2005;5:1120–5.
6. Kniesel B, Huth J, Bauer G, Mauch F. Systematic diagnosis and therapy of lateral elbow pain with emphasis on elbow instability. Arch Orthop Trauma Surg. 2014;134(12):1641–7.
7. Haahr J, Andersen J. Physical and psychosocial risk factors for lateral epicondylitis: a population based case-referent study. Occup Environ Med. 2003;60(5):322–9.
8. Clinch J, Deere K, Sayers A, Palmer S, Riddoch C, Tobias JH, Clark EM. Epidemiology of generalized joint laxity (hypermobility) in fourteen-year-old children from the UK: a population-based evaluation. Arthrits Rheum. 2011;63(9):2819–27.
9. O'Driscoll S. Elbow instability. Acta Orthop Belg. 1999;65(4):404–15.
10. Lee RK, Griffith JF, Yuen BT, Ng AW, Yeung DK. Elbow MR arthrography with traction. Br J Radiol. 2016;89(1064):20160378.
11. O'driscoll S, Bell D, Morrey B. Posterolateral rotatory instability of the elbow. J Bone Joint Surg Am. 1991;73(3):440–6.
12. Bot SD, van der Waal JM, Terwee C, Van der Windt D, Bouter LM, Dekker J. Course and prognosis of elbow complaints: a cohort study in general practice. Ann Rheum Dis. 2005;64(9):1331–6.
13. Degen RM, Cancienne JM, Camp CL, Altchek DW, Dines JS, Werner BC. Three or more preoperative injections is the most significant risk factor for revision surgery after operative treatment of lateral epicondylitis: an analysis of 3863 patients. J Shoulder Elb Surg. 2017;26(4):704–9.
14. Smidt N, Lewis M, Windt DAVD, Hay EM, Bouter LM, Croft P. Lateral epicondylitis in general practice: course and prognostic indicators of outcome. J Rheumatol. 2006;33(10):2053–9.
15. Solheim E, Hegna J, Øyen J. Extensor tendon release in tennis elbow: results and prognostic factors in 80 elbows. Knee Surg Sports Traumatol Arthrosc. 2011;19(6):1023–7.
16. Cohen MS. Lateral collateral ligament instability of the elbow. Hand Clin. 2008;24(1):69–77.
17. Potter HG, Hannafin JA, Morwessel RM, DiCarlo EF, O'Brien SJ, Altchek DW. Lateral epicondylitis: correlation of MR imaging, surgical, and histopathologic findings. Radiology. 1995;196(1):43–6.
18. Potter HG, Weiland AJ, Schatz JA, Paletta GA, Hotchkiss RN. Posterolateral rotatory instability of the elbow: usefulness of MR imaging in diagnosis. Radiology. 1997;204(1):185–9.
19. Ring D, Jupiter JB. Reconstruction of posttraumatic elbow instability. Clin Orthop Relat Res. 2000;370:44–56.
20. Aoki M, Wada T, Isogai S, Kanaya K, Aiki H, Yamashita T. Magnetic resonance imaging findings of refractory tennis elbows and their relationship to surgical treatment. J Shoulder Elb Surg. 2005;14(2):172–7.
21. Coleman B, Quinlan JF, Matheson JA. Surgical treatment for lateral epicondylitis: a long-term follow-up of results. J Shoulder Elb Surg. 2010;19(3):363–7.
22. Fedorka CJ, Oh LS. Posterolateral rotatory instability of the elbow. Curr Rev Musculoskelet Med. 2016;9(2):240–6.
23. Charalambous C, Stanley J. Posterolateral rotatory instability of the elbow. J Bone Joint Surg Br. 2008;90(3):272–9.
24. Sanchez-Sotelo J, Morrey B, O'driscoll S. Ligamentous repair and reconstruction for posterolateral rotatory instability of the elbow. J Bone Joint Surg Br. 2005;87(1):54–61.
25. Svernlöv B, Adolfsson L. Outcome of release of the lateral extensor muscle origin for epicondylitis. Scand J Plast Reconstr Surg Hand Surg. 2006;40(3):161–5.
26. Jones KJ, Dodson CC, Osbahr DC, Parisien RL, Weiland AJ, Altchek DW, Allen AA. The docking technique for lateral ulnar collateral ligament reconstruction: surgical technique and clinical outcomes. J Shoulder Elb Surg. 2012;21(3):389–95.

5

Genetic polymorphisms in bone morphogenetic protein receptor type IA gene predisposes individuals to ossification of the posterior longitudinal ligament of the cervical spine via the smad signaling pathway

Hao Wang[1*], Weitao Jin[1] and Haibin Li[2]

Abstract

Background: The present study investigated the molecular mechanisms underlying the 4A > C and -349C > T single nucleotide polymorphisms (SNPs) in bone morphogenetic protein receptor type IA (*BMPR-IA*) gene, which significantly associated with the occurrence and the extent of ossification of the posterior longitudinal ligament (OPLL) in the cervical spine.

Methods: The SNPs in *BMPR-IA* gene were genotyped, and the association with the occurrence and severity of OPLL were evaluated in 356 OPLL patients and 617 non-OPLL controls. In stably transfected mouse embryonic mesenchymal stem cells (C3H10T1/2), the expression levels of the *BMPR-IA* gene and Smad4 protein as well as phosphorylated Smad1/5/8 were detected by Western blotting. In addition, the alkaline phosphatase (ALP) and osteocalcin (OC) activity of osteogenesis specificity protein was assessed using the ALP quantitation and osteocalcin radioimmunoassay kit, respectively.

Results: The 4A > C and the -349C > T polymorphisms of *BMPR-IA* gene were significantly associated with the development of OPLL in the cervical spine. The C allele type in 4A > C polymorphism significantly increases the occurrence and the extent of OPLL. The T allele type in -349C > T polymorphism significantly increases the susceptibility to OPLL, but not the extent of OPLL. The current results further validate our previous observations. The expression levels of *BMPR-IA* gene were significantly increased in pcDNA3.1/BMPR-IA (mutation type, MT -349C > T; MT 4A > C; MT -349C > T and 4A > C) vector-transfected C3H10T1/2 cells compared to the wild type (WT) vector-transfected cells. The levels of phosphorylated Smad1/5/8 and ALP activity were significantly increased in pcDNA3.1/BMPR-IA (MT -349C > T) vector-transfected C3H10T1/2 cells compared to the WT vector-transfected cells. However, no significant differences were observed in the protein levels of phosphorylated Smad1/5/8 and the ALP activity between MT A/C and WT vector-transfected cells. In addition, no significant differences were observed in the Smad4 protein levels among the experimental groups, as well as in the OC activity between WT vector-transfected and MT C/T, MT A/C, MT C/T and MT A/C vector-transfected cells.

(Continued on next page)

* Correspondence: wanghao1980@ccmu.edu.cn
[1]Department of Orthopaedics, Beijing Tiantan Hospital, Capital Medical University, 6 TiantanXili, Dongcheng District, Beijing 100050, China
Full list of author information is available at the end of the article

(Continued from previous page)

Conclusions: Our results suggest that Smad signaling pathway may play important roles in the pathological process of OPLL induced by SNPs in BMPR-IA gene. These results will help to clarify the molecular mechanisms underlying the SNP and gene susceptibility to OPLL.

Keywords: Ossification of the posterior longitudinal ligament, Bone morphogenetic protein receptor type IA, Single nucleotide polymorphisms, Gene transfection, Smad signaling pathway

Background

Ossification of the posterior longitudinal ligament (OPLL) of the spine is characterized by abnormal ossification of the posterior longitudinal ligament in the spinal canal. This results in the compression of the spinal cord and nerve root, leading to serious neurological deficits as well as paralysis. Several studies have demonstrated that OPLL is a complicated multifactorial disease common in the Asian population with a prevalence of 2–4% [1]. Although a large number of genetic and environmental factors may be involved in OPLL, the etiology and pathogenesis are yet to be deciphered. Previous studies have shown that genetic factors play a crucial role in the development of OPLL [2–4]. The single nucleotide polymorphisms (SNPs) of bone morphogenetic protein (BMP) 2, 4, and 9, collagen 6A1, angiotensin I converting enzyme gene, BH3 interacting domain death agonist, nucleotide pyrophosphatase, and vitamin K epoxide reductase complex subunit 1 are significantly associated with the occurrence and development of OPLL [4–9]. These studies also suggested that the SNPs of the candidate genes increase the incidence of OPLL of an individual in an environmental specific manner. However, the molecular mechanisms underlying the activity of these susceptible genetic polymorphisms are unclear.

The bone morphogenetic protein receptors (BMPRs) are a family of transmembrane serine/threonine kinases, including three type I receptors (*BMPR-IA*, BMPR-IB, ActR-IA) and three type II receptors (BMPR-II, ActR-II, ActR-IIB) [10]. The receptor-ligand BMPs belong to the transforming growth factor-beta superfamily, and play significant roles in bone and cartilage development. Furthermore, BMP signaling is mediated by type I and type II BMP receptors. Although both types of BMP receptors are indispensable for signal transduction, the type I receptors are the high-affinity binding receptors [11]. The substrates of type I BMP receptors including the Smad protein family play a central role in BMPs signal transduction via the Smad signaling pathway. Activation of the Smad pathway leads to the expression of osteoblast-specific proteins including alkaline phosphatase (ALP), osteocalcin (OC) and collagen type I (COL1) [12–14].

Several pieces of evidence have demonstrated that *BMPR-IA* gene is a subtype of type I BMP receptors and responsible for the initiation of osteogenic differentiation [15–17]. Previous studies using immunohistochemistry staining and RT-PCR analysis have demonstrated that the expression of *BMPR-IA* mRNA and protein was elevated in the ossified ligaments of OPLL patients compared with controls. *BMPR-IA* is highly expressed in chondrocytes at the fibrocartilage tissue around the calcified zone and in fibroblast-like spindle cells at non-ossified ligaments. However, in non-OPLL patients, BMPR-IA is not expressed in the posterior longitudinal ligaments [18, 19]. In the absence of BMP2 expression, the fibroblast osteoblast activity of *BMPR-IA* gene overexpression was significantly enhanced compared to normal fibroblasts [20]. These results suggested that *BMPR-IA* gene plays an important role in the pathological ossification of OPLL. In our previous study, we demonstrated that the 4A > C and the -349C > T polymorphisms of *BMPR-IA* gene were significantly associated with the development of OPLL in the cervical spine in a Chinese Han cohort [21]. However, the molecular mechanisms underlying the 4A > C and -349C > T polymorphisms in *BMPR-IA* gene have not yet been fully deciphered. Therefore, the present study aimed to investigate the molecular mechanisms underlying the two SNPs in *BMPR-IA* gene and whether the Smad signaling pathway may be involved in the development of SNPs-induced OPLL in the cervical spine.

Methods

Subjects and disease criteria

The study protocol was approved by the Institutional Review Board (IRB) of Beijing Tiantan Hospital Capital Medical University. Informed consent was obtained from all the participants before the study. Study participants were recruited between January 2011 and January 2016, and consisted of 356 patients with OPLL and 617 control subjects without OPLL satisfying the inclusion criteria. The authors had access to information that could identify individual participants during or after data collection. All 973 participants were of the Han Chinese from the Beijing Tiantan Hospital Capital Medical University and resided in the northern region of mainland, China. The average age of the patients that included 199 males and 157 females was 55 years old. The control participants were age and gender matched (346 males and 271 females, 56% vs 44%). The case-control subjects were genetically homogenous. The diagnosis of OPLL was based on the criteria reported by Tsuyama [22]. Of the 356 patients with cervical spine OPLL, 131 were diagnosed as continuous type, 75 with mixed type, 118 with segmental type, and 32 with localized type. The ossification extent of OPLL was determined by the number of ossified cervical vertebrae based on lateral radiograph films. The study excluded participants with bone fluorosis, diffuse idiopathic skeletal hyperostosis, ankylosing spondylitis, and other bone metabolism diseases associated with OPLL.

Genotyping and SNPs in BMPR-IA gene

Genomic DNA was isolated from peripheral blood of participants using the Wizard Genomic DNA Purification Kit(Promega, Madison, WI, USA). The complete coding sequence of human BMPR-IA gene (GenBank Accession No: NM004329.2) was amplified by polymerase chain reaction (PCR) using a standard protocol [23]. The DNA fragments containing the exon sequences of BMPR-IA gene was then respectively amplified using ten pairs of specific primers (Table 1). The PCR products were analyzed by direct sequencing using BigDye Terminator cycle sequencing on an ABI 3730XL POP7 DNA sequencing analysis 5.2 (Applied Biosystems, Carlsbad, CA, USA).

Construction of *BMPR-IA* gene expression plasmids

The single-stranded (ss) DNA oligos of human *BMPR-IA* gene (wild type, WT) encoding sequence was synthesized by BioSia, Co., Ltd., Shanghai, China. Equivalent amounts of each pair of ss DNA oligos were annealed to generate double-stranded (ds) oligos. The ds-oligos were inserted into the pGEM-T vector (Invitrogen, Carlsbad, CA, USA) using T4 DNA ligase. The construct was transformed into chemically competent *E.coli* DH5α (Invitrogen). The pGEM-T/BMPR-IA (WT) plasmid was amplified and digested with Hind III/Bam HI enzyme. The BMPR-IA cDNA (1599 bp) and the pGEM-T vector (3000 bp) were found in all the PCR products as analyzed by 4% agarose gel electrophoresis and directly sequencing, respectively. Then, the BMPR-IA cDNA (1599 bp) was inserted into the pcDNA3.1 vector (Invitrogen) using T4 DNA ligase, and the construct was transformed into DH5α cells. Using pcDNA3.1/BMPR-IA (WT) plasmid as the template, the *BMPR-IA* gene of the mutation type (MT) was amplified by PCR, using four pairs of primers (Table 2) according to the Site-Directed Mutagenesis Kit (Invitrogen). The PCR products were cloned into the pcDNA3.1 (+) plasmid. The pcDNA3.1 plasmid with the target gene and the transformants were verified by PCR and direct sequencing. The recombinant plasmid was transformed into the DH5α strain. The positive clones were designated as pcDNA3.1/BMPR-IA (WT) plasmid, pcDNA3.1/BMPR-IA (MT -349C > T) plasmid, pcDNA3.1/BMPRIA (MT 4A > C) plasmid, and pcDNA3.1/BMPR-IA (MT -349C > T and 4A > C) plasmid, respectively.

Cell culture

Mouse embryonic mesenchymal stem cell line (C3H10T1/2 cells) was obtained from the American Type Culture Collection (ATCC, Maryland Rockefeller,USA). The cells were cultured in basal medium eagle (BME, Gibco BRL, Grand Island, NY, USA) medium supplemented with 10% fetal bovine serum (FBS, Gibco BRL, Grand Island, NY, USA). For osteogenic differentiation, cells were seeded at a density of 4.5×10^5 cells/well in 6-well plates and maintained in BME containing 10% FBS. Cells at 80% confluence

Table 1 Ten pairs of primers were used to amplify the complete exon sequences of human *BMPR-IA* gene by PCR using a standard protocol

Primer	Forward	Reverse	Annealing temperature (°C)
Primer1	GCGTTGGATGGGAGCGATAA	GGAAGCTGCGCACAGTGTTG	58
Primer2	CTCACGTCGGTCCTGTCC	CCCTGCTCCATGCCTCAC	61
Primer3	CGGAGGAGTTTATCACCTCAGCAGAGC	TTCCATCATGGCCAAAAGTTACTAGCA	60
Primer4	AGAGATTGGAATCCGCCTGCCGGGCTT	ACCCGCGAGTGGGAGACAAAAGAGG	55
Primer5	GGACTATTGAGATTGTTTAATATAC	GAAAGAACAGAAGCAAGAAATAGTG	55
Primer6	GGACTATTGAGATTGTTTAATATAC	GAAAGAACAGAAGCAAGAAATAGTG	55
Primer7	CCACAATGCATCTGGCCCCAAGGAG	TGTGATTATTACACATGGCATGCCTGTATC	55
Primer8	ACATCAGATTACTGGGAGCC	TATAGCAAAGCAGCTGGAG	52
Primer9	AAGCCTTAAGAAGATAAATGA	ATTACCCTAATGAAGTTTTTG	62
Primer10	TGATTAGTGTCTCCAGTCAAGC	TCTCAGGTAAAAGGCAAAGTC	50

Table 2 Four pairs of primers were used to amplify and synthesize the human *BMPR-IA* gene for the following mutations (MT -349C > T, MT 4A > C) by PCR using pcDNA3.1/BMPR-IA wild type plasmid as the template

SNPs	Primer	Forward	Reverse	Annealing Temperature (°C)
-349C > T	Primer 1	CCGGAATTCACCATGGTGGCCGGGACC	CCGACGCCGCCGCCGCGAACTT	60
	Primer 2	TCGCGGCGGCGGCGTCGG	CCGCTCGAGCTAGCGACACCCACAACCCTCCA	60
4A > C	Primer 1	CCGGAATTCACCATGGTGGCCGGGACC	CTGGTGTCCAAAAGTCTGGTCACGGG	60
	Primer 2	CCCCGTGACCAGACTTTTGGACACC	CCGCTCGAGCTAGCGACACCCACAACCCTCCA	60

were induced by osteogenic medium containing 100 nM dexamethasone (Sigma), 10 mM β-glycerophosphate (Sigma) and 0.2 mM ascorbic acid (Sigma) for 7–21 days. The culture medium was changed every 3 days and cells were grown at 37 °C in a humidified atmosphere containing 5% CO_2.

Transfection and stable selection

C3H10T1/2 cells were transfected with empty pcDNA3.1 (+) vector, pcDNA3.1/BMPR-IA (WT) vector, pcDNA3.1/BMPR-IA (MT -349C > T) vector, pcDNA3.1/BMPR-IA (MT 4A > C) vector, and pcDNA3.1/BMPR-IA (MT -349C > T and 4A > C) vector, respectively. For stable transfection, cells were seeded at 4.5×10^5 cells/well in 6-well plates pre-coated with poly-l-lysine (Sigma, St Louis, MO, USA) and maintained in BME containing 10% FBS. After cells were grown to confluence, the gene transfections were performed using lipofectamine (Invitrogen) according to the manufacturer's instructions. 4–6 h post-transfection, the transfected cells were cultured in osteogenic differentiation conditions with 200 ng/mL recombinant human BMP2 (rhBMP2, BioSia, Co., Ltd., Shanghai, China) for 72 h. The following day, the cells were trypsinized (Gibco) and plated into a large cell culture dish. Stably transfected C3H10T1/2 cells were selected with 800 μg/mL G418 media for 2 weeks and subsequently maintained at 200 μg/mL G418 media (Gibco), following which, G418-resistant clones were selected and expanded. After 6 weeks of G418 selection, the stably transfected cells were collected for subsequent experiments.

Western blotting

Lysates from stably transfected C3H10T1/2 cells were obtained using the total protein extraction kit (Applygen Technologies Inc., Beijing, China). The concentrations of protein were measured using the bicinchoninic acid (BCA) assay and quantified using bovine serum albumin (BSA) protein standards according to the manufacturer's instructions (Pierce, Rockford, IL, USA). The whole cell protein extracts were resolved by SDS-PAGE and transferred to nitrocellulose membrane. Pre-stained protein standards were used for determining the relative molecular mass of the proteins. The membranes were blocked in 5% nonfat dry milk in Tris-buffered saline, followed by incubation with the BMPR-IA (1:1000, Santa Cruz, CA, USA) or GAPDH monoclonal antibodies (1:1000, Santa Cruz) at 4 °C overnight, followed by incubation with a mouse anti-human HRP-conjugated secondary antibody (1:2000, Zhongshan Jinqiao, Beijing, China) for 1 h at room temperature. The protein levels of Smad4 and phosphorylated Smad1/5/8 were detected using specific monoclonal antibodies (1:000, Cell Signaling Technology; CST, Danvers, MA, USA), respectively, or GAPDH monoclonal antibody (1:1000, Santa Cruz) at 4 °C overnight, followed by 1 h incubation with a mouse anti-human HRP-conjugated secondary antibody (1:2000, Zhongshan Jinqiao, Beijing, China) at room temperature. The blots were washed and subjected to immuno-detection by chemiluminescence using SuperSignal (Pierce). The blots were scanned using the Kodak Image Station (440 CF; Kodak, Rochester, MN, USA), and the optical densities of the bands in each lane were analyzed to assess the variations in protein levels relative to GADPH.

ALP activity assay

The ALP activity was detected using the alkaline phosphatase quantitative kit (Jiancheng, Nanjing, China). The stably transfected C3H10T1/2 cells were scraped off the culture dish using 50 mmol Tris-HCl and lysed by sonication. The sample tube (30 μL cell lysis solution, 0.5 mL buffer solution, and 0.5 mL matrix liquid), Standard tube (30 μL phenol standard solution 0.1 mg/mL, 0.5 mL buffer solution, and 0.5 mL matrix liquid), and blank tube (30 μL double-distilled water, 0.5 mL buffer solution, and 0.5 mL matrix liquid) were thoroughly mixed and incubated in a 37 °C water bath for 15 min, followed by the addition of 1.5 mL color reagent. The reaction mixtures were then agitated, and the absorbance measured at 520 nm. The ALP activity for each samples was measure by the following equation; the activity of ALP (U/gprot) = (determination tube absorbance/

standard tube absorbance) × standard tube containing phenol (0.003 mg)/number of proteins in the sample.

OC activity assay

The OC activity was detected using the Osteocalcin Radioimmunoassay Kit (Dongya, Beijing, China) according to the principle of the competition of radiation immunity. The stably transfected C3H10T1/2 cells were scraped off the cell culture plate using 50 mmol Tris-HCl and lysed by sonication. ^{125}I- labeled OC and OC antibody were mixed for 24 h, followed by precipitation using the separation agent. After centrifugation at 4 °C, the radiation dose of the precipitate was detected using a γ-scintillation counter. The OC content of the sample was obtained based on the standard curve and presented as ng/mL.

Statistical analysis

The Pearson Chi-square test was performed to assess the difference in the genotypic and allelic distribution between OPLL patients and control subjects. The Student unpaired t-test was used to compare the number of ossified cervical vertebrae between the two groups. A p-value < 0.05 was considered to be statistically significant (two-sided). ANOVA followed by Bonferroni post hoc multiple comparison was used to examine significant differences among the experimental groups. A adjust p-value< 0.003 was considered to be significant [24]. All data was expressed as means ± standard deviation and analyzed with SPSS 13.0 software (SPSS, Chicago, IL).

Results

Typing and analysis of SNP loci in the BMPR-IA gene

The SNPs in the coding regions of *BMPR-IA* gene were detected by direct DNA sequencing (Figs. 1 and 2). The four SNPs analyzed in the exon regions of *BMPR-IA* gene included -349C > T in exon 1, the 4A > C in exon 3, the 1327C > T in exon 11, and the 1395G > C in exon 12. The genotypic and allelic distributions of the four SNP loci in *BMPR-IA* gene between OPLL patients and non-OPLL controls are shown in Table 3. The results showed that the -349C > T and the 4A > C polymorphisms in the coding region of *BMPR-IA* gene were significantly associated with the development of OPLL in the cervical spine. We observed that there was a significant difference between the 4A > C polymorphism in exon 3 of *BMPR-IA* gene and the occurrence and the extent of OPLL in the cervical spine (P < 0.001). The C allele type in 4A > C polymorphism significantly increased the occurrence and the extent of OPLL in the cervical spine (Fig. 3). In addition, there was a significant allelic frequency difference between the -349C > T polymorphism in exon 1 of *BMPR-IA* gene and the susceptibility to OPLL (P < 0.001), but did not affect the extent of OPLL in the cervical spine. The T allele type in -349C > T polymorphism significantly

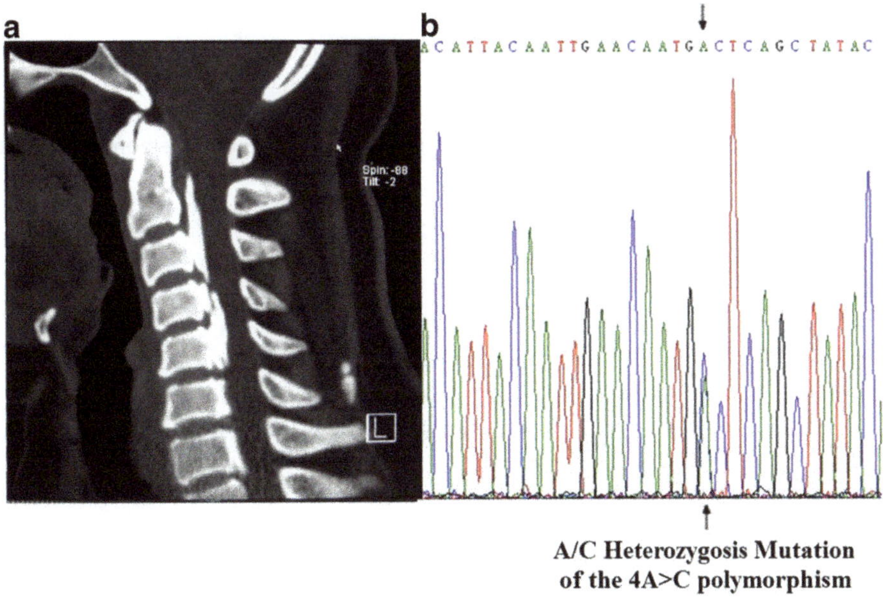

Fig. 1 The 2-dimensional (2D) CT and sequencing results of a 43 year old woman with OPLL in the cervical spine. **a** The 2D CT showed that the patient had OPLL (C2–C3, C4-C5, C6, and C7 mixed type). **b** The direct sequencing results of the PCR products showing the A/C heterozygous mutation of 4A > C polymorphism in *BMPR-IA* gene. A allele: green line; T allele: red line; C allele: blue line; G allele: black line

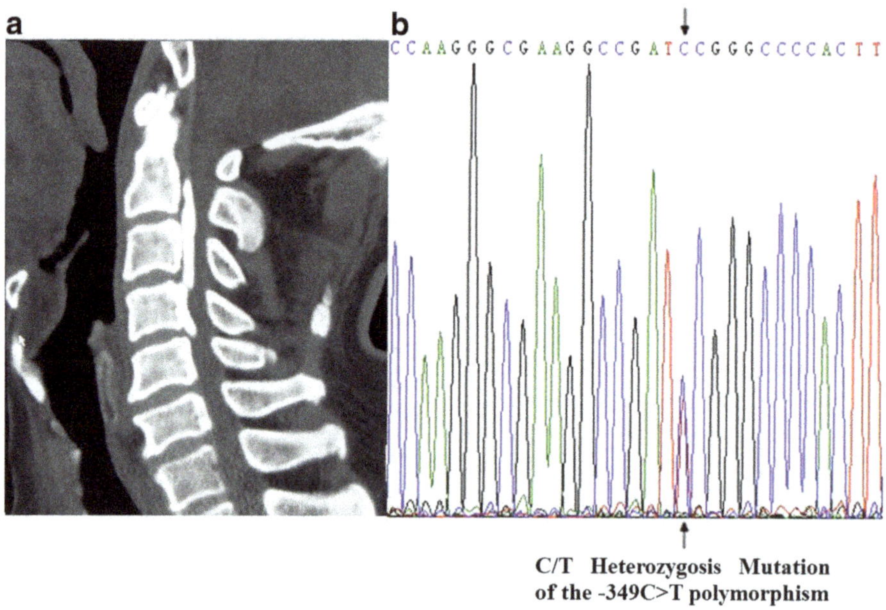

Fig. 2 The 2-dimensional (2D) CT and sequencing results of a 68 year old man with OPLL in the cervical spine. **a** The 2D CT showed the patient had OPLL (C2–C3, C4, C5, and C6, mixed type). **b**The direct sequencing results of the PCR products showing the C/T heterozygous mutation of -349C > T polymorphism in *BMPR-IA* gene. A allele: green line; T allele: red line; C allele: blue line; G allele: black line

increased the susceptibility to OPLL, but not the extent of OPLL in the cervical spine.

Construction of the *BMPR-IA* gene expression plasmids

The annealing efficiency of the ss oligos was analyzed by 4% agarose gel electrophoresis (Fig. 4a). The expected size of the ds oligos was 1599 bp. Each pair of ss oligos of the BMPR-IA gene encoding sequence was effectively annealed to form ds oligos, which were then ligated to linearized pGEM-T vector. The recombinant plasmid was then validated by digesting with Hind III-Bam H I enzyme. This generated two fragments, the *BMPR-IA* gene coding sequence (1599 bp) and the pGEM-T vector (3000 bp) (Fig. 4b). The BMPR-IA cDNA (1599 bp) was inserted into the pcDNA3.1 vector using T4 DNA ligase and transformed into DH5α. Analysis of the positive clones confirmed the orientation and sequence of the inserted ds-oligos.

BMPR-IA gene expression in transfected C3H10T1/2 cells

The expression of *BMPR-IA* gene in the transfected C3H10T1/2 cells was determined by Western blotting (Fig. 5). The results demonstrated that the BMPR-IA

Table 3 Genotypic and allelic distribution of four SNP loci in the exon regions of *BMPR-IA* gene between OPLL patients and non-OPLL Controls

SNPs	-349C > T			4A > C			1327C > T			1395G > C		
	exon1			exon3, Pro2Thr			exon11, Arg443Cys			exon12, Pro465Pro		
Genotype	CC	CT	TT	AA	AC	CC	CC	CT	TT	GG	GC	CC
OPLL (*n* = 356)	83	190	83	145	143	68	206	85	65	120	156	80
Control (*n* = 617)	297	246	74	283	284	50	370	148	99	240	222	155
Pearson Chi-Square Test	*P* < 0.001			*P* < 0.001			*P* = 0.662			*P* = 0.436		
Allele	C	T		A	C		C	T		G	C	
OPLL	356	356		433	279		497	215		396	316	
Control	840	394		850	384		888	346		702	532	
Pearson Chi-Square Test	*P* < 0.001			*P* < 0.001			*P* = 0.311			*P* = 0.586		

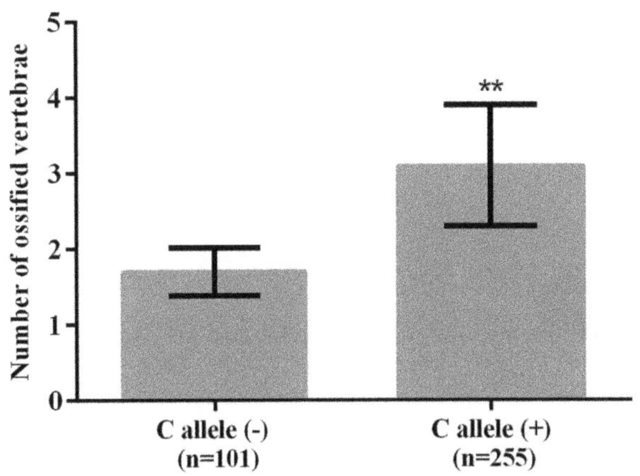

Fig. 3 The distribution of ossified cervical vertebrae of OPLL patients in each subgroup classified by C allele type in 4A > C polymorphism of *BMPR-IA* gene. The number of ossified vertebrae is shown under each bar. Data is expressed as means (bars) ± SD (error bars). The difference in the number of ossified vertebrae between the non-carriers and carriers of C allele type was statistically significant. ** $P < 0.001$

protein levels were significantly increased in pcDNA3.1/BMPR-IA (WT, MT -349C > T, MT 4A > C, MT -349C > T and 4A > C) vector-transfected C3H10T1/2 cells compared to the control cells and empty pcDNA3.1 (+) vector-transfected cells ($n = 5$, $^{*}p < 0.001$ C3H10T1/2/pcDNA3.1/BMPRIA WT cells compared with C3H10T1/2 cells, $^{*}p < 0.001$ C3H10T1/2/pcDNA3.1/BMPRIA WT cells compared with C3H10T1/2/pcDNA3.1 cells; $^{**}p < 0.001$ C3H10T1/2/pcDNA3.1/BMPRIA MT -349C > T cells compared with C3H10T1/2 cells, $^{**}p < 0.001$ C3H10T1/2/pcDNA3.1/BMPRIA MT -349C > T cells compared with C3H10T1/2/pcDNA3.1 cells; $^{**}p < 0.001$ C3H10T1/2/pcDNA3.1/BMPRIA MT 4A > C cells compared with C3H10T1/2 cells, $^{**}p < 0.001$ C3H10T1/2/pcDNA3.1/BMPRIA MT 4A > C cells compared with C3H10T1/2/pcDNA3.1 cells; $^{**}p < 0.001$ C3H10T1/2/pcDNA3.1/BMPRIA MT -349C > T and 4A > C cells compared with C3H10T1/2 cells, $^{**}p < 0.001$ C3H10T1/2/pcDNA3.1/BMPRIA MT -349C > T and 4A > C cells compared with C3H10T1/2/pcDNA3.1 cells). This demonstrated that pcDNA3.1/BMPR-IA (WT, MT) vectors were successfully transfected into C3H10T1/2 cells and stably expressed. In addition, the BMPR-IA protein levels in pcDNA3.1/BMPR-IA (MT -349C > T, MT 4A > C, MT -349C > T and 4A > C) vector-transfected C3H10T1/2 cells were higher than in pcDNA3.1/BMPR-IA (WT) vector-transfected C3H10T1/2 cells ($n = 5$, $^{**}p < 0.001$ C3H10T1/2/pcDNA3.1/BMPRIA MT -349C > T cells compared with C3H10T1/2/pcDNA3.1/BMPRIA WT cells, $^{**}p < 0.001$ C3H10T1/2/pcDNA3.1/BMPRIA MT 4A > C cells compared with C3H10T1/2/pcDNA3.1/BMPRIA WT cells, $^{**}p < 0.001$ C3H10T1/2/pcDNA3.1/BMPRIA MT -349C > T and 4A > C cells compared with C3H10T1/2/pcDNA3.1/BMPRIA WT cells).

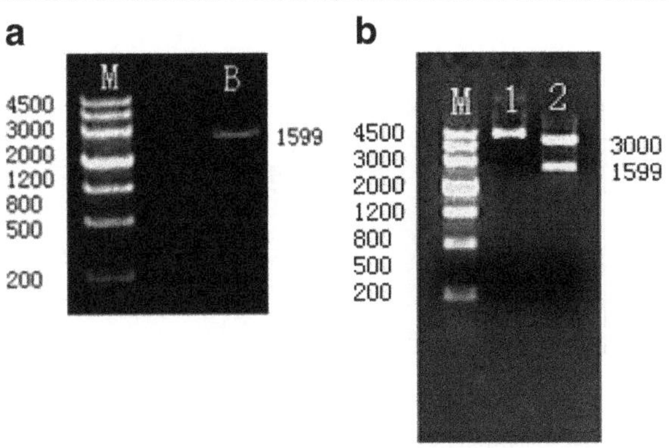

Fig. 4 The *BMPR-IA* gene coding sequence and pGEM-T/BMPR-IA (WT) vector digested with Hind III/Bam HI enzyme were analyzed by 4% agarose gel electrophoresis, respectively. **a** The annealed ds-oligos of *BMPR-IA* gene coding sequence was analyzed by 4% agarose gel electrophoresis. Each ds oligo annealing reactant showed a detectable molecular weight band around 1599 bp, as expected for the length of the designed ds-oligos of *BMPR-IA* gene. Lane M: Marker, Lane B: *BMPR-IA* gene.0020**b** After the pGEM-T/BMPR-IA (WT) vector had been digested with Hind III/Bam HI enzyme, the fragments for *BMPR-IA* cDNA (1599 bp) and the pGEM-T vector (3000 bp) were observed in all the PCR products as analyzed by 4% agarose gel electrophoresis, respectively. The results showed that the ds-oligos of the *BMPR-IA* gene cDNA were ligated into the pGEM-T vector. Lane M: Marker, Lane 1: pGEM-T/BMPR-IA (WT) vector, Lane 2: The pGEM-T vector and *BMPR-IA* cDNA

Phosphorylated Smad1/5/8 and Smad4 expression in transfected C3H10T1/2 cells

The proteins levels of Smad4 and phosphorylated Smad1/5/8 were determined by Western blotting (Figs. 6, 7). The phosphorylation levels of Smad1/5/8 were increased significantly in pcDNA3.1/BMPR-IA (WT, MT -349C > T, MT 4A > C, MT -349C > T and 4A > C) vector-transfected C3H10T1/2 cells compared to control C3H10T1/2 cells and empty pcDNA3.1 (+) vector-transfected C3H10T1/2 cells ($n = 5$, $^{*}p < 0.001$ C3H10T1/2/pcDNA3.1/BMPRIA WT cells compared with C3H10T1/2 cells, $^{*}p < 0.001$ C3H10T1/2/pcDNA3.1/BMPRIA WT cells compared with C3H10T1/2/pcDNA3.1 cells; $^{**}p < 0.001$ C3H10T1/2/pcDNA3.1/BMPRIA MT -349C > T cells compared with C3H10T1/2 cells, $^{**}p < 0.001$ C3H10T1/2/pcDNA3.1/BMPRIA MT -349C > T cells compared with C3H10T1/2/pcDNA3.1 cells; $^{*}p < 0.001$ C3H10T1/2/pcDNA3.1/BMPRIA MT 4A > C cells compared with C3H10T1/2 cells, $^{*}p < 0.001$ C3H10T1/2/pcDNA3.1/BMPRIA MT 4A > C cells compared with C3H10T1/2/pcDNA3.1 cells; $^{**}p < 0.001$ C3H10T1/2/pcDNA3.1/BMPRIA MT -349C > T cells compared with C3H10T1/2 cells, $^{**}p < 0.001$ C3H10T1/2/pcDNA3.1/BMPRIA MT -349C > T and 4A > C cells compared with C3H10T1/2/pcDNA3.1 cells). In

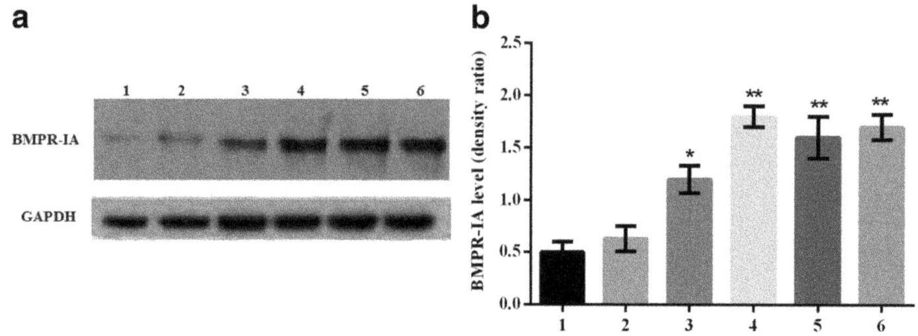

Fig. 5 The expression of *BMPR-IA* gene in the transfected C3H10T1/2 cells was detected by Western blotting. **a** Western blot analysis of *BMPR-IA* protein levels in transfected C3H10T1/2 cells. Lane 1: C3H10T1/2 cells; Lane 2: C3H10T1/2/pcDNA3.1 cells; Lane 3: C3H10T1/2/pcDNA3.1/BMPR-IA (WT) cell; Lane 4 C3H10T1/2/pcDNA3.1/BMPR-IA (MT -349C > T) cells; Lane 5 C3H10T1/2/pcDNA3.1/BMPR-IA (MT 4A > C) cells; Lane 6 C3H10T1/2/pcDNA3.1/BMPR-IA (MT -349C > T and 4A > C) cells. **b** Statistical analysis of *BMPR-IA* protein expression levels in transfected C3H10T1/2 cells using the linear density ratio of BMPR-IA/GAPDH. The protein expression levels of *BMPR-IA* gene were significantly increased in C3H10T1/2/pcDNA3.1/BMPRIA (MT -349C > T, MT 4A > C, MT -349C > T and 4A > C) cells compared to the C3H10T1/2/pcDNA3.1/BMPRIA (WT) cells, C3H10T1/2/pcDNA3.1 cells, and C3H10T1/2 cells. $n = 5$, *$p < 0.001$ C3H10T1/2/pcDNA3.1/BMPRIA WT cells compared with C3H10T1/2 cells, *$p < 0.001$ C3H10T1/2/pcDNA3.1/BMPRIA WT cells compared with C3H10T1/2/pcDNA3.1 cells; **$p < 0.001$ C3H10T1/2/pcDNA3.1/BMPRIA MT -349C > T cells compared with C3H10T1/2 cells, **$p < 0.001$ C3H10T1/2/pcDNA3.1/BMPRIA MT -349C > T cells compared with C3H10T1/2/pcDNA3.1 cells; **$p < 0.001$ C3H10T1/2/pcDNA3.1/BMPRIA MT 4A > C cells compared with C3H10T1/2 cells, **$p < 0.001$ C3H10T1/2/pcDNA3.1/BMPRIA MT 4A > C cells compared with C3H10T1/2/pcDNA3.1 cells; **$p < 0.001$ C3H10T1/2/pcDNA3.1/BMPRIA MT -349C > T and 4A > C cells compared with C3H10T1/2 cells, **$p < 0.001$ C3H10T1/2/pcDNA3.1/BMPRIA MT -349C > T and 4A > C cells compared with C3H10T1/2/pcDNA3.1 cells; **$p < 0.001$ C3H10T1/2/pcDNA3.1/BMPRIA MT -349C > T cells compared with C3H10T1/2/pcDNA3.1/BMPRIA WT cells, **$p < 0.001$ C3H10T1/2/pcDNA3.1/BMPRIA MT 4A > C cells compared with C3H10T1/2/pcDNA3.1/BMPRIA WT cells, **$p < 0.001$ C3H10T1/2/pcDNA3.1/BMPRIA MT -349C > T and 4A > C cells compared with C3H10T1/2/pcDNA3.1/BMPRIA WT cells

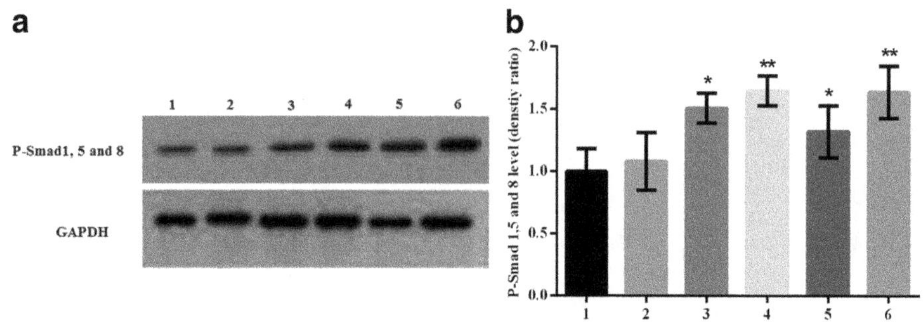

Fig. 6 The proteins levels of phosphorylated Smad1/5/8 in the transfected C3H10T1/2 cells were detected by Western blotting. **a** Western blot analysis of phosphorylated Smad1/5/8 proteins levels in transfected C3H10T1/2 cells. Lane 1 C3H10T1/2 cells; Lane 2 C3H10T1/2/pcDNA3.1 cells; Lane 3 C3H10T1/2/pcDNA3.1/BMPRIA (WT) cells; Lane 4 C3H10T1/2/pcDNA3.1/BMPR-IA (MT -349C > T) cells; Lane 5 C3H10T1/2/pcDNA3.1/BMPR-IA (MT 4A > C) cells; Lane 6 C3H10T1/2/pcDNA3.1/BMPR-IA (MT -349C > T and 4A > C) cells. **b** Statistical analysis of phosphorylated Smad1/5/8 proteins levels in C3H10T1/2 cells, C3H10T1/2/pcDNA3.1 cells, C3H10T1/2/pcDNA3.1/BMPR-IA (WT) cells, and C3H10T1/2/pcDNA3.1/BMPR-IA (MT -349C > T, MT 4A > C, MT -349C > T and 4A > C) cells using the linear density ratio of phosphorylated Smad1/5/8/GAPDH. The phosphorylated Smad1/5/8 proteins levels were significantly increased in C3H10T1/2/pcDNA3.1/BMPR-IA (MT -349C > T, MT -349C > T and 4A > C) cells compared to C3H10T1/2/pcDNA3.1/BMPR-IA (WT) cells, C3H10T1/2/pcDNA3.1 cells, and C3H10T1/2 cells. $n = 5$, *$p < 0.001$ C3H10T1/2/pcDNA3.1/BMPRIA WT cells compared with C3H10T1/2 cells, *$p < 0.001$ C3H10T1/2/pcDNA3.1/BMPRIA WT cells compared with C3H10T1/2/pcDNA3.1 cells; **$p < 0.001$ C3H10T1/2/pcDNA3.1/BMPRIA MT -349C > T cells compared with C3H10T1/2 cells, **$p < 0.001$ C3H10T1/2/pcDNA3.1/BMPRIA MT -349C > T cells compared with C3H10T1/2/pcDNA3.1 cells; *$p < 0.001$ C3H10T1/2/pcDNA3.1/BMPRIA MT 4A > C cells compared with C3H10T1/2 cells, *$p < 0.001$ C3H10T1/2/pcDNA3.1/BMPRIA MT 4A > C cells compared with C3H10T1/2/pcDNA3.1 cells; **$p < 0.001$ C3H10T1/2/pcDNA3.1/BMPRIA MT -349C > T cells compared with C3H10T1/2 cells, **$p < 0.001$ C3H10T1/2/pcDNA3.1/BMPRIA MT -349C > T and 4A > C cells compared with C3H10T1/2/pcDNA3.1 cells; **$p < 0.001$ C3H10T1/2/pcDNA3.1/BMPRIA MT -349C > T cells compared with C3H10T1/2/pcDNA3.1/BMPRIA WT cells, **$p < 0.001$ C3H10T1/2/pcDNA3.1/BMPRIA MT -349C > T and 4A > C cells compared with C3H10T1/2/pcDNA3.1/BMPRIA WT cells. The protein levels of phosphorylated Smad1/5/8 were not increased significantly in C3H10T1/2/pcDNA3.1/BMPR-IA (MT 4A > C) cells compared to the C3H10T1/2/pcDNA3.1/BMPR-IA (WT) cells ($n = 5$)

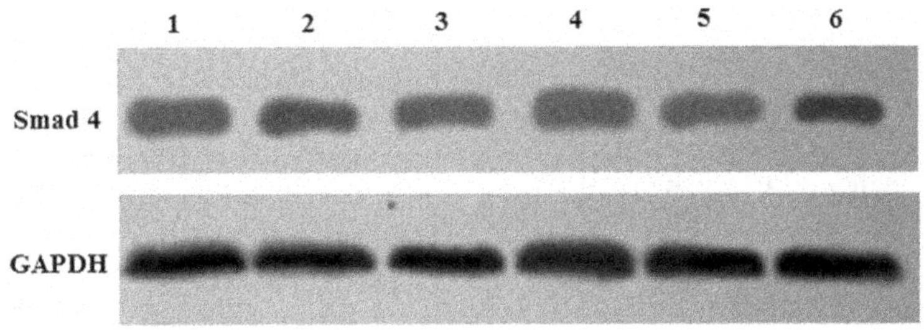

Fig. 7 Western blot analysis of Smad4 protein levels in the transfected C3H10T1/2 cells. Lane 1 C3H10T1/2 cells; Lane 2 C3H10T1/2/pcDNA3.1 cells; Lane 3 C3H10T1/2/pcDNA3.1/BMPR-IA (WT) cells; Lane 4 C3H10T1/2/pcDNA3.1/BMPR-IA (MT -349C > T) cells; Lane 5 C3H10T1/2/pcDNA3.1/BMPR-IA (MT 4A > C) cells; Lane 6 C3H10T1/2/pcDNA3.1/BMPR-IA (MT -349C > T and 4A > C) cells. There was no significant differences in Smad4 protein levels among the experimental groups ($n = 5$)

addition, the phosphorylation levels of Smad1/5/8 were significantly increased in pcDNA3.1/BMPR-IA (MT -349C > T, MT -349C > T and 4A > C) vector-transfected C3H10T1/2 cells compared to pcDNA3.1/BMPR-IA (WT) vector-transfected C3H10T1/2 cells ($n = 5$, $^{**}p < 0.001$ C3H10T1/2/pcDNA3.1/BMPRIA MT -349C > T cells compared with C3H10T1/2/pcDNA3.1/BMPRIA WT cells, $^{**}p < 0.001$ C3H10T1/2/pcDNA3.1/BMPRIA MT -349C > T and 4A > C cells compared with C3H10T1/2/pcDNA3.1/BMPRIA WT cells). However, no significant differences were observed in the phosphorylation levels of Smad1/5/8 between pcDNA3.1/BMPR-IA (MT 4A > C) and pcDNA3.1/BMPR-IA (WT) vector-transfected cells (n = 5). The Smad4 protein levels also did not differ significantly among the experimental groups ($n = 5$).

ALP and OC activity in transfected C3H10T1/2 cells

The activities of ALP and OC were determined in stably transfected C3H10T1/2 cells by ALP quantitation and osteocalcin radioimmunoassay kits, respectively (Figs. 8, 9). The ALP activity was increased in pcDNA3.1/BMPR-IA (WT 23.67 ± 0.42 U/gprot, MT -349C > T 30.56 ± 0.44 U/gprot, MT 4A > C 23.84 ± 0.42 U/gprot, MT -349C > T and 4A > C 26.91 ± 0.41 U/gprot) vector-transfected C3H10T1/2 cells compared to control C3H10T1/2 cells (14.74 ± 0.46 U/gprot) and empty pcDNA3.1 (+) vector-transfected C3H10T1/2 cells (15.08 ± 0.51 U/gprot) ($n = 5$). ALP activity was significantly higher in pcDNA3.1/BMPR-IA (MT -349C > T 30.56 ± 0.44 U/gprot, MT -349C > T and 4A > C 29.91 ± 0.41 U/gprot) vectors-transfected C3H10T1/2 cells compared to pcDNA3.1/BMPR-IA (WT 23.67 ± 0.42 U/gprot) vector-transfected C3H10T1/2 cells ($n = 5$). However, no significant differences were observed in the ALP activity between pcDNA3.1/BMPR-IA (MT 4A > C 23.84 ± 0.42 U/gprot) and pcDNA3.1/BMPR-IA (WT 23.67 ± 0.42 U/gprot) vector-transfected C3H10T1/2 cells ($n = 5$). In addition, the OC activity increased in pcDNA3.1/BMPRIA (WT 1.01 ± 0.10 ng/mL, MT -349C > T 1.04 ± 0.12 ng/mL, MT 4A > C 1.02 ± 0.09 ng/mL, MT -349C > T and 4A > C 1.03 ± 0.13 ng/ml) vector-transfected C3H10T1/2 cells compared to the control C3H10T1/2 (0.72 ± 0.11 ng/mL) cells and empty pcDNA3.1 (+) (0.79 ± 0.12 ng/mL) vector-transfected C3H10T1/2 cells (n = 5). In addition, no significant

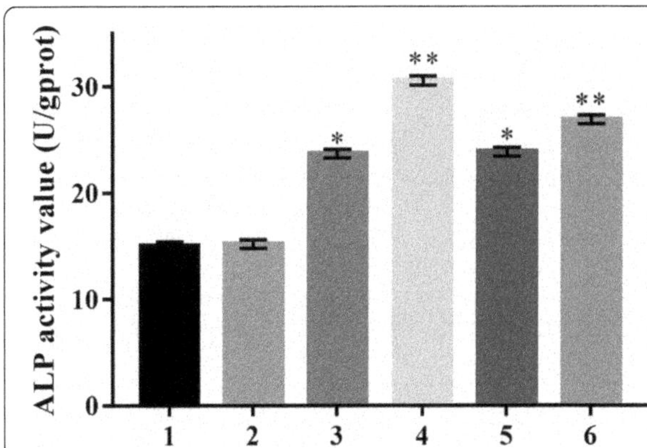

Fig. 8 The ALP activity in transfected C3H10T1/2 cells. The ALP activity levels were significantly increased in C3H10T1/2/pcDNA3.1/BMPR-IA (MT -349C > T 30.56 ± 0.44 U/gprot, MT -349C > T and 4A > C 26.91 ± 0.41 U/gprot) cells compared to C3H10T1/2/pcDNA3.1/BMPR-IA (WT 23.67 ± 0.42 U/gprot) cells. n = 5, $^{*}p < 0.001$ C3H10T1/2/pcDNA3.1/BMPRIA WT cells compared with C3H10T1/2 cells, $^{*}p < 0.001$ C3H10T1/2/pcDNA3.1/BMPRIA WT cells compared with C3H10T1/2/pcDNA3.1 cells; $^{**}p < 0.001$ C3H10T1/2/pcDNA3.1/BMPRIA MT -349C > T cells compared with C3H10T1/2 cells, $^{**}p < 0.001$ C3H10T1/2/pcDNA3.1/BMPRIA MT -349C > T cells compared with C3H10T1/2/pcDNA3.1 cells; $^{*}p < 0.001$ C3H10T1/2/pcDNA3.1/BMPRIA MT 4A > C cells compared with C3H10T1/2 cells, $^{*}p < 0.001$ C3H10T1/2/pcDNA3.1/BMPRIA MT 4A > C cells compared with C3H10T1/2/pcDNA3.1 cells; $^{**}p < 0.001$ C3H10T1/2/pcDNA3.1/BMPRIA MT -349C > T and 4A > C cells compared with C3H10T1/2 cells, $^{**}p < 0.001$ C3H10T1/2/pcDNA3.1/BMPRIA MT -349C > T and 4A > C cells compared with C3H10T1/2/pcDNA3.1 cells; $^{**}p < 0.001$ C3H10T1/2/pcDNA3.1/BMPRIA MT -349C > T cells compared with C3H10T1/2/pcDNA3.1/BMPRIA WT cells, $^{**}p < 0.001$ C3H10T1/2/pcDNA3.1/BMPRIA MT -349C > T and 4A > C cells compared with C3H10T1/2/pcDNA3.1/BMPRIA WT cells. No differences in ALP activity in C3H10T1/2/pcDNA3.1/BMPR-IA (MT 4A > C 23.84 ± 0.42 U/gprot) cells were observed compared to the C3H10T1/2/pcDNA3.1/BMPR-IA (WT 23.67 ± 0.42 U/gprot) cells ($n = 5$)

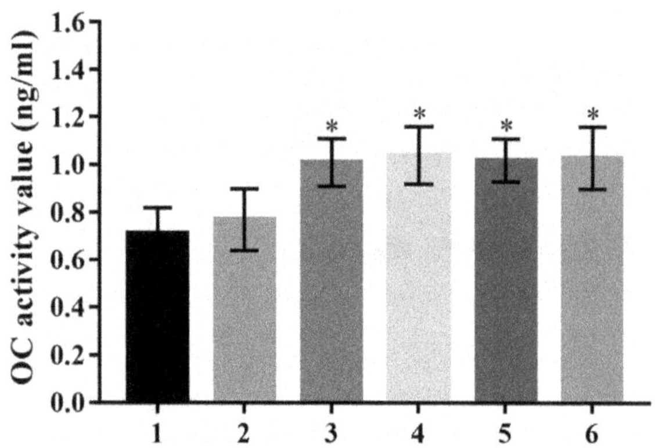

Fig. 9 The OC activity in transfected C3H10T1/2 cells. The OC activity levels were significantly increased in C3H10T1/2/pcDNA3.1/BMPR-IA (WT 1.01 ± 0.10 ng/mL, MT -349C > T 1.04 ± 0.12 ng/mL, MT 4A > C 1.02 ± 0.09 ng/mL, MT -349C > T and 4A > C 1.03 ± 0.13 ng/mL) cells compared to the control groups. n = 5, *$p < 0.001$ C3H10T1/2/pcDNA3.1/BMPRIA WT cells compared with C3H10T1/2 cells, *$p < 0.001$ C3H10T1/2/pcDNA3.1/BMPRIA WT cells compared with C3H10T1/2/pcDNA3.1 cells; *$p < 0.001$ C3H10T1/2/pcDNA3.1/BMPRIA MT -349C > T cells compared with C3H10T1/2 cells, *$p < 0.001$ C3H10T1/2/pcDNA3.1/BMPRIA MT -349C > T cells compared with C3H10T1/2/pcDNA3.1 cells; *$p < 0.001$ C3H10T1/2/pcDNA3.1/BMPRIA MT 4A > C cells compared with C3H10T1/2 cells, *$p < 0.001$ C3H10T1/2/pcDNA3.1/BMPRIA MT 4A > C cells compared with C3H10T1/2/pcDNA3.1 cells; *$p < 0.001$ C3H10T1/2/pcDNA3.1/BMPRIA MT -349C > T and 4A > C cells compared with C3H10T1/2 cells, *$p < 0.001$ C3H10T1/2/pcDNA3.1/BMPRIA MT -349C > T and 4A > C cells compared with C3H10T1/2/pcDNA3.1 cells. However, no significant differences were observed in OC activity between C3H10T1/2/pcDNA3.1/BMPRIA (WT 1.01 ± 0.10 ng/ml) cells and C3H10T1/2/pcDNA3.1/BMPRIA (MT -349C > T 1.04 ± 0.12 ng/mL, MT 4A > C 1.02 ± 0.09 ng/mL, MT -349C > T and 4A > C 1.03 ± 0.13 ng/mL) cells (n = 5)

differences in the OC activity were observed between pcDNA3.1/BMPRIA (WT 1.01 ± 0.10 ng/mL) vector-transfected C3H10T1/2 cells and pcDNA3.1/BMPRIA (MT -349C > T 1.04 ± 0.12 ng/mL, MT 4A > C 1.02 ± 0.09 ng/mL, MT -349C > T and 4A > C 1.03 ± 0.13 ng/mL) vector-transfected C3H10T1/2 cells (n = 5).

Discussion

OPLL of the spine is a pathological condition that causes ossification in the posterior longitudinal ligament of the spine with the formation of ectopic bone primarily through endochondral ossification [25, 26]. The ossification of the spinal ligament causes myelopathy, radiculopathy, or both and leads to severe neurological deficits and paralysis. Although the incidence of OPLL is higher in Asian countries than non-Asian [1], the pathogenesis is unclear. OPLL is a multifactorial disease and may result from genetic, gene interactions and various environmental factors. Epidemiological studies have demonstrated that genetic susceptibility may be a critical factor for the development of OPLL, and genetic components appear to play a crucial role in its pathogenesis [2–4]. Previous studies have indicated that SNPs in BMP2, 4, and 9, collagen 6A1, angiotensin I converting enzyme gene, BH3 interacting domain death agonist, nucleotide pyrophosphatase, and vitamin K epoxide reductase complex subunit 1 are associated with the development of OPLL. The occurrence and development of OPLL are regulated by various factors and several genes [4–9]. However, identifying all the susceptible genes for OPLL, especially the molecular machinery underlying these genetic polymorphisms is challenging.

BMPRs are the receptor binding proteins of BMPs, and include type I and II serine/threonine kinase receptors. Receptor-ligand BMPs are involved in the formation of new bone and cartilage, and play a vital role in bone formation during different developmental stages. The binding of BMP to at least one type I and one type II serine/threonine kinase receptor is essential for the activation of BMP signaling [27]. BMPs exert their effects via hetero-oligomeric complexes of type I and II receptors. There are three type I receptors: BMPR-IA, BMPR-IB, and ActR-IA and three type II receptors: BMPR- II, ActR-II, and ActR-IIB. BMPR-IA, IB, and II are specific for BMPs, as well as for ActR-IA, II, and IIB, which are also signaling receptors for activins [10]. BMP bind with different affinities to specific type I and II receptors. The type I BMP receptors have been reported as the high-affinity binding receptors, whereas type II BMP receptors bind BMPs directly with low affinity [11]. The affinity of the BMPs to receptors is crucial for signal transduction activity [28]. The type I BMP receptors play a central role in BMP signal transduction from the receptor to target genes in the nucleus.

The *BMPR-IA* gene on chromosome 10 is a subtype of type I BMP receptors and contains 13 exons. Previous studies have suggested that the levels of protein and mRNA of *BMPR-IA* gene were highly expressed in chondrocytes of fibrocartilage tissue around the calcified zone and fibroblast-like spindle cells in non-ossified ligaments of OPLL patients. However, the gene was not expressed in ligament tissues in non-OPLL patients [18, 20]. Our present study demonstrates that BMPR-IA, which transduces signals for BMPs, plays an important role in the pathological ossification of OPLL.

Previously, we reported that the 4A > C and the -349C > T polymorphisms of *BMPR-IA* gene was associated with OPLL in the cervical spine [21]. In this study, we further validated our findings using a larger cohort. The C allele type in the 4A > C polymorphism was significantly associated with the occurrence and extent of OPLL in the cervical spine. The T allele type in the -349C > T polymorphism increased the susceptibility to OPLL of the cervical spine but not the extent. However, the molecular mechanisms underlying the two SNPs in the *BMPR-IA* gene have not yet been elucidated. Based on our preliminary data, a series of in vitro experiments were performed to determine whether Smad signaling pathway may be involved in the increased susceptibility and severity to OPLL via these *BMPR-IA* gene polymorphisms.

Signal transduction studies have demonstrated that the immediate downstream molecules of BMP receptors are Smad proteins, especially Smad1, 5 and 8, which play a central role in BMP signal transduction. Binding of BMP ligand to at least one type I and one type II BMP receptors results in the type II BMP receptor phosphorylating the type I receptor [29], which subsequently leads to the recruitment of the receptor-activated Smads (R-Smads, Smads 1, 5 and 8). The activation of type I BMP receptor is required for the direct interaction between type I receptor and R-Smads (Smads 1, 5 and 8). R-Smads associate directly and transiently with activated type I BMP receptors and undergo direct phosphorylation at the C-terminal SSXS motif of Smad in a ligand-dependent manner [30, 31]. R-Smads are the only Smads that have an SSXS motif in their C-terminal region. After rapid release from the type I receptor, the phosphorylated R-Smads proteins form hetero-oligomeric complexes with the common-mediator Smads (Co-Smads, Smad4), which acts as a shared partner. The R-Smads and Co-Smad complexes then translocate into the nucleus to regulate the transcription of specific target genes with other transcription factors. In the nucleus, the Smads 1 and 5 proteins exert their transcriptional activity by direct interaction with DNA and association with other DNA-binding proteins [32]. ALP, OC, and type I collagen are osteogenesis-specific protein factors in the downstream regulation of the BMP signaling pathway. Moreover, ALP is essential for the osteogenic phenotype and is critical for bone formation mediated by the regulation of the mineralization of bone matrix [33, 34].

In order to determine the role of the -349C > T and 4A > C polymorphisms of *BMPR-IA* gene in the osteogenesis mechanism during the development of OPLL, we examined whether these two SNPs affected *BMPR-IA* gene expression and signal transduction of the Smad signaling pathway. The present study demonstrated that the expression levels of *BMPR-IA* gene were significantly increased in pcDNA3.1/BMPR-IA (MT -349C > T, MT 4A > C, MT -349C > T and 4A > C) vector-transfected C3H10T1/2 cells compared to the pcDNA3.1/BMPR-IA (WT) vector-transfected C3H10T1/2 cells. These data suggest that *BMPR-IA* gene may be overexpressed in pcDNA3.1/BMPR-IA (MT -349C > T, MT 4A > C, MT -349C > T and 4A > C) vector-transfected C3H10T1/2 cells. The phosphorylation levels of Smad1/5/8 were significantly increased in pcDNA3.1/BMPR-IA (MT -349C > T) vector-transfected C3H10T1/2 cells compared to the pcDNA3.1/BMPR-IA (WT) vector-transfected cells. This may indicate that the -349C > T polymorphism of *BMPR-IA* gene is positively associated with the phosphorylation of Smad1/5/8 expression levels. In addition, the ALP activity was significantly higher in the pcDNA3.1/BMPR-IA (MT -349C > T) vector-transfected C3H10T1/2 cells compared to the pcDNA3.1/BMPR-IA (WT) vector-transfected. These observations demonstrate that the -349C > T polymorphism of *BMPR-IA* gene is significantly associated with ALP activity, and suggest that the -349C > T polymorphism of *BMPR-IA* gene can enhance ALP activity via the Smad signaling pathway. Moreover, our results demonstrated that the overexpression of the *BMPR-IA* gene induced by the -349C > T polymorphism could increase the phosphorylation levels of Smad1/5/8, and further lead to the increase in ALP activity of osteogenesis-specific protein factors. Based on previous BMP receptor signal transduction studies, we propose that the -349C > T polymorphism of the BMPR-IA gene may play an important role in mediating susceptibility to OPLL via Smad signaling pathway. However, no significant differences were observed in the levels of Co-Smad4 protein among the experimental groups. There were no significant differences in the OC activity between pcDNA3.1/BMPRIA (WT) vector-transfected C3H10T1/2 cells and pcDNA3.1/BMPRIA (MT -349C > T, MT 4A > C, MT -349C > T and 4A > C) vector-transfected C3H10T1/2 cells. These results indicate that the -349C > T and 4A > C polymorphisms of BMPR-IA gene do not affect genetic predisposition to OPLL that is mediated through the increased levels of the Co-Smad4 protein and OC activity. In addition, we found that the protein levels of phosphorylated Smad1/5/8 and the ALP activity were not increased significantly in pcDNA3.1/BMPR-IA (MT 4A > C) vector-transfected C3H10T1/2 cells compared to the pcDNA3.1/BMPR-IA (WT) vector-transfected C3H10T1/2 cells. This result led us to hypothesize that the 4A > C polymorphism in the BMPR-IA gene may increase the susceptibility and severity of OPLL through another signaling pathway in addition to Smads. Based on previous studies, in addition to Smad signaling pathway, BMP binding to a homomeric type I or II BMPR leads to secondary formation of heterotetrameric complexes that activates non-Smad signaling pathways such as mitogen-activated protein kinase (MAPK) family of molecules including p38 and ERK1/2.

Finally, we would like to highlight some limitations in our study. We did not examine the protein levels of TAB1/TAK1, p38, and ERK1/2 in C3H10T1/2 cells and hence unable to state whether non-Smad signaling pathways are involved in the pathogenesis of OPLL. Future studies are necessary to examine if non-Smad signaling pathways are involved in the development of OPLL.

Conclusions

The present results demonstrate that the expression levels of BMPR-IA gene, the levels of phosphorylated Smad1/5/8 and ALP activity were significantly increased in pcDNA3.1/BMPR-IA (MT -349C > T) vector-transfected C3H10T1/2 cells than the WT vector-transfected cells. Our data suggest that Smad signaling pathway may play important roles in the pathological process of OPLL induced by SNPs in BMPR-IA gene. The current study may help to clarify the molecular mechanisms underlying the susceptibility of the gene to OPLL, thereby providing a novel potential target for the diagnosis and therapy for OPLL.

Abbreviations

ALP: Alkaline phosphatase; BME: Basal medium eagle; BMP: Bone morphogenetic protein; *BMPR-IA*: Bone morphogenetic protein receptor type IA; BMPRs: Bone morphogenetic protein receptors; C3H10T1/2: The mouse embryonic mesenchymal stem cells; DNA: Deoxyribonucleic acid; DS: Double-stranded; FBS: Fetal bovine serum; MT: Mutation type; OC: Osteocalcin; OPLL: Ossification of the posterior longitudinal ligament; PCR: Polymerase chain reaction; SNPs: Single nucleotide polymorphisms; SS: Single-stranded; WT: Wild type

Acknowledgements

The authors would like to thank all the patients and participants in this study, as well as the basic research clinic foundation of Capital Medical University (No.2011JL45 and No.15JL50) for making this study possible.

Funding

This study was supported by grants from the basic research clinic foundation of Capital Medical University (No.2011JL45 and No.15JL50).

Authors' contributions

HW designed the study, analyzed and interpreted the data, helped perform the experiments, and wrote the manuscript. WTJ helped to design the study, perform the experiments, analyze and interpret the data. HBL helped to analyze, interpret the data and perform the statistical analysis. All authors read and approved the final manuscript.

Consent for publication

Not applicable.

Competing interests

The authors declare that they have no competing interests.

Author details

[1]Department of Orthopaedics, Beijing Tiantan Hospital, Capital Medical University, 6 TiantanXili, Dongcheng District, Beijing 100050, China. [2]Department of Epidemiology and Biostatistics, School of Public Health, Capital Medical University, Beijing 100069, China.

References

1. Matsunaga S, Sakou T. Ossification of the posterior longitudinal ligament of the cervical spine: etiology and natural history. Spine (Phila Pa 1976). 2012; 37(5):E309–14.
2. Ikegawa S. Genomic study of ossification of the posterior longitudinal ligament of the spine. Proc Jpn A cad Ser B Phys Biol Sci. 2014;90(10):405–12.
3. Nakajima M, Takahashi A, Tsuji T, Karasugi T, Baba H, Uchida K, Kawabata S, Okawa A, Shindo S, Takeuchi K, Taniguchi Y, Maeda S, Kashii M, Seichi A, Nakajima H, Kawaguchi Y, Fujibayashi S, Takahata M, Tanaka T, Watanabe K, Kida K, Kanchiku T, Ito Z, Mori K, Kaito T, Kobayashi S, Yamada K, Takahashi M, Chiba K, Matsumoto M, Furukawa K, Kubo M, Toyama Y, Genetic Study Group of Investigation Committee on ossification of the spinal ligaments, Ikegawa S. A genome-wide association study identifies susceptibility loci for ossification of the posterior longitudinal ligament of the spine. Nat Genet. 2014;46(9):1012–6.
4. Kim KH, Kuh SU, Park JY, Lee SJ, Park HS, Chin DK, Kim KS, Cho YE. Association between BMP-2 and COL6A1 gene polymorphisms with susceptibility to ossification of the posterior longitudinal ligament of the cervical spine in Korean patients and family members. Genet Mol Res. 2014; 13(1):2240–7.
5. Wang H, Liu D, Yang Z, Tian B, Li J, Meng X, Wang Z, Yang H, Lin X. Association of bone morphogenetic protein-2 gene polymorphisms with susceptibility to ossification of the posterior longitudinal ligament of the spine and its severity in Chinese patients. Eur Spine J. 2008;17(7):956–64.
6. Ren Y, Liu ZZ, Feng J, Wan H, Li JH, WANG H, Lin X. Association of a BMP9 haplotype with ossification of the posterior longitudinal ligament (OPLL) in a Chinese population. PLoS One. 2012;7(7):e40587.
7. Kim DH, Yun DH, Kim HS, Min SK, Yoo SD, Lee KH, Kim KT, Jo DJ, Kim SK, Chung JH, Ban JY, Lee SY. The insertion/deletion polymorphism of angiotensin I converting enzyme gene is associated with ossification of the posterior longitudinal ligament in the Korean population. Ann Rehabil Med. 2014;38(1):1–5.
8. He Z, Zhu H, Ding L, Xiao H, Chen D, Xue F. Association of NPP1 polymorphism with postoperative progression of ossification of the posterior longitudinal ligament in Chinese patients. Genet Mol Res. 2013; 12(4):4648–55.
9. Chin DK, Han IB, Ropper AE, Jeon YJ, Kim DH, Kim YS, Park Y, Teng YD, Kim NK, Kuh SU. Association of VKORC1-1639 G>A polymorphism with susceptibility to ossification of the posterior longitudinal ligament of the spine: a Korean study. Acta Neurochir. 2013;155(10):1937–42.
10. Miyazono K, Kamiya Y, Morikawa M. Bone morphogenetic protein receptors and signal transduction. J Biochem. 2010;147(1):35–51.
11. Rosenzweig BL, Imamura T, Okadome T, Cox GN, Yamashita H, ten Dijke P, Heldin CH, Miyazono K. Cloning and characterization of a human type II receptor for bone morphogenetic proteins. Proc Natl Acad Sci U S A. 1995; 92(17):7632–6.
12. Moustakas A, Heldin CH. From mono- to oligo-Smads: the heart of the matter in TGF-beta signal transduction. Genes Dev. 2002;16(15):1867–71.
13. Xu WP, Shiba H, Mizuno N, Uchida Y, Mouri Y, Kawaguchi H, Kurihara H. Effect of bone morphogenetic proteins-4, –5 and –6 on DNA synthesis and expression of bone-related proteins in cultured human periodontal ligament cells. Cell Biol Int. 2004;28:675–82.
14. Ye G, Li C, Xiang X, Chen C, Zhang R, Yang X, Yu X, Wang J, Wang L, Shi Q, Weng Y. Bone morphogenetic protein-9 induces PDLSCs osteogenic differentiation through the ERK and p38 signal pathways. Int J Med Sci. 2014;11(10):1065–72.
15. Kaps C, Hoffmann A, Zilberman Y, Pelled G, Häupl T, Sittinger M, Burmester G, Gazit D, Gross G. Distinct roles of BMP receptors type IA and IB in osteo –/chondrogenic differentiation in mesenchymal progenitors (C3H10T1/2). BioFactors. 2004;20(2):71–84.
16. Fujii M, Takeda K, Imamura T, Aoki H, Sampath TK, Enomoto S, Kawabata M, Kato M, Ichijo H, Miyazono K. Roles of bone morphogenetic protein type I receptors and Smad proteins in osteoblast and chondroblast differentiation. Mol Biol Cell. 1999;10(11):3801–13.
17. Yeh LC, Unda R, Lee JC. Osteogenic protein-1 differentially regulates the mRNA expression of bone morphogenetic proteins and their receptors in primary cultures of osteoblasts. J Cell Physiol. 2000;185(1):87–97.
18. Kawa-Uchi T, Furuya K, Shinomiya K, Yama-Ura I, Kurosa Y, Wozney JM, Ueno N, Noda M. Messenger RNA expression of the genes encoding receptors for bone morphogenetic protein (BMP) and transforming growth factor-B (TGF-B) in the cells from the posterior longitudinal ligament in cervical spine. Endocrine. 1996;5:307–14.

19. Yonemori K, Imamura T, Ishidou Y, Okano T, Matsunaga S, Yoshida H, Kato M, Sampath TK, Miyazono K, ten Dijke P, Sakou T. Bone morphogenetic protein receptors and activin receptors are highly expressed in ossified ligament tissues of patients with ossification of the posterior longitudinal ligament. Am J Pathol. 1997;150(4):1335–47.
20. Liu R, Ginn SL, Lek M, North KN, Alexander IE, Little DG, Schindeler A. Myoblast sensitivity and fibroblast insensitivity to osteogenic conversion by BMP-2 correlates with the expression of Bmpr-1a. BMC Musculoskelet Disord. 2009;10:51.
21. Jin W, Yang H, Yan L, Zhao C, Lin X, Wang H. Association of Bone Morphogenic Protein Receptor IA (BMPRIA) gene polymorphism with ossification of posterior longitudinal ligament (OPLL) of the cervical spine in a Chinese Han population. J Spine. 2013;2:131–6.
22. Tsuyama N. Ossification of the posterior longitudinal ligament of the spine. Clin Orthop Relat Res. 1984;(184):71–84.
23. Oste C. Polymerase Chain reaction. BioTechniques. 1988;6(2):162–7.
24. Kim HY. Statistical notes for clinical researchers: post-hoc multiple comparisons. Restor Dent Endod. 2015;40(2):172–6.
25. Onji Y, Akiyama H, Shimomura Y, Ono K, Hukuda S, Mizuno S. Posterior paravertebral ossification causing cervical myelopathy: a report of eighteen cases. J Bone Joint Surg. 1967;49:1314–28.
26. Ono K, Ota H, Tada K. Ossified Posterior longitudinal ligament: a clinicopathological study. Spine. 1977;2:126–38.
27. Ten Dijke P, Miyazono K, Heldin CH. Signaling via hetero-oligomeric complexes of type I and type II serine/threonine kinase receptors. Curr Opin Cell Biol. 1996;8(2):139–45.
28. Macías-Silva M, Hoodless PA, Tang SJ, Buchwald M, Wrana JL. Specific activation of Smad1 signaling pathways by the BMP7 type I receptor, ALK2. J Biolumin Chemilumin. 1998;273(40):25628–36.
29. Wrana JL, Attisano L, Wieser R, Ventura F, Massague J. Mechanism of activation of the TGF-beta receptor. Nature. 1994;370(6488):341–7.
30. Hoodless PA, Haerry T, Abdollah S, Stapleton M, O'Connor MB, Attisano L, Wrana JL. MADR1, a MAD-related protein that functions in BMP2 signaling pathways. Cell. 1996;85(4):489–500.
31. Nishimura R, Kato Y, Chen D, Harris SE, Mundy GR, Yoneda T. Smad5 and DPC4 are key molecules in mediating BMP-2-induced osteoblastic differentiation of the pluripotent mesenchymal precursor cell line C2C12. J Biolumin Chemilumin. 1998;273(4):1872–9.
32. Derynck R, Zhang Y, Feng XH. Smads: transcriptional activators of TGF-beta responses. Cell. 1998;95(6):737–40.
33. Hessle L, Johnson KA, Anderson HC, Narisawa S, Sali A, Goding JW, Terkeltaub R, Millan JL. Tissue-nonspecific alkaline phosphatase and plasma cell membrane glycoprotein-1 are central antagonistic regulators of bone mineralization. Proc Natl Acad Sci U S A. 2002;99(14):9445–9.
34. Anderson HC, Sipe JB, Hessle L, Dhanyamraju R, Atti E, Camacho NP, Millan JL, Dhamyamraju R. Impaired calcification around matrix vesicles of growth plate and bone in alkaline phosphatase-deficient mice. Am J Pathol. 2004; 164(3):841–7.

6

Correlation between the sagittal spinopelvic alignment and degenerative lumbar spondylolisthesis

Qi Lai†, Tian Gao†, Xin Lv, Xuqiang Liu, Zongmiao Wan, Min Dai, Bin Zhang* and Tao Nie*

Abstract

Background: Pain and disability associated with degenerative lumbar spondylolisthesis (DLS) results in significant burden on both the patients' quality of life and healthcare costs. Currently, there is controversy regarding the specificity of spinopelvic measures of sagittal plane alignment with respect to DLS. Moreover, the correlation among spinopelvic parameters of sagittal plane alignment remains to be clarified. Our aim in this study was to compare these measurements between patients with single-segment DLS at L5 and a control group with no history of DLS.

Methods: Our study group was formed of 132 patients who underwent full length lateral view radiographs of the spine in a relaxed standing posture. Among these, DLS at L5 was identified in 72 patients, forming the DLS group, with no radiographic evidence of lumbar spine disease in the remaining 60 patients, forming the control group. The patient and control groups were balanced with regard to age and sex distribution. The following spinopelvic parameters of sagittal plane alignment were measured: angle of incidence (PI) and tilt (PT) of the pelvis; sacral slope (SS); thoracic kyphosis (TK); lumbar lordosis (LL); and the spinal sagittal vertical axis (SVA). The Meyerding grade of L5 slippage was quantified for each patient in the DLS group.

Results: Measures of TK, PI, SS, and LL were significantly greater in the DLS than control group ($P < 0.05$), with no between-group difference in SVA and PT. In the DLS group, the grade of L5 slippage correlated with SS ($r = 0.873$, $P < 0.0001$), PI ($r = 0.791$, $P < 0.0001$) and LL ($r = 0.790$, $P < 0.0001$). Moreover, the measurement for SS correlated more strongly with the PI ($r = 0.94$, $P < 0.01$) than the LL ($r = 0.69$, $P < 0.01$).

Conclusion: Measurements of SS, PI, and LL were specifically associated with DLS, with measurements correlating positively with the grade of slippage.

Keywords: Lumbar degenerative spondylolisthesis, Sagittal alignment, Lumbar lordosis, Pelvic incidence, L5

Background

The definition of DLS has been gradually refined over time, from a simple slippage of the vertebral body, described in 1930, to a slippage due to the absence of the pedicle isthmus, known as a pseudo spondylolisthesis and described by MacNab [1] in 1950. In 1963, Newman [2] introduced the concept of degenerative spondylolisthesis, with an estimated 4.1% incidence rate of DLS [3]. The incidence of DLS among women is 400% greater than among men [4], with DLS being most prevalent among women over the age of 50 years, and usually affecting the L4-L5 segment, with a grade of slippage of I-III [5].

The pain and disability associated with degenerative lumbar spondylolisthesis (DLS) cause a significant burden both at the level of patients' quality of life and healthcare costs. The aetiology of DLS is complex and remains controversial, although some researchers have attributed DLS to age, trauma, sustained weight-bearing, and congenital malformation [6–8]. Barrey et al. [9, 10]

* Correspondence: acker11@126.com; 18702508157@163.com
†Equal contributors
Department of Orthopedics, The First Affiliated Hospital of Nanchang University, Artificial Joints Engineering and Technology Research Center of Jiangxi Province, Nanchang, Jiangxi 330006, People's Republic of China

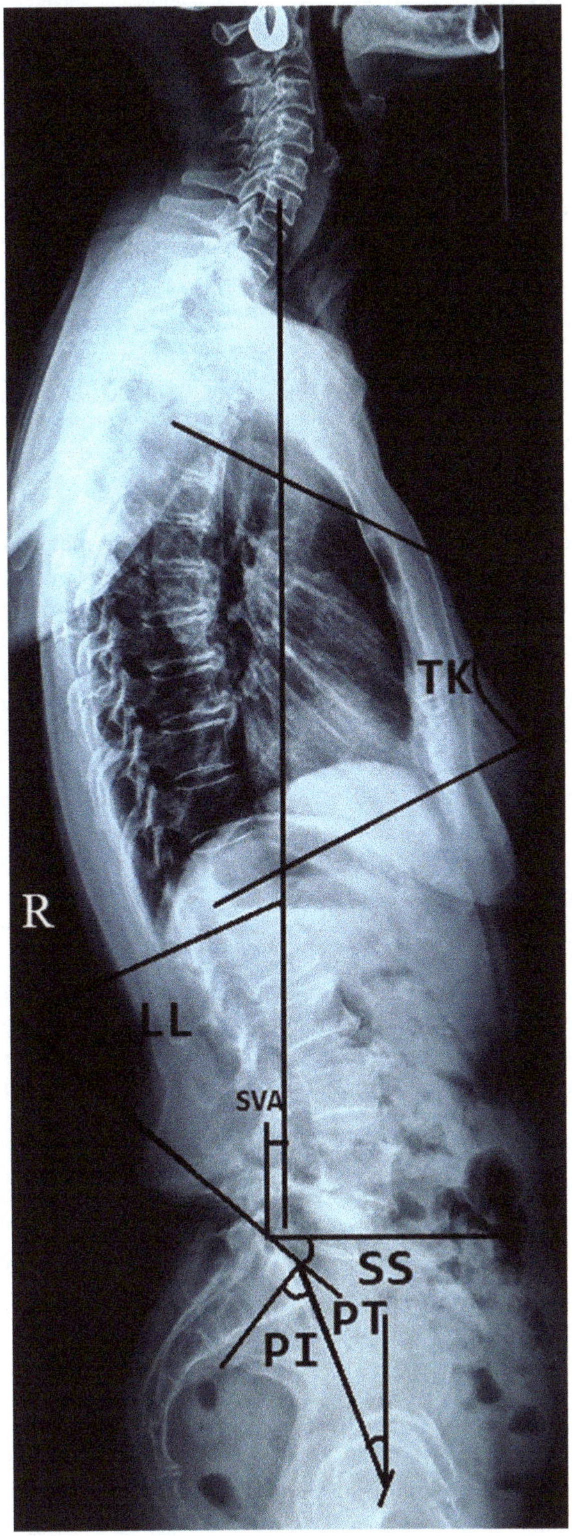

Fig. 1 TK: The angle between the upper endplate of T4 and the lower endplate of T12; LL was measured using the Cobb angle between the superior end plate of the L1 and S1. PT was defined as the angle between a straight line connecting the midpoint of the bilateral femoral head centre to the midpoint of the sacral plate and the plumb line. PI was defined as the angle between the perpendicular line of the sacral plate and the line of the midpoint of the superior endplate of S1 joining with the centre of the hip axis. SS was defined as the angle formed by the upper endplate of S1 and the horizontal plane; SVA:C7 vertebral body along the vertical line and the upper edge of the S1 vertebral body

reported an increase in the angle of incidence (PI) and tilt (PT) of the pelvis among patients with DLS in comparison to healthy volunteers, combined with a decrease in the slope of the sacrum (SS) and lumbar lordosis (LL). In their review of the spinopelvic alignment parameters for 65 patients with DLS, Barrey et al. concluded that PI was a causative factor of DLS. In their comparison of spinopelvic alignment between 50 patients with DLS and a control group without DLS, Fuano et al. [11] also reported the PI to be greater among patients with DLS compared to a control group, with an associated increase in SS, the slope of L4 and L5, thoracic kyphosis (TK) and LL. Therefore, although both studies identified an increase in PI, the association between DLS and other parameters of spinopelvic alignment (LL, PT, and SS) is controversial. Therefore, our aim in this study was to clarify this issue through a comparison of the spinopelvic parameters of sagittal plane alignment among patients with a DLS at L5 and a control group with no radiographic evidence of DLS.

Methods

Study group

Our study group included both patients with a single-segment DLS at L5 and individuals without DLS who underwent radiographic examination of the spine over the same period. All prospective participants underwent a lateral view radiograph of the spine in a relaxed standing position, including C7 and the hips. The inclusion criteria for participants in the control group were an absence of spondylolysis and scoliosis. The inclusion criteria for the DLS group was confirmation of a single-segment L5 spondylolisthesis. The Meyerding grade [12] of the DLS was defined based on the percentage of slippage of the L5 vertebral body (grade 0, no slip; grade I, a 1–25% slip; grade II, a 25–50% slip; grade III, a 51–75% slip; and grade IV, a 75–100% slip). Individuals with a previous history of spinal or pelvic surgery, as well as those with a lumbosacral transitional vertebra, spinal deformity, tumour, infection, fractures, Any condition that could affect the sagittal plane alignment of the spine, such as abnormal BMI, were excluded.

Over the study period from January 2015 to December 2016, 72 patients (35 males and 37 females) with a L5

DLS and meeting our inclusion/exclusion criteria were identified through the Department of Orthopaedics at our hospital and enrolled in our study. The distribution of DLS grades among this group was as follows: grade I, 28 cases; grade II, 22 cases; grade III, 15 cases; and grade IV, 7 cases. The average age of our patient group was 55.11 ± 2.567 years (range, 43–66 years). Our control group included 60 individuals (28 males and 32 females), with an average age of 55.38 ± 2.02 years (range, 40–65 years). The age and sex distribution was comparable between the patient and control group.

Measurement of the sagittal plane spinopelvic alignment parameters

Spinopelvic parameters of sagittal plane alignment were measured from full-length lateral radiographs, obtained in a relaxed standing position (Fig. 1) The following parameters were measured: thoracic kyphosis (TK), defined as the angle between the upper endplate of T4 and the lower endplate of T12; lumbar lordosis (LL), defined as the Cobb angle between the superior endplate of L1 and S1; pelvic tilt angle (PT), defined as the angle between a straight line connecting the midpoint of the femoral head, bilaterally, and the midpoint of the sacral plate and the plumb line; pelvic incidence angle (PI), defined as the angle between a line perpendicular to the sacral plate and a line joining the midpoint of the superior endplate of S1 to the centre of the hip axis; sacral slope (SS), defined as the angle formed by the upper endplate of S1 and the horizontal plane; and the sagittal vertical axis (SVA), defined by the position of a plumb line, drawn from the vertebral body of C7, relative to the upper edge of the S1 vertebral body, with positive values indicative of the line passing through the anterior margin of S1 and negative values indicative of the line passing through the posterior margin of S1. All measurements were performed using our department's Haitai Picture Archiving and Communication System (PACS). All parameters were measured by two physicians, to an accuracy of two decimals, with the average of the two measures used for analysis.

Statistical analysis

All analyses were performed using Graphpad 5.0 statistical software. All data were expressed as the mean ± standard deviation, with the between-group difference for each alignment parameter evaluated using Student's *t*-test. Correlations between two quantitative values were determined using the Pearson correlation coefficient. Additionally, One-way ANOVA could be performed to compare the value of PI, LL, SS, and TK in different DLS groups. If the value of these groups are different after the One-way ANOVA, Newman-Keuls test was used for post-hoc analysis. A *P*-value < 0.05 was considered statistically significant.

Table 1 Comparison of the spinopelvic parameters between the 72 DS and 60 non-DS group (x ± s)

	DLS group	Normal group	*P* value
n	72	60	–
age	55.11 ± 2.567	55.38 ± 2.022	0.8165
SVA(mm)	24.87 ± 0.6580	25.44 ± 0.7107	0.5598
TK(°)	43.08 ± 0.5601	38.39 ± 0.9947	<0.0001
LL(°)	46.76 ± 0.7212	42.14 ± 0.7796	<0.0001
SS(°)	39.55 ± 1.090	35.47 ± 1.077	<0.0095
PT(°)	24.88 ± 0.5968	25.62 ± 0.6490	0.4023
PI(°)	52.85 ± 1.026	46.75 ± 0.8269	<0.0001

DLS degenerative lumbar spondylolisthesis, *DS* degenerative spondylolisthesis, *LL* lumbar lordosis, *PI* pelvic incidence, *PT* pelvic tilt, *SS* sacral slope, *SVA* sagittal vertical axis, *TK* thoracic kyphosis

Results

Between-group differences in spinopelvic parameters are summarized in Table 1. Measures of PI, SS, TK, and LL were greater for the DLS than control group, with no between-group difference in PT and SVA. Then, the correlation between measured parameters and the DLS grade is reported in Table 2. PI, SS and LL correlated positively with the grade of L5 slippage as follows: SS ($r = 0.873$, $P < 0.001$); LL ($r = 0.79$, $P < 0.001$) and PI ($r = 0.7916$, $P < 0.001$). Additionally, via to One-way ANOVA analysis and Newman-Keuls as post-hoc test, the Fig. 2 displayed that the value of PI, SS and LL in grade I and II of DLS were obviously different compared to grade III or IV of DLS, with no between-group difference in TK. Finally, the correlation among spinopelvic parameters is summarised in Table 2. The degree of correlation among spinopelvic parameters differed between the DLS and control group, with SS being more strongly correlated with PI ($r = 0.94$, $P < 0.01$)

Table 2 Correlation coefficients among the spinopelvic parameters in the DLS

	DLS group (*n* = 72)		Non-DLS group (*n* = 60)	
	r value	*P* value	*r* value	*P* value
TK - % Slip	−0.03507	0.7699	–	–
LL - % Slip	0.7900	< 0.0001	–	–
SS - % Slip	0.8730	< 0.0001	–	–
PI - % Slip	0.7916	< 0.0001	–	–
LL - PI	0.6546	4.457	0.1511	0.5988
LL - SS	0.6881	< 0.0001	0.3763	< 0.01
LL - TK	0.0688	0.565	0.1435	0.2290
PI - SS	0.9367	< 0.0001	0.3313	< 0.01
PI - TK	−0.0555	0.6432	0.0692	0.5988
TK - SS	0.03055	0.7988	−0.0290	0.8085

DLS degenerative lumbar spondylolisthesis, *LL* lumbar lordosis, *PI* pelvic incidence, *SS* sacral slope, *TK* thoracic kyphosis

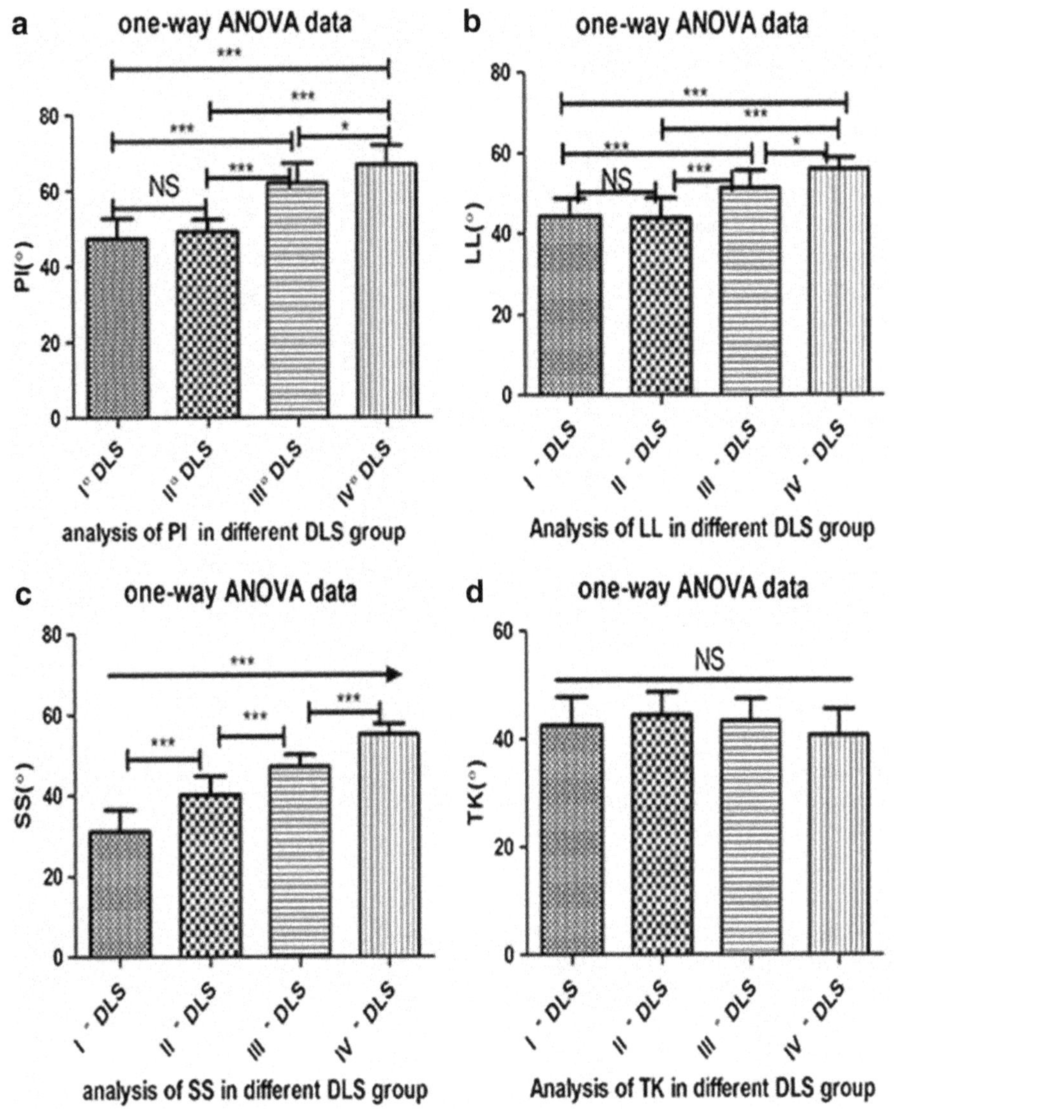

Fig. 2 **a** represented that analysis result of PI in different DLS group via to one-way ANOVA; **b** represented that analysis result of LL in different DLS group via to one-way ANOVA; **c** represented that analysis result of ss in different DLS group via to one-way ANOVA; **d** represented that analysis result of TK in different DLS group via to one-way ANOVA; Additionally, "***" represented that P <0.0001;"**" represented that P <0.01;"*" represented that P <0.05;"NS" represented that P >0.05

than LL ($r = 0.69$, $P < 0.01$) in the DLS group, compared to stronger correlation with LL ($r = 0.38$, $P < 0.01$) than PI ($r = 0.33$, $P < 0.01$) in the control group.

Discussion

Although the aetiology of DLS remains controversial, degenerative structural changes, including a decrease in intervertebral space, is commonly associated with a DLS. Specifically, these structural changes cause segmental instability which leads to a progressive slippage (or spondylolisthesis) of the affected vertebra. Progressive degenerative changes in the intervertebral disc, and associated changes in the structure and function of supporting muscles and ligaments of the spinal segment, may also play a role. More recently, changes in the line of force application on the spine, which cause changes in the sagittal plane alignment of the spine, have been implicated in the development and progression of DLS. In this regard, both anatomical measurements of alignment (PI) and postural measurements of alignment (LL, TK, PT, SS, and SVA) have been evaluated in relation to DLS [13–16]. Moreover, once a DLS develops, compensation in posture may lead to further change in spinopelvic parameters of sagittal plane balance and, consequently, progression of the DLS. Barrey et al. [9] proposed that an increase in the tilt angle of the L5 endplate, from normal reference values, was predictive of a spondylolisthesis, with an increase in PI being predictive of DLS. In agreement with these findings, Curylo et al. [17]

reported a significantly greater PI (mean, 76.4°) among 53 patients with a lumbar spondylolisthesis compared to a control group. Labelle et al. [18] also reported greater values of LL and PT among patients with a lumbar spondylolisthesis, with an increase in these parameter values being positively correlated to the grade of spondylolisthesis. These studies confirm a relationship between DLS and spinopelvic parameters of sagittal plane alignment, with an increase in PI being specifically associated with DLS.

Despite previous studies, an increase in PI, and the association between DLS and other parameters of spinopelvic alignment (LL, PT, and SS) remains controversial [9–11]. Through our research, we similarly found that PI was associated with DLS. In addition, we also showed that among patients with DLS, TK, SS, and LL had higher values compared to a control group; however there were no between-group differences in SVA and PT. We also report a positive correlation between the grade of L5 slippage and PI, SS and LL ($P < 0.01$), with these parameter values increasing as a function of the grade of slippage. However, LL and PI values did not vary significantly among patients with a grade I or II DLS (Fig. 2a, b). It is possible that the degenerative changes in grade I and II DLS are mild and, therefore, not sufficient to influence sagittal plane alignment. Due to the relatively low number of patients in each of these two categories in our study group, verification of our findings in a larger population of patients with a grade I or II DLS is warranted. We also identified a difference in the correlation among the measured spinopelvic parameters for the DLS and control group. Specifically, in the DLS group, SS correlated more strongly with PI ($r = 0.94$) than LL ($r = 0.69$), while in the control group, SS correlated more closely to LL ($r = 0.38$) than PI ($r = 0.33$). Based on our findings, which are supported by a published report [11], we propose that PI is consistently associated with a DLS, with greater values of PI being associated with a higher grade of slippage. Measured changes in SS, LL and TK are likely to evolve as a function of the primary slippage of a vertebra.

Static equations of force on the lumbar vertebrae demonstrate the association between PI and SS in the DLS group. While standing, the force exerted on L5 can be composed into two force vectors, F1 being a shear force, parallel to the end plate of the vertebra, F2 being a compression force exerted perpendicular to the end plate (Fig. 3). Considering F1 to be equal to G*cos α, where α is angle between F1 and G, then F1 will be positively correlated to SS. As such, as SS increases, the magnitude of the forward shear force (F1) will also increase. As SS also correlates positively with PI ($r = 0.94$), PI, which is an invariable morphologic parameter of lumbosacral sagittal plane alignment, can be used to predict DLS

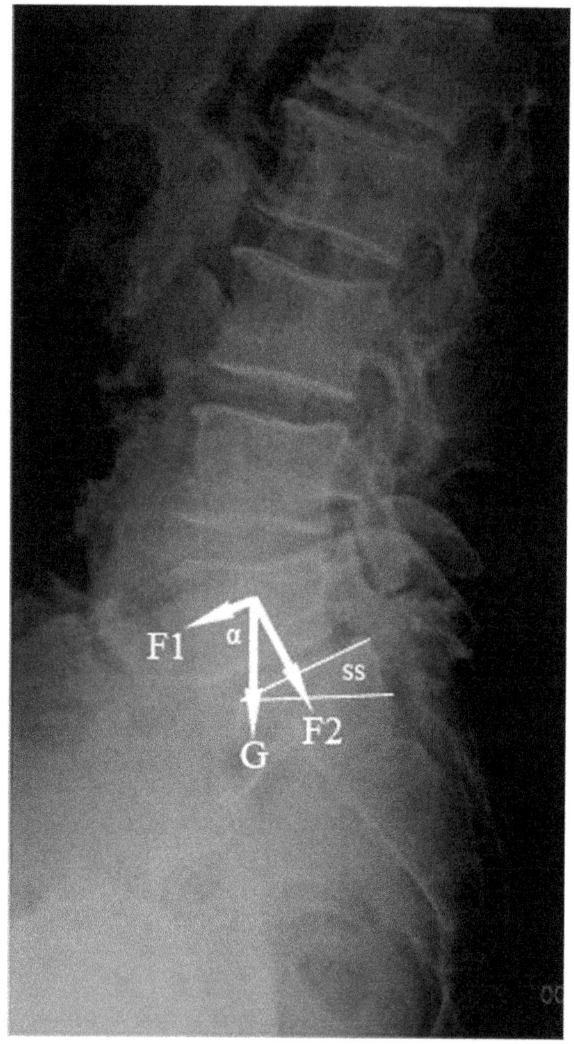

Fig. 3 Vertebral mechanics analysis. G, gravity; F1, forward shear force, parallel to the end plate; F2, compression force exerted perpendicular to the end plate

[19], where PI = SS + PT [20]. Therefore, an increase in PI is a risk factor for DLS. The anterior slippage of L5 will explicitly cause a posterior displacement of the line of gravity of the lumbosacral spine and, therefore, an increase in LL. Although the effect of LL on DLS has been debated [21], we propose that the increase in LL is a secondary consequence of an anterior slippage of L5, rather than being a causative factor of DLS.

The limitations of our study need to be acknowledged in the interpretation of our results. Foremost, this is a retrospective study, with implicit selection bias. Moreover, although we identified a positive correlation between an increase in PI and DSL, we did not evaluate if DLS was more prevalent in a group of individuals with a higher PI. Therefore, the specific cause cannot be attributed to a higher PI, which would require a longitudinal study design. As well, we only included single-segment DLS involving L5, with no comparison to L4 spondylolisthesis, which might differentially influence measured spinopelvic parameters.

Conclusions

Measurements of SS, PI, TK, and LL were specific to DLS, and were all significantly greater in the DLS group than in the control group. Moreover, measures of SS, PI, and LL positively correlated with the grade of L5 slippage in the DLS group. Among patients with a DLS, SS correlated strongly with PI, as well as with LL, albeit to a lower extent. This information should assist orthopaedic surgeons in the diagnosis and management of DLS.

Abbreviations

BMI: Body mass index; DLS: Degenerative lumbar spondylolisthesis; DS: Degenerative spondylolisthesis; LL: Lumbar lordosis; PI: Pelvic incidence; PT: Pelvic tilt; SS: Sacral slope; SVA: Sagittal vertical axis; TK: Thoracic kyphosis

Funding

This study was supported by grants from the Science and Technology Research Project of the Department of Education of Jiangxi Province (14043), [NSFC (No. 81460341)], Gan-Po Talents Project 555 of Jiangxi Province, Jiangxi Provincial Department of Science and Technology (20171BAB205059), Jiangxi Provincial Department of Education (GJJ160127), and Jiangxi Province Postgraduate Innovation Special Funds (YC2016-S107).

Authors' contributions

QL, MD, TN and BZ conceived and designed the study; QL, TG, and XL performed the experiments; ZMW and XQL analysed the data; QL and BZ wrote the paper; TG, XL, XQL, ZMW, TN MD, and BZ reviewed and edited the manuscript. TN performed major revision and minor revision. All authors read and approved the manuscript.

Competing interests

The authors declare that they have no competing interests.

References

1. Macnab I. Spondylolisthesis with an intact neural arch; the so-called pseudo-spondylolisthesis[J]. J Bone Joint Surg Br. 1950;32-B(3):325–33.
2. Newman PH, Stone KH. The etiology of spondylolisthesis [J]. Bone & Joint Journal. 1963;45-B(1):39-45.
3. Lim JK, Kim SM. Difference of sagittal spinopelvic alignmentsbetween degenerative spondylolisthesis and isthmicspondylolisthesis [J]. J Korean Neurosurg Soc. 2013;53(2):96–101.
4. Steiger F, Becker HJ, Standaert CJ, et al. Surgery in lumbar degenerative spondylolisthesis: indications, outcomes and complications. A systematic review[J]. Eur Spine J. 2014;23(5):945–73.
5. Gao T, Lai Q, Dai M, Zhang B, et al. Correlation between facet tropism and lumbar degenerative disease: a retrospective analysis. BMC Musculoskelet Disord. 2017;18(1):483.
6. Liu H, Li S, Zheng Z, et al. Pelvic retroversion is the key protective mechanism of L4–5 degenerative spondylolisthesis[J]. Eur Spine J. 2015; 24(6):1204–11.
7. Hosoe H, Ohmori K. Degenerative lumbosacral spondylolisthesis:possible factors which predispose the fifth lumbar vertebra to slip[J]. J Bone Joint Surg Br. 2008;90(3):356–9.
8. Sébastien S, Yann Philippe C, Jean-Paul S. Sagittal spinopelvic alignment and body mass index in patients with degenerative spondylolisthesis.[J]. Eur Spine J. 2011;20(5):713–9.
9. Barrey C, Jund J, Noseda O, et al. Sagittal balance of the pelvis - spine complex and lumbar degenerative diseases. A comparative study about 85 case [J]. Eur Spine J. 2007;16(9):1459–67.
10. Barrey C, Jund J, Perrin G, et al. Spinopelvic alignment of patients with degenerative spondylolisthesis[J]. Neurosurgery. 2007;61(5):981–6.
11. Funao H, Tsuji T, Hosogane N, et al. Comparative study of spinopelvic sagittal alignment between patients with and without degenerative spondylolisthesis. Eur Spine J. 2012;21:2181–7.
12. Merding HW. Spondylolisthesis; surgical fusion of lumbosacral portion of spinal column and interarticular facets; use of autogenous bone grafts for relief of disabling backache. J Int Coll Surg. 1956;26(5 Part 1):566–91.
13. Mac-Thiong JM, Berthonnaud E, Dimar JR 2nd, et al. Sagittal alignment of the spine and pelvis during growth [J]. Spine. 2004;29(15):1642–7.
14. Marty C, Boisaubert B, Descamps H, et al. The sagittalanatomy of the sacrum among young adults, infants, andspondylolisthesis patients[J]. Eur Spine J. 2002;11(2):119–25.
15. Mac-Thiong JM, Labelle H, Berthonnaud E, et al. Sagittalspinopelvic balance in normal children and adolescents[J]. Eur Spine J. 2007;16(2):227–34.
16. Vialle R, Ilharreborde B, Dauzac C, et al. Is there a sagittalimbalance of the spine in isthmic spondylolisthesis? Acorrelation study[J]. Eur Spine J. 2007; 16(10):1641–9.
17. Curylo LJ, Edwards C, DeWald RW. Radiographic markersin spondyloptosis: implications for spondylolisthesis progression[J]. Spine. 2002;27(18):2021–5.
18. Labelle H, Roussouly P, Berthonnaud E, et al. The importance of spino—pelvic balance in L5-S1 developmental spondylolisthesis:a review of pertinent radiologic measurements.[J]. Spine. 2005;30(6 Suppl):S27–34.
19. Duval-Beaupère G, Schmidt C, Cosson P. A barycentremetric study of the sagittal shape of spine and pelvis: the conditions required for an economic standing position. Ann Biomed Eng. 1992;20:451–62.
20. Roussouly P, Gollogly S, Berthonnaud E, Dimnet J. Classification of the normal variation in the sagittal alignment of the human lumbar spine and pelvis in the standing position. Spine. 2005;30:346–53.
21. Harroud A, Labelle H, Joncas J, et al. Global sagittal alignment and health-related quality of life in lumbosacral spondylolisthesis[J]. Eur Spine J. 2013; 22(4):849–56.

Characteristics of cervical sagittal parameters in healthy cervical spine adults and patients with cervical disc degeneration

Rong Xing[†], Wangmi Liu[†], Xilei Li, Libo Jiang, Mumingjiang Yishakea and Jian Dong[*]

Abstract

Background: The cervical sagittal parameters of the normal population and the impact of disc degeneration on cervical sagittal alignment have not been clearly defined yet. This study is applied to investigate the characteristics and relationships of cervical sagittal parameters in normal adults and patients with cervical disc degeneration.

Methods: We reviewed 50 normal control subjects (normal group, NG) and 50 patients with cervical disc degeneration (degeneration group, DG), who had both cervical MRI and radiographs obtained together, between January 2010 and September 2015. Data including C2–7 lordosis (CL), T1 slope (T1S), thoracic inlet angle (TIA), neck tilt (NT), C2–7 sagittal vertical axis (C2–7 SVA), cervical tilting, and cranial tilting on cervical radiographs were collected and analyzed.

Results: T1S in the NG was significantly greater than in the DG ($P < 0.05$), while NT and C2–7 SVA in the NG were significantly lower than in the DG ($P < 0.01$ and $P < 0.05$, respectively). T1S positively correlated with CL in both groups (Pearson correlation coefficients of 0.588 in the NG and 0.504 in the DG). No significant difference was seen in TIA between the NG and DG.

Conclusions: T1S was involved in the occurrence and development of cervical disc degeneration, and TIA could be considered as a constant morphological parameter in both the normal population and cervical disc degeneration patients.

Keywords: T1 slope, Cervical disc degeneration, Cervical sagittal alignment, Radiograph, Cervical sagittal parameter

Background

The sagittal alignment of the spine is an important factor involved in deformity, degenerative diseases, surgical planning, and postoperative recovery [1, 2]. Much research has focused on lumbosacral alignment, where the pelvic incidence (PI), a constant morphological parameter, plays a significant role. The influence of pelvic incidence on lumbar lordosis and thoracic kyphosis has been widely accepted [3, 4].

Recent studies have demonstrated the importance of cervical sagittal alignment, because neck pain and functional disability could be caused by loss of cervical lordosis, besides trauma, tumour, disc degeneration, soft tissue inflammation, etc. [5]. Further studies have showed that cervical sagittal alignment is not influenced solely by cervical lordosis. A close correlation exists between cervical lordosis and cervical sagittal parameters such as T1 slope (T1S), neck tilt (NT), and thoracic inlet angle (TIA) [6]. Some investigators have described TIA as the cervical spine equivalent of PI [7]. To preserve a physiological NT of around 44°, a large TIA led to both an increased T1 slope and cervical lordosis, and vice versa [8]. Therefore, accurate analysis of cervical sagittal parameters is critical to the study of cervical sagittal alignment. Previous studies have measured these parameters on cervical radiographs of asymptomatic adults. However, as MRI have not been applied to distinguish the status of their cervical discs, some asymptomatic subjects with cervical disc degeneration or herniation that cannot be shown on cervical radiographs were most

* Correspondence: dong.jian@zs-hospital.sh.cn
[†]Equal contributors
Department of Orthopaedic Surgery, Zhongshan Hospital, Fudan University, 180 Fenglin Road, Shanghai 200032, China

likely included. The prevalence of cervical disc degenerative changes in asymptomatic individuals has been reported as over 20% [9–11]. It suggests that previous studies of cervical sagittal alignment included subjects undiagnosed cervical disc degeneration or herniation, which makes the accurate data and correct relationship of cervical sagittal parameters of healthy cervical spine adults still unclear.

In the present study, all subjects underwent MRI to assess the condition of their cervical discs and select the healthy cervical spine adults. To our knowledge, this study is also the first study to compare data of cervical parameters on radiographs between the normal population and cervical disc degeneration patients. The purpose of the present study was to obtain accurate cervical sagittal parameters for both the healthy cervical spine adults and patients with cervical disc degeneration, and analyze the relationship and characteristics of the two groups.

Methods

A retrospective analysis was performed of data from 50 normal control subjects whose cervical spine are healthy (normal group, NG) and 50 patients with cervical disc degeneration (degeneration group, DG), who visited the outpatient department or physical examination center of our hospital between January 2010 and September 2015. Each individual had both a cervical MRI and cervical radiographs.

The inclusion criteria of the NG were as follows: (1) enrolled asymptomatic volunteers whose age are between 20 and 50 years; (2) no history of diagnosis or treatment related to any part of the spine, all of them underwent both MRI and cervical radiographs; (3) no evidence of degenerative cervical discs on MRI, according to the modified Matsumoto's classification [12] (Table 1); and (4) T1 vertebral body or upper end of sternum clearly visible on lateral radiograph (not obscured by the shoulder contour).

The subjects of the DG were selected by image data system in our hospital. We searched and selected subjects who had both a cervical MRI and cervical radiographs. The inclusion criteria of the DG were as follows: (1) age between 20 and 50 years; (2) no history of spinal surgery, trauma, deformities, or tumors; (3) symptomatic adults with degenerative cervical discs (≥1and ≤3) assessed via cervical MRI, according to the modified Matsumoto's classification (Table 1); and (4) T1 vertebral body or upper end of sternum clearly visible on lateral radiograph (not obscured by the shoulder contour).

The cervical intervertebral discs, including C2/3 to C7/T1, were evaluated. Each disc was assessed using MRI by two independent spine surgeons for: (1) decrease in signal intensity of intervertebral disc; (2)

Table 1 Grading system of the modified Matsumoto's classification

Decrease in signal intensity of intervertebral disc
0: As bright as or slightly less bright than healthy disc
1: Markedly darker than healthy disc
2: No signal
Posterior disc protrusion
0: No protrusion
1: Disc material protruding beyond the posterior margin of the vertebral body without cord compression
(less than one-third of dural sac)
2: Beyond vertebral body with cord compression (more than one-third of dural sac)
Disc space narrowing
0: 100–75% of height of upper healthy disc
1: 75–50% of height of upper healthy disc
2: Less than 50% of height of upper healthy disc

posterior disc protrusion; and (3) disc space narrowing, according to the modified Matsumoto's classification. Each reader evaluated twice at different time points. The final MRI result depended on their comprehensive opinions. A cervical disc was defined as normal if it is no more than grade 1 in all of the section of the modified Matsumoto's classification, and degenerative if it was more than grade 1 in any section of the modified Matsumoto's classification.

A standing lateral radiograph of the cervical spine was obtained with the subject in a neutral standing position, looking straight ahead. The parameters, including T1 slope, TIA, neck tilt, C2–C7 lordosis, sagittal vertical axis (SVA) C2–C7, cervical tilt, and cranial tilt were measured on the cervical radiograph.

Cervical parameters

C2–7 lordosis (CL): the Cobb angle between the lower endplates of C2 and C7 (Fig. 1a).

C2–7 sagittal vertical axis (C2–7 SVA): the distance from the posterosuperior corner of C7 to a vertical line from the center of the C2 vertebra (Fig. 1a).

T1 slope (T1S): the angle between the upper endplate of T1 (T1UEP) and the horizontal (Fig. 1b).

Thoracic inlet angle (TIA): an angle formed by a vertical line from the center of the T1UEP, and a line connecting the center of the T1UEP and the upper end of the sternum (Fig. 1b).

Neck tilt (NT): an angle formed by a vertical line from the sternum tip and a line connecting the center of the T1UEP and the upper end of the sternum (Fig. 1b).

Cervical tilting: an angle formed between the vertical line from the center of T1UEP and the line from the center of T1UEP to the center of C2 vertebra (Fig. 1b).

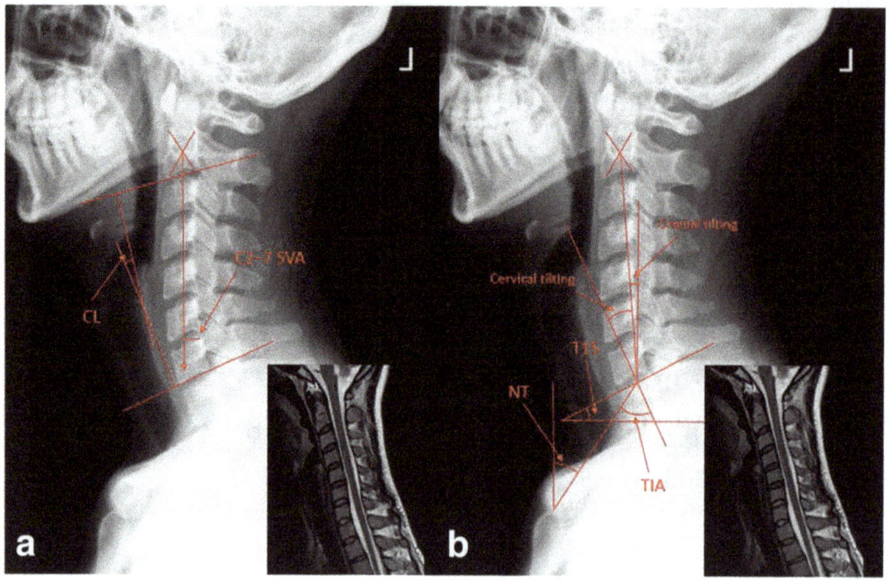

Fig. 1 Measurements of radiological parameters. **a**: C2–7 lordosis (CL), C2–7 sagittal vertical axis (C2–7 SVA). **b**: T1 slope (T1S), thoracic inlet angle (TIA), neck tilt (NT), cervical tilting, cranial tilting

Cranial tilting: an angle formed between the line from the center of the T1UEP to the dens and the SVA from the T1UEP (Fig. 1b).

T1S minus C2–7 lordosis (T1S-CL): the T1S angle minus the C2–7 lordosis.

Geometrically, TIA = T1S + NT while T1S = cervical tilting + cranial tilting.

Statistical analysis

All measurements were determined using the picture archiving and communication system in the hospital by two independent spine surgeons and their average value adopted. Quantitative data were analyzed using t test, and categorical data were analyzed using the chi-squared test. The correlations between parameters of the normal and degenerative groups were analyzed using the Pearson correlation coefficient. Statistical analyses were performed using SPSS 22.0 (SPSS Inc., Chicago, IL, USA) and $P < 0.05$ was considered significant.

Results

Comparison of the NG and DG (Additional files 1 and 2) yielded no significant differences in age, gender, C2–7 SVA, CL, TIA, cervical tilting, cranial tilting, or T1S-CL (Table 2). However, the mean T1S in the NG was 25.792 ± 5.13, significantly greater than in the DG, while the mean NT (44.6 ± 6.2) and the C2–7 SVA (12.0 ± 9.6) were significantly lower (Table 2).

There were significant relationships between C2–7 SVA and C2–7 lordosis, C2–7 SVA and T1S, C2–7 SVA and Cervical tilt,C2–7 SVA and Cranial tilt,C2–7 SVA and T1S-C2–7 lordosis, TIA and T1S, C2–7 lordosis and TIA, C2–7 lordosis and T1S, C2–7 lordosis and Cervical tilt, C2–7 lordosis and T1S-C2–7 lordosis, TIA and NT, TIA and T1S, TIA and Cervical tilt, T1S and NT, T1S and Cervical tilt, Cervical tilt and Cranial tilt, Cervical tilt and T1S-C2–7 lordosis, Cranial tilt T1S-C2–7 lordosis in both the NG and DG. (Tables 3 and 4).

T1 slope was the parameter that demonstrated significant correlations with most other parameters in both group, especially significantly correlated with TIA and C2–7 lordosis (Pearson correlation coefficients of 0.475 and 0.588 in the NG, 0.610 and 0.504 in the DG, Fig. 2).

Table 2 Data of normal group and degeneration group

	Normal group	Degeneration group	*P* value
No. of subjects (n)	50	50	
Age (years)	32.14 ± 9.19	35.02 ± 5.46	0.060
Gender (n)			
Male	25	30	0.315
Female	25	20	
C2–7 SVA (mm)	12.0 ± 9.6	16.7 ± 11.9	0.032*
CL (°)	19.2 ± 11.9	15.1 ± 12.2	0.093
TIA (°)	70.22 ± 6.8	71.5 ± 8.0	0.387
T1S (°)	25.8 ± 5.1	22.9 ± 7.0	0.020*
NT (°)	44.6 ± 6.2	48.6 ± 6.8	0.002*
Cervical tilt (°)	19.4 ± 6.9	16.7 ± 7.6	0.071
Cranial tilt (°)	5.4 ± 5.7	6.2 ± 6.5	0.824
T1S-CL (°)	6.6 ± 9.89	7.8 ± 10.5	0.569

*Indicates significant difference

Table 3 Pearson correlation of the parameters in the normal group

	C2–7 SVA	CL	TIA	T1S	NT	Cervical tilt	Cranial tilt	T1S-CL
Age	−0.345[a]	0.411[b]	0.268	0.194	0.128	0.320[a]	− 0.213	−0.397[b]
C2–7 SVA		−0.482[b]	− 0.074	0.310[a]	− 0.084	−0.638[b]	0.785[b]	0.592[b]
CL			0.303[a]	0.588[b]	− 0.166	0.600[b]	− 0.194	−0.906[b]
TIA				0.475[b]	0.681[b]	0.346[a]	0.010	−0.119
T1S					−0.320[a]	0.588[b]	0.193	−0.191
NT						−0.120	−0.145	0.035
Cervical tilt							−0.680[b]	− 0.420[b]
Cranial tilt								0.337[a]

[a]Significant correlation at the 0.05 level (2 tailed)
[b]Significant correlation at the 0.01 level (2 tailed)

Discussion

The previous studies of spinal sagittal alignment focused on the thoracolumbar or spinopelvic region. Little attention has been paid to cervical sagittal alignment until recently. Several parameters were proposed to have a critical effect on cervical sagittal alignment. Some researchers consider TIA as a constant morphologic parameter, which significantly correlates with cervical sagittal alignment. T1 slope correlates highly with the other cervical parameters and plays an important role in the cervical sagittal alignment [7, 8]. Previous studies of cervical sagittal alignment were concentrated on asymptomatic adults; however, selection by radiographs without MRI may have resulted in enrolment of some asymptomatic patients with disc degeneration. X-ray usually only demonstrated relatively severe disc degeneration, while the early stage of degenerative disc and mild disc degeneration could not be found in radiographs. As a result, the high prevalence (usually over 20%) of the cervical disc degenerative change in the asymptomatic individuals were reported in previous studies [10–12]. Therefore, the cervical sagittal parameters of normal population and the impact of disc degeneration in cervical sagittal alignment are still uncertain.

In the present study, all individuals who visited the outpatient department or physical examination center of the hospital were screened, and they had both cervical MRI and cervical radiographs obtained together in the last five years, and selected asymptomatic adults with normal imaging. To the best of our knowledge, this is the first study to investigate the cervical parameters of cervical radiographs of the normal population screened via MRI, as well as, the first comparative study of cervical parameters data on radiographs between the normal population and cervical disc degeneration patients.

In the present study, the mean TIA of the NG and DG were 70.22 ± 6.8 and 71.5 ± 8.0, respectively, similar to data in previous studies [4, 8]. There was no significant differences between the TIA in the two groups, indicating that TIA was not involved in the development of cervical disc degeneration, which could be considered a constant parameter of approximately 70°. The relationships between TIA, T1S, and NT in both groups were similar to previous studies. There were positive correlations between TIA and T1S, and TIA and NT.

Before the study, we suspected that the result of normal population might be different from previous studies of asymptomatic subjects since we excluded the disc degeneration asymptomatic subjects. However, most parameters including T1S (25.8 ± 5.1) in the NG was similar to asymptomatic subjects in previous studies, [13] even though asymptomatic subjects in previous

Table 4 Pearson correlation of the parameters in the degeneration group

	C2–7 SVA	CL	TIA	T1S	NT	Cervical tilt	Cranial tilt	T1S-CL
Age	0.053	0.210	−0.003	0.063	−0.070	0.038	0.024	−0.200
C2–7 SVA		−0.475[b]	0.021	0.320[a]	− 0.144	−0.601[b]	0.875[b]	0.654[b]
CL			0.432[b]	0.504[b]	− 0.018	0.646[b]	− 0.212	−0.817[b]
TIA				0.610[b]	0.546[b]	0.434[b]	0.151	−0.091
T1S					−0.330[a]	0.607[b]	0.369[b]	0.087
NT						−0.124	− 0.211	−0.200
Cervical tilt							−0.515[b]	− 0.340[a]
Cranial tilt								0.491[b]

[a]Significant correlation at the 0.05 level (2 tailed)
[b]Significant correlation at the 0.01 level (2 tailed)

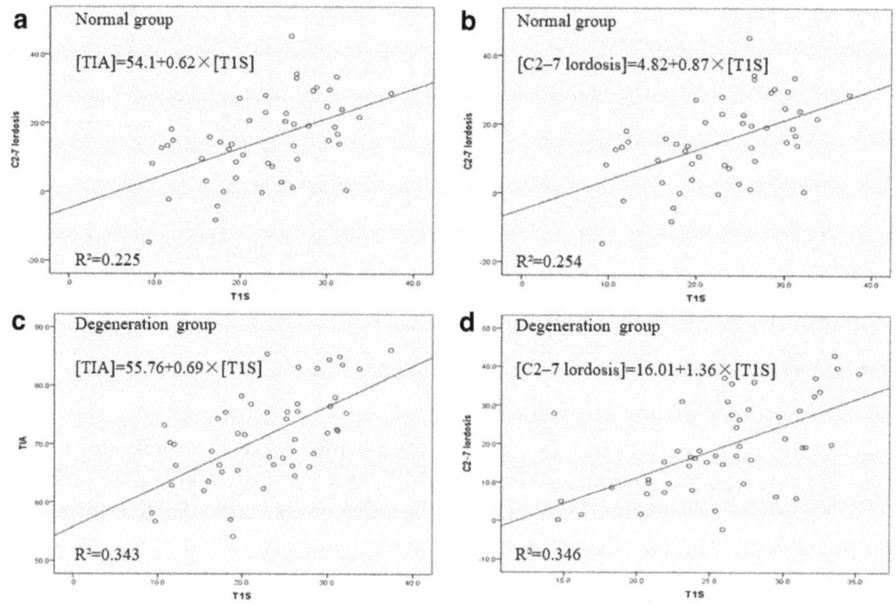

Fig. 2 Linear regression analysis model of the parameters showed statistically significant relationships. **a**: T1 slope versus Thoracic inlet angle in NG; **b**: T1 slope versus C2–7 lordosis in NG; **c**: T1 slope versus Thoracic inlet angle in DG; **d**: T1 slope versus C2–7 lordosis in DG

studies might have contained some subjects with disc degeneration. We considered that the number of degenerative cervical discs generally was small and the level of degeneration was mild while the subjects with cervical disc degeneration were asymptomatic; therefore, we infer that a small number of degenerative discs and mild disc degeneration might not cause an obvious impact on T1S.

Since subjects in DG were selected with at least one degenerative disc, usually relatively severe degeneration in our study, the degeneration level of disc in DG was obviously more serious than the asymptomatic subjects with disc degeneration in previous studies, there were significant difference between some parameters in the NG and DG. C2–7 SVA and T1S in the DG were significantly lower than in the NG (16.7 ± 11.9 vs 12.0 ± 9.6, and 22.9 ± 7.0 vs 25.8 ± 5.1, respectively) and NT in the DG was significantly greater than in the NG (48.6 ± 6.8 vs 44.6 ± 6.2). We speculated a possible pathological process of cervical disc degeneration according to our findings. As the T1S positively correlated to CL (Pearson correlation coefficients of 0.588 in the NG and 0.504 in the DG), lower T1S decreased the CL to obtain a sagittally balanced cervical spine, and led to a relatively straight cervical spine. This mechanism might increase the stress due to gravity and accelerate cervical disc degeneration, which could explain why T1S in the DG was lower than in the NG (22.9 ± 7.0 vs25.8 ± 5.1). However, as the effect of T1S on cervical disc degeneration, degenerative discs might also have an impact on T1S and other cervical parameters which could be gradually changed due to the development of disc degeneration. Although we could define that lower T1S was a risk of the occurrence or development of cervical disc degeneration according to our finding that significantly different T1S in the normal population and cervical disc degeneration patients, we could not determine the causal relationship between T1S and cervical disc degeneration without a longitudinal study, they might interact with each other. However, this study could provide a new finding that some cervical parameters including T1S were significantly different in normal population and degeneration patients, and also a new research direction of the relationship between cervical alignment and cervical disc degeneration that we need more researches especially longitudinal studies to determine.

Cervical sagittal balance was important and had regulatory mechanism. We speculated a possible compensatory principle according to our result: high T1 slope in either group increased the CL, which correlated with a lower SVA C2–7 (Pearson correlation coefficients of − 0.482 in the NG and − 0.475 in the DG). We considered that T1S-CL was a better parameter than T1S to demonstrate the compensatory mechanism of the cervical spine, analogous to PI-LL in the lumbopelvic spine [14, 15]. In our study, T1S-CL significantly correlated with C2–7 SVA (Pearson correlation coefficients of 0.592 in the NG and 0.654 in the DG). A large T1S-CL increased the C2–7 SVA and an excessively large C2–7 SVA that caused cervical spine decompensation would contribute to imbalance in the cervical spine. In addition, as some researchers found that T1S-CL significantly correlated with postoperative neck disability index scores in posterior cervical fusion surgery, [16, 17] future studies could estimate the value of T1S-CL in predicting and preventing cervical axial symptoms.

However, there are several limitations in this study. Firstly, the relatively small sample size prevented division of the DG into subgroups according to the amount and level of disc degeneration. Secondly, there was a relatively narrow age distribution; further studies should enroll normal volunteers with a wider distribution. Finally, this is a cross-sectional comparative study that lacked longitudinal data to demonstrate an association between T1S and the occurrence and development of cervical disc degeneration.

Conclusion

The findings indicate that lower T1S might be a risk of the occurrence and development of cervical disc degeneration and provide a new thought about the relationship between T1S and cervical disc degeneration. Our findings also demonstrate that TIA could be considered as a constant morphological parameter in the normal population and in cervical disc degeneration patients.

Acknowledgments

We are grateful to Dr. Guofeng Zhou (Department of Radiology, Zhongshan Hospital, Fudan University) for his kindly assistance in MRI evaluation.

Funding

This work was sponsored by Natural Science Foundation of China (81372002, 31170925), Natural Science Foundation of Shanghai (16ZR1405500).

Authors' contributions

RX and JD were in charge and contributed to all stages of the present study. LJ and MY was responsible for the original data collection. WL contributed to interpreting the data and writing the final manuscript. XL contributed to reviewing the accuracy of the data. All authors read and approved the final manuscript.

Consent for publication

Not applicable.

Competing interest

We declare that we do not have any competing interest.

References

1. Vialle R, Levassor N, Rillardon L, Templier A, Skalli W, Guigui P. Radiographic analysis of the sagittal alignment and balance of the spine in asymptomatic subjects. J Bone Joint Surg. 2005;87:260–7.
2. Schuller S, Charles YP, Steib JP. Sagittal spinopelvic alignment and body mass index in patients with degenerative spondylolisthesis. Eur Spine J. 2011;20:713–9.
3. Boulay C, Tardieu C, Hecquet J, Benaim C, Mouilleseaux B, Marty C, et al. Sagittal alignment of spine and pelvis regulated by pelvic incidence: standard values and prediction of lordosis. Eur Spine J. 2006;15:415–22.
4. Jang JS, Lee SH, Min JH, Kim SK, Han KM, Maeng DH. Surgical treatment of failed back surgery syndrome due to sagittal imbalance. Spine. 2007;32:3081–7.
5. Tang JA, Scheer JK, Smith JS, Deviren V, Bess S, Hart RA, et al. The impact of standing regional cervical sagittal alignment on outcomes in posterior cervical fusion surgery. Neurosurgery. 2012;71:662–9.
6. Knott PT, Mardjetko SM, Techy F. The use of the T1 sagittal angle in predicting overall sagittal balance of the spine. Spine J. 2010;10:994–8.
7. Lee SH, Son ES, Seo EM, Suk KS, Kim KT. Factors determining cervical spine sagittal balance in asymptomatic adults: correlation with spinopelvic balance and thoracic inlet alignment. Spine J. 2015;15:705–12.
8. Lee SH, Kim KT, Seo EM, Suk KS, Kwack YH, Son ES. The influence of thoracic inlet alignment on the craniocervical sagittal balance in asymptomatic adults. J Spinal Disord Tech. 2012;25:E41–7.
9. Teresi LM, Lufkin RB, Reicher MA, Moffit BJ, Vinuela FV, Wilson GM, et al. Asymptomatic degenerative disk disease and spondylosis of the cervical spine: MR imaging. Radiology. 1987;164:83–8.
10. Lao LF, Zhong GB, Li QY, Liu ZD. Kinetic magnetic resonance imaging analysis of spinal degeneration: a systematic review. Orthop Surg. 2014;6:294–9.
11. Matsumoto M, Fujimura Y, Suzuki N, Nishi Y, Nakamura M, Yabe Y, et al. MRI of cervical intervertebral discs in asymptomatic subjects. J Bone Joint Surg Br. 1998;80:19–24.
12. Matsumoto M, Okada E, Toyama Y, Fujiwara H, Momoshima S, Takahata T. Tandem age-related lumbar and cervical intervertebral disc changes in asymptomatic subjects. Eur Spine J. 2013;22:708–13.
13. Janusz P, Tyrakowski M, Glowka P, Offoha R, Siemionow K. Influence of cervical spine position on the radiographic parameters of the thoracic inlet alignment. Eur Spine J. 2015;24:2880–4.
14. Kim YJ, Bridwell KH, Lenke LG, Cheh G, Baldus C. Results of lumbar pedicle subtraction osteotomies for fixed sagittal imbalance: a minimum 5-year follow-up study. Spine. 2007;32:2189–97.
15. Lafage V, Ames C, Schwab F, Klineberg E, Akbarnia B, Smith J, et al. Changes in thoracic kyphosis negatively impact sagittal alignment after lumbar pedicle subtraction osteotomy: a comprehensive radiographic analysis. Spine. 2012;37:E180–7.
16. Iyer S, Nemani VM, Nguyen J, Elysee J, Burapachaisri A, Ames CP, et al. Impact of cervical sagittal alignment parameters on neck disability. Spine. 2016;41:371–7.
17. Hyun SJ, Kim KJ, Jahng TA, Kim HJ. Relationship between T1 slope and cervical alignment following multilevel posterior cervical fusion surgery: impact of T1 slope minus cervical lordosis. Spine. 2016;41:E396–402.

Fatigue and disturbances of sleep in patients with osteogenesis imperfecta

Heidi Arponen[1*], Janna Waltimo-Sirén[1,2], Helena Valta[3] and Outi Mäkitie[3,4,5]

Abstract

Background: Persisting fatigue has been reported to be a common complaint by individuals with connective tissue disorders, including Osteogenesis imperfecta (OI). This controlled study evaluated in an adult OI population the subjective experience of fatigue, affecting daily life. Sleep disturbances and chronic pain were examined as hypothesized underlying factors.

Methods: This cross-sectional study analyzed the answers of 56 OI patients and 56 matched healthy controls to a questionnaire, designed to evaluate levels of experienced fatigue and bodily pain, as well as the presence or absence of symptoms related to sleep disturbances or sleep apnea. The relationships between fatigue, pain, and sleep disturbances were evaluated with correlation analysis and regression analysis.

Results: Fatigue was reported by 96%, and daily pain by 87% of the individuals with OI. Notably, the level of fatigue was similarly experienced by patient respondents and controls. In total, 95% of the patients and 77% of the controls reported one to several sleep disturbance symptoms. These symptoms as well as previously diagnosed sleep apnea were statistically significantly more prevalent in the patient group than in the controls ($p < 0.05$). Likewise, the experienced bodily pain was statistically highly significantly more severe among the respondents with OI ($p < 0.001$), and correlated with the reported fatigue.

Conclusions: In comparison with age-matched controls, adults with OI do not differ in experienced fatigue, unlike hypothesized. Therefore, sleep disturbances, which based on the frequency of reported related symptoms and previous sleep apnea diagnoses appear to be common in OI patients, may remain undiagnosed.

Keywords: Osteogenesis imperfecta, Fatigue, Sleep disturbances, Quality of life

Background

Osteogenesis imperfecta (OI) is a group of genetic disorders of collagen synthesis, characterized by osteoporosis and increased fracture tendency. OI affects approximately one in 10,000 people [1]. The clinical phenotype of OI ranges from mild to severe, the mild type being the most common. The original Sillence classification designated the mild type as type I, the perinatally lethal as type II, the severe, progressively deforming one as type III, and the moderate one as type IV OI. [2, 3]. Despite the subsequent addition of histologically, radiologically, and genetically distinct OI types, autosomal dominant mutations in COL1A1 and COL1A2 still account for approximately 90% of OI cases, and the patients can be classified according to phenotypic severity into the originally defined four types [4, 5]. Particularly in the moderate and severe forms of OI, recurrent long-bone fractures and vertebral compression fractures commonly result in skeletal deformities and scoliosis, leading to short stature and physical disability. Potential extra-skeletal manifestations of OI include cardiovascular complications, pulmonary dysfunction, neurologic problems, hearing loss, dental and occlusal problems, pain, and fatigue. These co-morbidities, or a fear of them, affect in several ways the patients' quality of life and functional ability [6–9].

* Correspondence: heidi.arponen@helsinki.fi
[1]Department of Oral and Maxillofacial Diseases, University of Helsinki, P.O. Box 41, FI-00014 Helsinki, Finland

The Constitution of World Health Organization (WHO) defines quality of life (QoL) as " individuals' perception of their position in life in the context of the culture and value systems in which they live and in relation to their goals, expectations, standards and concerns". QoL is a broad, multidimensional concept that includes subjective evaluations of both positive and negative aspects of life. OI affects not only the QoL of the patient, but also that of a caregiver. [8, 10, 11]. Previous research indicates that QoL of individuals with OI is negatively influenced by reduced function due to tiredness and fatigue [8, 9]. Yet, the prevalence and experience of fatigue in patients with OI remains largely unexplored.

The aim of this cross-sectional study was to examine in an adult OI population the subjective experience of fatigue, affecting the patients' everyday life, and to evaluate in particular the level of pain and prevalence of self-reported sleep disturbances, in order to assess their role in excessive daytime sleepiness and fatigue. The hypothesis is that patients with OI in comparison to healthy controls report higher levels of both fatigue and pain, and that pain, poor quality of sleep, and fatigue form a vicious circle, impairing the QoL in OI.

Methods

The study was approved by the Research Ethics Committee, Helsinki University Hospital. We constructed a custom questionnaire to assess the subjective perception of fatigue, bodily pain, and sleep disturbance symptoms. The questionnaire was posted to the unselected 151 individuals, registered as patient members of the Finnish Osteogenesis Imperfecta Association. Inclusion criteria were diagnosis of OI, and age of 16 years or above. Data were unavailable of those Association members who did not return the study questionnaire.

The survey was presented in the following sequence: (1) Collection of general demographic and anthropometric information, and subjective assessments on experienced daily pain and fatigue (Table 1); (2) collection of specific information on symptoms related to fatigue and sleep disturbances (Table 2); and (3) qualitative analysis of subjective reports on sleep related problems. Demographic data included age and gender. Height and weight were enquired as anthropometric information, and were used to calculate the body mass index (BMI). Medical information addressed OI type according to Sillence classification, primary means of mobility, medical diagnosis of sleep apnea confirmed by a polysomnography, and sleep disturbance symptoms. Pain and fatigue were evaluated with a visual analogue scale (VAS) from 0 to 10, where 0 is no pain/fatigue and 10 is the worst possible pain/fatigue a person can imagine. To establish the level of general physical impairment and functional performance, ambulation was assessed as walking without aid, walking with crutches, or wheelchair as a primary mode of mobility. The other variables, presented in Table 2, were dichotomous (yes/no). This study used additional qualitative analysis in order to gain insight into any factor affecting sleep. Qualitative data were collected with one open-ended question:" Do you have other sleep-related problems?". The same questionnaire, excluding anthropometric information to increase unidentifiability of the participants, was completed by 56 age- and gender-matched volunteer controls without OI.

Descriptive data are given as means, ranges, frequencies, and percentages. Height Z-score, reflecting the general severity of the disorder [12], was calculated and used in the statistical analysis. Pearson and Spearman correlation coefficients were computed, according to the distribution of the data, to assess the relationship between the variables in SPSS (IBM Corp. Released 2015. IBM SPSS Statistics for Windows, Version 23.0. Armonk, NY: IBM Corp.) The relationship between sleep disturbance symptoms and fatigue was evaluated by means of logistic regression analysis. Explanatory variables were: diagnosed sleep apnea, snoring, pauses of breathing during sleep, restless sleep, grinding of teeth during sleep, recurrent nightmares, daytime sleepiness, likelihood of dozing, dysphagia, difficulties of concentration, nocturia, and restless legs. Two-sample t-test and chi-square test were used to compare the responses of the patients and controls.

Results

The study group comprised 56 individuals with OI completing the survey (37% of those who received the questionnaire), and 56 healthy controls. Of the respondents, 39 had a classified OI, and of them 22 had type I (mild), 7 had type IV (moderate), and 10 had type III OI (severe) (Table 1). Altogether 17 reported OI type to be unknown. Of the respondents, 41 were females and 15 males. Their age distribution showed that middle-aged and older individuals were active participants. In total, 20% of the respondents were in the age range of 16–29 years old, 32% were in the age range of 30–49 years, and 48% were aged 50 years or more. Mean age was somewhat lower in those with severe OI (34 years) compared to those with mild OI type (48 years). The majority of the respondents walked unaided (55%). Those with a more severe OI type utilized more often mobility aids. Wheelchair was the primary means of mobility for 19 patients (34%).

Table 1 outlines the notable variation in the reported current bodily pain and fatigue, with an average score of 5 for fatigue and 4 for pain for the patient group, corresponding to a moderate intensity of fatigue and pain. Fatigue and bodily pain were positively correlated [$r(55) = 0.29$, $p = 0.034$]. No correlation between bodily

Table 1 Characteristics of the Osteogenesis imperfecta (OI) patient cohort, sub-grouped by OI type, and of the healthy controls

	All	Mild type	Moderate type	Severe type	Unknown type	Controls
Number of participants	56	22	7	10	17	56
Age range in years (mean)	16–75 (47)	19–75 (48)	26–55 (43)	18–52 (33)	16–71 (54)	16–75 (44)
Females/males	41/15	19/3	7/0	5/5	10/7	41/15
Height range in meters (mean)	0.80–1.75 (1.45)	1.47–1.75 (1.6)	0.80–1.65 (1.3)	0.80–1.33 (1.1)	1.10–1.75 (1.5)	NA
Body mass index, mean	29	27	28	36	29	NA
Ambulation (no aid/crutches/wheelchair)	31/5/19	19/2/1	3/0/3	0/0/8	9/3/8	56/0/0
Bodily pain range (mean)	0–10 (4)	0–9 (4)	0–10 (4)	0–5 (2.3)	0–9 (4)	0–9(2)[a]
Fatigue range (mean)	0–10 (5)	2–10 (6)	2–8 (5.8)	1–7 (2.9)	0–8 (5)	0–8 (4)
Diagnosed sleep apnea	8	2	1	2	3	1

NA data not requested
[a]the difference, as compared to patient group mean, is statistically highly significant as $p < 0.001$

pain and severity of OI was found, whereas fatigue and severity of OI were negatively correlated [$r_s(38) = -0.34$, $p = 0.037$], indicating more reports of severe fatigue among those with a mild OI type. In the youngest patient age-group, the average score was 2 for pain and 4 for fatigue. In the age-group of 30–49 year-olds, the average score was 4 for pain and 5 for fatigue. In the oldest age group, the average scores for pain and fatigue were 5.

Of the 54 participants with OI, who responded to the dichotomous question about the presence or absence of sleep apnea, eight (15%) had diagnosed sleep apnea and used a positive airway pressure ventilator during sleep. Yet of the remaining 46 without diagnosis of sleep apnea, as many as 44 (96%) reported one or more sleep disturbance related symptoms, daytime sleepiness (in 81%) being the most common one (Table 2). BMI and height Z-score showed a negative correlation [$r(56) = -0.38$, $p = 0.004$], implying that the more severe the OI is, the higher the BMI. No correlation was found between height Z-score and presence of sleep apnea. In contrast, BMI correlated positively with sleep apnea [$r_s(54) = 0.28$, $p = 0.043$]. The average scores for fatigue and pain were similar in the eight patients with sleep apnea diagnosis and those without a diagnosis (5 for fatigue and 4 for pain).

Logistic regression analysis showed that in patients with OI, a risk of higher levels of fatigue correlated with daytime sleepiness (OR 3.8; 95%CI: 1.77–6.01; $p = 0.001$) but the risk was not associated with the other sleep disturbance symptoms. Those OI respondents with pauses of breathing during sleep had significantly more frequently diagnosed sleep apnea [$r_s(42) = 0.46$, $p = 0.002$], habit of snoring [$r_s(42) = 0.51$, p = 0.001], and high likelihood of dozing [$r_s(41) = 0.47$, p = 0.002], as can be anticipated. In contrast, pauses of breathing and daytime sleepiness did not show a correlation [$r_s(40) = 0.25$, $p = 0.117$].

Table 2 Prevalence of self-reported symptoms related to sleep-disturbances and sleep apnea among the respondents in the Osteogenesis imperfecta patient cohort and controls

	Number of patients with symptoms (%) *N* = 56	Number of controls with symptoms (%) *N* = 56	Significance of difference between the study groups (Chi-Square test)
Snoring	32/52 (62)	15/54 (28)	11.1 $p = 0.001$
Pauses of breathing during sleep	13/42 (31)	3/54 (6)	9.9 $p = 0.002$
Restless sleep	43/55 (78)	23/54 (43)	12.9 $p < 0.001$
Grinding of teeth during sleep	22/52 (42)	23/55 (42)	Non-significant
Recurrent nightmares	16/50 (32)	2/55 (4)	13.3 $p < 0.001$
Daytime sleepiness	43/53 (81)	34/56 (61)	5.6 $p = 0.018$
Likelihood of dozing	14/52 (27)	5/56 (9)	6.3 $p = 0.012$
Dysphagia	17/51 (33)	1/55(2)	20.0 $p < 0.001$
Difficulties of concentration	24/50 (48)	6/54 (11)	16.6 $p < 0.001$
Nocturia	15/51 (29)	5/54 (9)	5.8 $p = 0.016$
Restless legs	19/51 (37)	8/54 (15)	10.0 $p = 0.002$
Diagnosed sleep apnea	8/54 (15)	1/55 (2)	5.4 $p = 0.020$

OI patients were afflicted by statistically significantly more severe bodily pain than the controls ($t_{102} = 4.6$, $p < 0.001$), whereas the level of experienced fatigue did not differ significantly between the patient and control groups. Among the controls, the average scores for fatigue were similar in all age groups; 3.4 for those aged 29 years or below, 3.8 for those between 30 and 49 years, and 3.7 for those aged 50 years or above. Of the controls, 73% reported symptoms related to sleep disturbances. Statistically significantly more common in the OI patient group than in the controls were snoring, pauses of breathing during sleep, restless sleep, recurrent nightmares, daytime sleepiness, likelihood of dozing, dysphagia, difficulties of concentration, nocturia, and restless legs, whereas grinding of teeth during sleep was equally prevalent (Table 2).

In addition, answers to the open-ended question revealed that eleven respondents with OI suffered from frequent awakenings and four from difficulties in falling asleep. Other reported sleep disturbances among the OI patients were insomnia, nocturnal sweating, pain-induced awakening, numbness of limbs and cranium, depression, anxiety, and awakening by a feeling of falling or choking. One healthy control detailed nocturnal sweating, and another foot spasms as sleep-related disruptive events.

Discussion

This study found self-reported fatigue of various severity in 96% of individuals with OI. Fatigue was similarly experienced by respondents of all ages. Altogether 76% of the patients also reported symptoms that suggest the presence of a sleep disturbance such as sleep apnea. Daily pain was reported by 87% in the patient cohort. The older patients reported more severe pain than the younger ones. A subjective feeling of fatigue was interestingly an equally current complaint in the control group. Among the control respondents experiencing fatigue, 86% also reported at least one symptom related to sleep disturbances.

Fatigue is considered a more long-term condition than somnolence [13]. It can have multiple physical and mental causes. Fatigue appears to be a common finding in patients with connective tissue disorders when compared to the general population [14]. In patients with Marfan and Ehlers-Danlos syndromes higher levels of fatigue have been shown to be associated with chronic pain [14, 15]. Similarly, in our patient cohort, the severities of fatigue and pain were expectedly positively correlated. To our knowledge, the underlying causes of fatigue, apart from physical fitness, had not previously been studied in OI population.

Presumably low muscle function and level of physical activity contribute to fatigue. Restrictions of physical activity due to recurrent fractures, skeletal deformities and pulmonary dysfunction may lead to decreased functional ability, and furthermore aggravate fatigue in individuals with OI. In patients with mild OI (type I), no pulmonary or cardiac symptoms at rest are normally present. Previous studies, however, show that muscle size, exercise tolerance and muscle strength are significantly reduced in patients with OI [16–20]. On the other hand, training has been shown to improve aerobic capacity and muscle force, and to reduce the level of subjective fatigue in children with mild and moderate OI types [21]. In the light of previous studies, our finding of lower average fatigue score in the individuals with severe OI type, in contrast to those with mild type, was unexpected. It is still unclear how the fatigue and severity of OI relate to each other. One possible explanation for our seemingly contradictory finding could be that those individuals with mild OI type might have higher social participation level than those with severe type. The following hypothetical assumption would be that for instance occupational participation alongside general population demands considerable effort, leading to exhaustion. In addition, importantly, respondents with mild OI were on average 14 years older than those with severe type, which might contribute to their fatigue level - although the reported fatigue among the control group did not correlate with respondents' age, emphasizing the subjective aspect of fatigability. In patients with OI, we found the severity of fatigue not correlating with the presence of sleep disturbance symptoms other than daytime sleepiness.

Chronic pain is intertwined with insomnia, psychological distress, difficulties in falling asleep, and frequent arousal [22, 23]. Our results agree with these findings. Insomnia, defined as a difficulty of falling asleep or staying asleep, was reported by 25% of the patient respondents in our cohort in the answers to the open-ended question. All of them were also suffering from a generalized pain. Interestingly however, the two patients who declared having anxiety and depression reported low scores for fatigue and pain. The answers obtained from the open-ended question are consistent with the trend of the quantitative data results, indicating a considerable variability and subjectivity of the experience of pain and fatigue.

Individuals with varying severity of OI face several QoL challenges across their lifespan. OI is conjoint with high prevalence of co-morbidities in musculoskeletal, auditory, pulmonary, and endocrine systems, as well as dental problems and physical appearance alterations, all of which are factors that can affect individuals' QoL [9]. Earlier studies have revealed that adults with OI experience lower physical QoL but similar or higher levels of mental QoL than the general population [24].

The severity of OI has been found to correlate with worsening of QoL. Experiencing pain, isolation, activity limitations and participation limitations have been shown to negatively affect QoL in OI. High scholastic competence has been found in children and adults with OI. The risk of fractures is an important concern faced by both adults and children [11, 24]. This study found several of the previously mentioned QoL risk factors, such as experienced pain and activity limitations in the OI population.

Sleep apnea is a sleep disorder characterized by pauses in breathing or instances of shallow or infrequent breathing during sleep. Sleep apnea is classified as central, obstructive, or mixed. The diagnosis of sleep apnea is based on the conjoint evaluation of clinical symptoms and of the results of a polysomnography as apneic events per hour of sleep [25]. Many of the symptoms of sleep apnea are non-specific and can have other possible causes. Sleep apnea affects roughly 3% of middle-aged men and 2% of women in Finland [26]. In comparison, a self-reported 14% prevalence of sleep apnea in an adult OI population in US has been reported [9]. Similarly, in our cohort, 15% of the respondents had a diagnosed sleep apnea, confirmed by a polysomnography. General factors predisposing to sleep apnea are obesity, snoring, male gender, advanced age, structural abnormalities in the nose and pharynx, nasal obstruction, small or receding lower jaw, functional factors such as small lung capacity, and unstable ventilatory control during sleep [27, 28]. In our OI cohort, BMI exceeded the WHO diagnostic threshold for obesity (30 kg/m^2) in 33%. The use of BMI-measure can be misleading in individuals with scoliosis and lower extremity deformities that lead to loss of height, since the index is a height-related measure. Location of fat deposition, especially anterolateral to the upper airway, is more important than BMI in regard to risk for obstructive sleep apnea (OSA) [29]. Findings on the association between BMI and excessive daytime sleepiness are inconsistent in the literature when the effect of OSA is not considered [30, 31]. Daytime sleepiness has been associated with depression, nocturia, and metabolic factors more strongly than with sleep-disordered breathing or sleep disruption per se. Individuals with sleep apnea are not always pathologically sleepy [30, 32].

Snoring was reported by 62% of the OI respondents. Snoring is a poor predictor of sleep apnea due to its commonness in the general population. Of men 35–45% and of women 15–28% report habitual snoring. The absence of snoring, however, makes apnea unlikely; only 6% of apnea patients do not snore [29]. Insomnia and restless legs syndrome are each clinically significant in 5–10% of adults in general population, and an average incidence of 23% of respiratory-related leg movements has been documented in a sleep apnea cohort [33–35]. According to this study, insomnia and restless legs are more frequent in OI population than among unaffected peers.

This study presented with several strengths and limitations. We used a mixed-method subjective self-evaluation approach, using a non-validated detailed questionnaire for not to miss any data that might help us to understand the subjective experience of fatigue. The visual analogue scale (VAS) is a simple and frequently used method for assessment of intensity of pain [36]. Similarly, VAS has been shown to be a valid and reliable instrument for the quantitative assessment of fatigue in both healthy subjects and in patients who complain of poor-quality sleep [37]. The possible use of psychoactive drugs affecting sleep was not documented. Without knowledge of the pharmaceutical history of the patients, the association of possible bisphosphonate treatment and experienced bodily pain could not be evaluated. The younger patients and those with severe OI are more likely to have been treated with bisphosphonates that have been shown to be effective in reducing bone pain and fatigue [38, 39]. The study population was limited due to the rarity of OI. Although the disease equally affects both genders, females were more active than males in participating. Possible response bias cannot be evaluated, as the investigators did not have access to the entire target population's characteristics and medical history. It is likely that those with more symptoms were more likely to participate. However, more than one third of the target population responded and the frequency of symptoms was very high, indicating that the studied symptoms involve a significant proportion of the entire OI population.

Conclusions

From the outcome of our investigation it is possible to conclude that sleep disturbances are relatively common symptoms in adults with OI, and more prevalent in adults with OI than in the general population. Subjective feeling of fatigue was equally experienced among the healthy controls and in patients with OI. There are several possible explanations for this result. Persistent fatigue that affects day-to-day life was experienced by respondents of all ages. The data gathered show that 76% of those OI patients suffering from fatigue also reported symptoms that suggest the presence of a sleep disturbance such as sleep apnea. However, only 15% of the respondents with OI had a sleep apnea diagnosis. Therefore, further studies of the true prevalence, causes, and characteristics of sleep disturbances in OI population would be of interest.

Abbreviations

OI: Osteogenesis imperfecta; OSA: Obstructive sleep apnea; QoL: Quality of life

Acknowledgements
The authors thank Finnish Osteogenesis imperfecta Association for the collaboration.

Funding
This study was financially supported by Academy of Finland, Sigrid Jusélius Foundation, Novo Nordisk Foundation, and Folkhälsan Research Foundation. None of the funding bodies had any role in the design of the study and collection, analysis, and interpretation of data and in writing the manuscript.

Authors' contributions
Study design: HA, HV, JWS, and OM. Acquisition of data: HA. Data analysis: HA and JWS. Interpretation of data: HA, HV, JWS, and OM. Drafting manuscript: HA. Revising manuscript content: HV, JWS, and OM. All authors read and approved the final manuscript.

Consent for publication
Not applicable

Competing interests
The authors declare that they have no competing interests.

Author details
[1]Department of Oral and Maxillofacial Diseases, University of Helsinki, P.O. Box 41, FI-00014 Helsinki, Finland. [2]Department of Oral and Maxillofacial Diseases, Helsinki University Hospital, Helsinki, Finland. [3]Children's Hospital, University of Helsinki and Helsinki University Hospital, Helsinki, Finland. [4]Folkhälsan Research Center, Helsinki, Finland. [5]Center for Molecular Medicine, Karolinska Institutet, and Department of Clinical Genetics, Karolinska University Hospital, Stockholm, Sweden.

References

1. Rauch F, Glorieux FH. Osteogenesis imperfecta. Lancet. 2004;363(9418):1377–85.
2. Sillence DO, Rimoin DL, Danks DM. Clinical variability in osteogenesis imperfecta-variable expressivity or genetic heterogeneity. Birth Defects. 1979;15:113–29.
3. Sillence DO, Senn A, Danks DM. Genetic heterogeneity in osteogenesis imperfecta. J Med Genet. 1979;16:101–16.
4. Thomas IH, DiMeglio LA. Advances in the classification and treatment of osteogenesis imperfecta. Curr Osteopor Rep. 2016;14(1):1–9.
5. Van Dijk FS, Byers PH, Dalgleish R, Malfait F, Maugeri A, Rohrbach M, et al. EMQN best practice guidelines for the laboratory diagnosis of osteogenesis imperfecta. Eur J Hum Genet. 2012;20:11–9.
6. Basel D, Steiner RD. Osteogenesis imperfecta: recent findings shed new light on this once well-understood condition. Genet Med. 2009;11(6):375–85.
7. Wekre LL, Kjensli A, Aasand K, Falch JA, Eriksen EF. Spinal deformities and lung function in adults with osteogenesis imperfecta. Clin Respir J. 2014;8:437–43.
8. Hill CL, Baird WO, Walters SJ. Quality of life in children and adolescents with osteogenesis imperfecta: a qualitative interview based study. Health Qual Life Out. 2014;12:54.
9. Tosi LL, Oetgen ME, Floor MK, Huber MB, Kennelly AM, McCarter RJ, et al. Initial report of the osteogenesis imperfecta adult natural history initiative. Orphanet J Rare Dis. 2015;10:146.
10. Vanz AP, Félix TM, Rocha NS, Schwartz IVD. Quality of life in caregivers of children and adolescents with osteogenesis imperfecta. Health Qual Life Out. 2015;13:41.
11. Tsimicalis A, Denis-Larocque G, Michalovic A, Lepage C, Williams K, Yao TR, et al. The psychosocial experience of individuals living with osteogenesis imperfecta: a mixed-methods systematic review. Qual Life Res. 2016;25(8):1877–96.
12. Borodulin K, Levälahti E, Saarikoski L, Lund L, Juolevi A, Grönholm M, et al. National Finriski health study. National Institute for Health and Welfare. Report. 2013;022:2.
13. Shen J, Barbera J, Shapiro CM. Distinguishing sleepiness and fatigue: focus on definition and measurement. Sleep Med Rev. 2006;10(1):63–76.
14. Scheper MC, Juul-Kristensen B, Rombaut L, Rameckers EA, Verbunt J, Engelbert RH. Disability in adolescents and adults diagnosed with hypermobility related disorders: a meta-analysis. Arch Phys Med Rehab. 2016;97:2174–87.
15. Bathen T, Velvin G, Rand-Hendriksen S, Robinson HS. Fatigue in adults with Marfan syndrome, occurrence and associations to pain and other factors. Am J Med Genet. 2014;164A:1931–9.
16. Takken T, Terlingen HC, Helders PJ, Pruijs H, Van der Ent CK, Engelbert RH. Cardiopulmonary fitness and muscle strength in patients with osteogenesis imperfecta type I. J Pediatr. 2004;145(6):813–8.
17. Gentry BA, Ferreira JA, McCambridge AJ, Brown M, Phillips CL. Skeletal muscle weakness in osteogeneis imperfecta mice. Matrix Biol. 2010;29:638–44.
18. Veilleux L-N, Lemay M, Pouliot-Laforte A, Cheung MS, Glorieux FH, Rauch F. Muscle anatomy and dynamic muscle function in osteogenesis imperfecta type I. J Clin Endocrinol Metab. 2014;99(2):E356–62.
19. Pouliot-Laforte A, Veilleux L-N, Rauch F, Lemay M. Physical activity in youth with osteogenesis imperfecta type I. J Musculoskel Neuron Interact. 2015;15(2):171–6.
20. Palomo T, Glorieux FH, Schoenau E, Rauch F. Body composition in children and adolescents with osteogenesis imperfect. J Pediatr. 2016;169:232–7.
21. Van Brussel M, Takken T, Uiterwaal CS, Pruijs HJ, Van der Net J, Helders PJ, Engelbert RH. Physical training in children with osteogenesis imperfecta. J Pediatr. 2008;152:111–6.
22. Taylor DJ, Mallory LJ, Lichstein KL, Durrence HH, Riedel BW, Bush AJ. Comorbidity of chronic insomnia with medical problems. Sleep. 2007;30(2):213–8.
23. Morphy H, Dunn KM, Lewis M, Boardman HF, Croft PR. Epidemiology of insomnia: a longitudinal study in a UK population. Sleep. 2007;30(3):274–80.
24. Dahan-Oliel N, Oliel S, Tsimicalis A, Montpetit K, Rauch F, Dogba MJ. Quality of life in osteogenesis imperfecta: a mixed-methods systematic review. Am J Med Genet. 2016;170A:62–76.
25. McNicholas WT. Diagnosis of obstructive sleep apnea in adults. Proc Am Thorac Soc. 2008;5:154–60.
26. Laitinen LA, Anttalainen U, Pietinalho A, Hämäläinen P, Koskela K. Expert advisory group listed in foreword. Sleep apnoea: Finnish national guidelines for prevention and treatment 2002-2012. Respir Med. 2003;97(4):337–65.
27. Solow B, Siersbaek-Nielsen S, Greve E. Airway adequacy, head posture, and craniofacial morphology. Am J Orthod. 1984;86:214–23.
28. Al Lawati NM, Patel SR, Ayas NT. Epidemiology, risk factors, and consequences of obstructive sleep apnea and short sleep duration. Prog Cardiovasc Dis. 2009; 51:285–93.
29. Schlosshan D, Elliott MW. Review: clinical presentation and diagnosis of the obstructive sleep apnoea hypopnoea syndrome. Thorax. 2004;59:347–52.
30. Bixler EO, Vgontzas AN, Lin HM, Calhoun SL, Vela-Bueno A, Kales A. Excessive daytime sleepiness in a general population sample: the role of sleep apnea, age, obesity, diabetes, and depression. J Clin Endocrinol Metab. 2005;90(8):4510–5.
31. Vgontzas AN, Bixler EO, Chrousos GP. Obesity-related sleepiness and fatigue: the role of the stress system and cytokines. Ann N.Y. Acad Sci. 2006;1083:329–44.
32. Adams RJ, Appleton SL, Vakulin A, Lang C, Martin SA, Taylor AW, et al. Association of daytime sleepiness with obstructive sleep apnoea and comorbidities varies by sleepiness definition in a population cohort of men. Respirology. 2016;21(7):1314–21.
33. Riemann D, Spiegelhalder K, Espe C, Pollmächer T, Léger D, Bassetti C, et al. Chronic insomnia: clinical and research challenges–an agenda. Pharmacopsychiatry. 2011;44:1–14.

34. Innes KE, Selfe TK, Agarwal P. Prevalence of restless legs syndrome in north American and western European populations: a systematic review. Sleep Med. 2011;12:623–34.
35. Aritake S, Blackwell T, Peters KW, Rueschman M, Mobley D, Morrical MG, et al. Osteoporotic fractures in men (MrOS) study research group. Prevalence and associations of respiratory-related leg movements: the MrOS sleep study. Sleep Med. 2015;16(10):1236–44.
36. Ferreira-Valente MA, Pais-Ribeiro JL, Jensen MP. Validity of four pain intensity rating scales. Pain. 2011;152(10):2399–404.
37. Lee KA, Hicks G, Nino-Murcia G. Validity and reliability of a scale to assess fatigue. Psychiatry Res. 1991;36:291–8.
38. Bishop N, Adami S, Ahmed SF, Antón J, Arundel P, Burren CP, et al. Risedronate in children with osteogenesis imperfecta: a randomised, double-blind, placebo-controlled trial. Lancet. 2013;382:1424–32.
39. Salehpour S, Tavakkoli S. Cyclic pamidronate therapy in children with osteogenesis imperfecta. J Pediatr Endocrinol Metab. 2010;23:73–80.

9

Musculoskeletal disorders among preschool teachers: analyzing the relationships among relational demands, work meaning, and intention to leave the job

Daniela Converso[1], Sara Viotti[1*], Ilaria Sottimano[1], Vincenza Cascio[2] and Gloria Guidetti[1]

Abstract

Background: Based on the conservation of resource (COR) theory by Hobfoll, the aim of the present study was to test whether the relationships among relational demands, work meaning, and intention to leave vary as a function of the presence of musculoskeletal disorders (MSDs).

Method: The study was cross-sectional and non-randomized. Analyses were carried out on a dataset consisting of 429 preschool teachers, who filled out a self-report questionnaire. Of them, 238 reported a MSD diagnosis and 191 were free form MSDs.

Results: As expected, among those who reported MSDs, relational demands were significantly associated to intention to leave, and this relationship was mediated by work meaning; moreover, among those free from MSDs, no significant paths among the three variables were found.

Conclusion: In general, results showed that suffering from MSDs impairs workers' ability to face to relational demands, thus activating a spiral that encompasses diminished work meaning and intention to leave. Practical implications of results will be discussed in the paper.

Keywords: Musculoskeletal disorders, Relational demands, Preschool teachers, Conservation of resources theory

Background

Preschool services are essential in the modern societies since they have a strategic role, in concert with families, in sustaining children's whole development (e.g., emotional, social, physical, and cognitive). In this context preschool teachers, who are professionals, mostly women, properly trained to fulfill these aims, carry out a job primarily of a relational nature, consisting of nurturing and teaching children under the age of six years, as well as constantly interacting with their parents [1, 2].

However, an under-considered aspect of preschool teaching profession is that the job requires the mobilization not only of emotional, but also of physical resources. Teachers are constantly required to lift, bend, or carry children as well as sit on small furniture or on the floor to take care of, play with, and interact with children [3]. Wortman [4] described teachers' tasks as requiring constant interaction with active (sometimes hyperactive), spontaneous, impulsive, heavy (sometimes very heavy) children. Previous studies have clearly demonstrated how these kinds of physical demands negatively impact on preschool teacher musculoskeletal system [5–8]. According to the literature review carried out by Erick and Smith [9], the incidence rate of musculoskeletal disorders (MSDs) among such workers is quite high, varying from 39 to 95%. MSDs involve various body regions, particularly the back, neck, and shoulders.

MSDs may involve a wide range of inflammatory and degenerative conditions affecting the muscles, ligaments, tendons, nerves, bones, and joints. MSDs negatively impact individual well-being, having consequences on all facets of their existence, including work life [10]. Studies

* Correspondence: sara.viotti@unito.it; sara.viotti@gmail.com
[1]Department of Psychology, University of Turin, Via Giuseppe Verdi 8, 10124 Turin, Italy

carried out in many occupational contexts but rarely among preschool teachers, have focused on the practical repercussions of MSDs, highlighting the loss for individuals and organizations in terms of absenteeism [11], presenteeism [12], work inability [13], and compensation claims [14]. Previous studies have also ascertained the role of MSDs in the exacerbation of perceived physical demands [15–17]. However, a clear gap of the current literature is the little attention paid to understand whether suffering from MSDs may affect the perception of other types of demands, e.g., relational demands. Different from the physical component of the job, which definitely represent a risk factor among preschool teachers, the relational nature can be seen as a double-edged sword. On one hand, the relational nature of the job may be perceived as demanding: Kelly and Berthelsen [18] showed in a qualitative study that preschool teachers felt stressed due to their high expectations about meeting the needs of the children and their parents. On the other hand, this aspect of the job may be perceived as meaningful and stimulating: Li Grining et al. [19] found that emotional demands did not necessarily negatively affect preschool teachers' ability to implement particular management strategies. In this view, the identification of the conditions in which, among preschool teachers, this "core demand" represents a risk factor is of importance because this knowledge may help to develop preventive measures aimed at supporting workers' health and well-being and hence maintaining a high standard of service quality.

A further gap in the literature is that whereas it was largely demonstrated that job demands may be associated with negative consequences both for workers and organizations [20], few studies have tried to understand, either among preschool teachers or among other working populations, whether and how poor health conditions, such as in the presence of MSDs, may affect this mechanism. Moreover, the literature to date has mostly focused on the buffering factors of job demands on workers' well-being, identifying the moderating role of some job and personal resources [20], but mostly neglecting to look for the "exacerbators" of job demands. The present study may contribute to advance the literature as it is aimed to identify the psychological processes that suffering from MSDs may set in motion in workers, examining whether and how it may lead to a change in workers' attitudes toward their job.

In particular, using the conservation of resources theory (COR) [21] as a theoretical framework, we propose that suffering from MSDs represents a condition in which relational demands may turn into a risk factor, being associated with negative attitudes toward work, i.e., perceiving their work as less meaningful and the desire to leave their job. Equally, we propose that, among preschool teachers free from MSDs, relational demands do not represent a risk factor, not showing associations with both meaning of work and intention to leave.

Work meaning refers to the degree to which the work is perceived as meaningful, important, and constructive [22]. In COR terms, work meaning may be defined as a positive motivational-affective state of fulfillment that may enhance the energetic process and thus favor the gaining of further resources. On the other hand, COR theory suggests that intention to leave represents a withdrawal strategy that individuals may plan to put into action to interrupt the loss spiral experienced [23].

COR [21] is a motivational theory based on the idea that individuals strive to obtain, retain, foster, and protect resources. Primary resources are those related to basic and survival aspects. Examples are health, shelter, and basic social needs [21]. People may instinctively seek such primary resources. Secondary resources are culturally defined and may aid people in gaining or protecting their primary resources (e.g., social status, money, and professional identity). A basic tenet of this theory is the concept of the loss spiral, which refers to the process of the depletion of resources that makes people unable to cope with future loss, thus potentially leading to further resource loss. Conversely, a strong armamentarium of resources tends to generate other resources, thus creating resource caravans, which may result in positive outcomes such as greater well-being and less job-related strain symptoms [24].

In personal as well as in professional life, a key aspect that considerably affects these processes is an individual's intrinsic energetic state. According to Hobfoll and Shirom [25], the energetic state helps the body to stay in line with the activities people are undertaking to effectively respond to demands they face. At work, an excellent health status can be considered a resource functioning to keep the energetic process activated. On the other hand, the emergence of MSDs may be accompanied by an alteration of the energetic state, impairing workers' ability to adapt to their work environment. According to the COR theory [21], individuals have a limited amount/pool of personal resources (including physical/emotional/cognitive) and dealing with MSDs could drain them, leaving worker fewer resources to cope with relational demands. For instance, in the case of preschool teachers, MSDs may seriously impair their interaction with children. This may occur because the mobilization of additional effort to compensate for workers' limited ability due to MSDs may contribute to the acumination of pain and fatigue.

Moreover, COR theory [21] states that a condition of depleted resources may be associated with secondary costs. For example, overwhelming relational demands may lead workers to raise doubts about the usefulness and meaningfulness of the job carried out and, in turn, to foster their desire to leave the job. This mechanism may be favored by the perception of a mismatch from what teachers believe users expect and what they can actually offer [26].

From an empirical point of view, studies have provided evidence for the significance of the relationships among job demands, work meaning, and intention to leave [27, 28]. Moreover, previous literature suggests the plausibility of the mediating role of work meaning between relational demands and intention to leave [29, 30]. However, no study argued that these relationships may vary as a function of the health status of the musculoskeletal system.

Therefore, based on the COR theory (Hobfoll, 1989, 21), the present paper proposes that the health status of the musculoskeletal system represents a crucial variable among preschool teachers that differentiates those who experience a loss spiral from those who do not. In particular, we identified two subgroups, based on the presence of the MSDs, i.e., "MSDs free" and "diagnosed MSDs," and building on what was explained above, we expect that the significance of the relationship among variables under study vary as a function of the presence of the MSDs. In particular, we expected that in the group free from MSDs, relational demands, work meaning and the intention to leave will not be significantly associated each other; on the other hand, in the group reporting MSDs, we expected that work meaning will mediate the relationship between relational demands and intention to leave.

Method

Data collection

Data were collected by a survey conducted in 2013 and involved all the preschool teachers employed in the Educational Municipal Public Services of Turin (Italy). A self-report pencil-and-paper questionnaire was administered individually to the teachers. The data collection took place during work hours in sessions expressly organized in each school, in which a researcher from the Department of Psychology of the University of Turin was available to assist teachers in the questionnaire completion. The voluntary nature of participation and the anonymity of the data processing were ensured.

In accordance with the legal requirements of the study country (Italy), no additional ethical approval was required because no patients were involved. Moreover, no treatment, including medical, invasive diagnostics, or procedures causing psychological or social discomfort, was administered to the participants. The research also conforms to the requirements of the 1995 Declaration of Helsinki (as revised in Edinburgh in 2000).

Eight-hundred and 84 questionnaires were distributed, 776 were returned to the research group, and 677 were correctly filled out. Male teachers were excluded because of their small number ($n = 7$).

Measures

The self-reported questionnaire included two sections. The first was dedicated to collecting socio-demographic data (age and gender).The second section included scales aimed at measuring relational demands, work meaning, and the intention to leave as well as MSDs measures. As explained below, all the scales employed in the present study were already used or validated in previous study.

Relational demands (RDs) were measured with five items referring to relationships with children and families (e.g., "the demands of our recipients are exorbitant", m = 2.82, sd = .67) from the Customer-Related Social Stressors (CSS) inventory developed by Dormann and Zapf [31] and adapted for the preschool context in a previous study [32]. Responses were given on a four-point scale ranging from 1 ("strongly disagree") to 4 ("strongly agree").

Work meaning was measured with the scale from the Copenhagen Psychosocial Questionnaire by Kristensen et al. [22][1]. It consisted of three items (e.g., "Is your work meaningful?," m = 3.58, sd = .42) and responses to all sub-scales were given on a four-point scale ranging from 1 ("strongly disagree") to 4 ("strongly agree").

Intention to leave the job was measured by three item by Cammann et al. [33] aimed at assessing the employee desire to quit the job (e.g., "I often think about quitting", m = 1.71, sd = .61). Responses were given on five-point Likert type scales ranging from 1 "strongly disagree" to 4 "strongly agree."

MSD symptoms were assessed using a section from the Nordic Musculoskeletal Questionnaire [34] which included nine forced-choice items (yes/no) identifying areas of the body causing musculoskeletal problems focusing on the following sites of the body: the neck, shoulders, upper back, elbows, low back, wrist/hands, hips/thighs, knees, and ankles/feet. Respondents were asked if they had musculoskeletal pain in any of these sites in the previous 12 months, lasting at least four days in a week (including the current week).

The section regarding MSDs also included questions aimed at collecting the following information: having received a medical diagnosis to which any of the symptoms suffered were attributed (yes/no); having consulted with a specialist (e.g., a physician, a physical therapist) in the last 12 months because of musculoskeletal pain (yes/no); having used drugs because of musculoskeletal symptoms (yes/no) in the past 12 months.

Statistical analyses

Analyses were performed using SPSS 21 and MPLUS 8.

For the purpose of the present study, respondents were included in the study dataset only if eligible to be incorporated in one of the following two categories: "MSDs free" and "MSDs diagnosed." A respondent was classified as "MSDs free" if she had never experienced musculoskeletal pain in the last 12 months (including the week in which the questionnaire was administered) and no medical diagnosis (e.g., back pain, hernias, arthrosis) was reported.

On the other hand, a respondent was included in the group "diagnosed MSDs" if both the following conditions were satisfied: (a) having experienced in the last 12 months, musculoskeletal pain in at least one site (neck, shoulders, upper back, elbows, low back, wrist/hands, hips/thighs, knees, and ankles/feet), for at least four days in a week; (b) having reported a medical diagnosis (e.g., back pain, hernias, arthrosis) to which any of the symptoms suffered were attributed.

Those who did not fall into any of these two categories were excluded from the present study. The choice to exclude from the subgroup "diagnosed MSDs" people not reporting a diagnosis, despite reporting musculoskeletal pains (measured with the Nordic questionnaire, [34]), was made in order to minimize the risk related to have used a self-report method in collecting MSDs [35], which may consist in overestimating or underestimating impairments and diseases.

As the percentage rate of missing values on each study variable was very low (less than 10%), missing values were handled by a listwise deletion procedure (i.e., an entire record is excluded from analysis if any single value is missing).

To ascertain the adequacy of the psychometric properties and the reliability of the research instruments, Cronbach's alpha and confirmatory factor analyses (CFAs) were performed. Cronbach's alpha was used to determine the internal consistency of each scale. On the other hand, to determine that the best structure for the data was the one hypothesized (i.e., no other latent structures underlie the data) and that measures used did not overlap each other, three models were compared with a series of CFA. The first model consisted of a one-factor model in which all items loaded on one factor. The second was a two-factor model in which the items of relational demands loaded on one factor and the rest of the items on the other factor. Finally, in the three-factor model (hypothesized factor structure), items from relational demands and work meaning and the intention to leave loaded on their corresponding factors. Because no serious violations of the normal distribution were found (all the skewness and kurtosis values of the variables considered were within ±1), maximum likelihood (ML) was employed as an estimation method. The fit of the model was assessed with the ratio of χ^2 to the degrees of freedom (df), the comparative fit index (CFI), the Tucker-Lewis index (TLI), the standardized root mean square residual (SRMR), and the root mean square error of approximation (RMSEA). According to Kline [36], a χ^2/df ratio of 3 or less indicates a good model fit and less than 2 indicates an excellent model fit. For TLI and CFI indices, values higher than .90 are considered indicators for good model fit [37, 38]. A value of the SRMR equal to or less than .09 indicates good fit [39]. Finally, a RMSEA value lower than .08 indicates acceptable model fit [40].

To test whether the strength of the relationships among the variables under study (i.e., relational demands, work meaning, and the intention to leave) vary as a function of MSDs, multi-group structural equation modeling (SEM) was conducted using ML. Age was included in the model as a control variable and regressed on the three major study variables [41]. The fit of the model was assessed with the ratio of $\chi 2$/df, the CFI, the TLI, the SRMR, and the RMSEA.

The mediating effects of work meaning on the relationships between relational demands and the intention to leave was assessed through both the Baron and Kenny's method [42] and the bootstrapping procedure [43]. According to Baron and Kenny [42], the significance ($p \leq .05$) of the following relationships suggest the presence of a mediation: (a) between the independent variable (X, i.e., relational demands) and the dependent variable (Y, i.e., intention to leave), (b) between the independent variable (X, i.e., relational demands) and the mediator (M, i.e., work meaning), and (c) between the mediator and the dependent variable (M and X, i.e., work meaning and intention to leave).

However, because several recent statistical simulation studies showed that the ability to detect mediated effects using the Baron and Kenny [42] method can be very low [44], the bootstrapping procedure was employed in order to calculate the indirect effect of relational demands on intention to leave through work meaning. In particular, the bootstrapping procedure extracted, from the original sample, 1000 bootstrap samples of the same size as the original one and estimate the indirect effect (IE) and its confidence interval (CI). A significant *p* value associated to the indirect effect and CI (95%) not including zero were both considered proves for significant mediation.

Results

Descriptive statistics

According to the criteria identified above, 191 preschool teachers were assigned to the category "MSDs free" and 238 to the category "diagnosed MSDs." On the other hand, 241 were excluded by the present study.

Whereas in the MSDs-free group ($n = 191$), the average age was 47.24 (sd = 8.87; min = 29, max = 67), in the group with MSDs, the average age was 52.10 (sd = 6.35; min = 31, max = 62). ANOVA revealed significant differences among two groups on age ($F = 40.91$, $p = .001$).

In the group with MSDs, 84% reported pain in the upper back, 75.6% reported pain in the neck, 70.6% in the low back, 56.3% in the shoulders, 49.6% in the hips/

thighs, 49.6% in the knees, 38.7% in the wrist/hands, 16. 8% in the ankles/feet, and 16% in the elbows. In this group, 6.3% reported pain at only one site, 10.9% at two sites, 14.3% at three sites, 22.3% at four sites, 19.3% at five sites, 12.6% at six sites, and 14.5% at seven sites or more. Finally, 32.8% reported the regular use of drugs because of MSDs, 76.5% had consulted with a specialist (e.g., a physician, a physical therapist) in the last 12 months because of musculoskeletal pain, and 100% had received a medical diagnosis to which they attributed some or all the symptoms suffered.

The measurement model: Multi-group CFA

Table 1 shows the goodness-of-fit indices of the three alternative measurement models estimated trough multi-group CFA on the two subgroups involved in the present study. The hypothesized model (M3) was the only one that showed an acceptable fit to the data. Moreover, $\Delta\chi^2$ tests confirmed that this three-factor model fits the data significantly better, if compared with the alternative models with two and one factors, respectively. All items in the three-factor model loaded significantly on their corresponding latent factors in the two sub-samples. In the subgroup reporting MSDs, all correlations between factors were significant ($\phi_{\text{relational demands-work meaning}} = -.18$, $p = .02$; $\phi_{\text{relational demands-intention to leave}} = .39$, $p = .001$; $\phi_{\text{work meaning -intention to leave}} = -.26$, $p = .001$). In the subgroup free from MSDs, factors did not significantly correlate with each other ($\phi_{\text{relational demands-work meaning}} = .11$, $p = .22$; $\phi_{\text{relational demands-intention to leave}} = .05$, $p = .59$; $\phi_{\text{work meaning -intention to leave}} = -.08$, $p = .41$).

Cronbach's alpha was found to be satisfactory since values of the scales in each group were always above .70.

Multi-group SEM

The multi-group SEM performed across the two subgroups (MSDs Free $N_{\text{listwise}} = 182$, MSDs diagnosed $N_{\text{listwise}} = 221$) showed an acceptable fit: $\chi^2 = 229.49$, df = 114, CFI = .92, TLI = .91, SRMR = .07, RMSEA = .07 [.06–.08].

As showed in Fig. 1, in the subgroup MSDs free, nor the path from relational demands to work meaning ($\beta = .10$ $p = .20$) or the path from work meaning to intention to leave ($\beta = -.09$, $p = .33$) or the path from relational demands to intention to leave ($\beta = .06$, $p = .53$) showed significant values. In addition, age was found not to significantly affect any of the major study variables ($\gamma_{\text{age-relational demands}} = .07$ $p = .39$; $\gamma_{\text{age-work meaning}} = .14$ $p = .08$; $\gamma_{\text{age-intention to leave}} = .07$ $p = .41$).

In the subgroup with MSDs, the path from relational demands to work meaning ($\beta = -.21$, $p = .01$), the path from work meaning to intention to leave ($\beta = -.23$, $p = .003$) and the path from relational demands to intention to leave ($\beta = .35$, $p = .0001$) were all significant. In this subgroup age significantly predicted relational demands ($\beta = .17$, $p = .02$), intention to leave ($\beta = .19$, p = .02), and not work meaning ($\gamma = .04$, $p = .54$).

Moreover, in the subgroup reporting MSDs, the bootstrap test indicated the presence of a significant indirect effect of relational demands on intention to leave via work meaning in the subgroup (Standardized IE = .05, $p = .04$; CI(95%) = .01–.08).

Discussion

Based on the COR theory [21], the aim of the present study was to test whether MSDs exacerbate the role of relational demands in lessening work meaning and, in turn, in determining intention to leave in a sample of preschool teachers. To accomplish this, from a dataset including 670 female preschool teachers employed in the educational system of the Municipality of Turin (Italy), two subgroups were selected based on the presence of the MSDs (i.e., MSDs free = 191 and diagnosed MSDs =238) and the patterns of relationships among the variables under study were examined and compared across these groups.

Overall, findings obtained confirms our expectations. In the subgroup not reporting MSDs, relational demands, work meaning, and intention to leave were found not to be significantly associated. On the other hand, in the subgroup reporting MSDs, work meaning mediated the relationship between relational demands and intention to leave.

Generally speaking, the results confirmed what was postulated based on the COR theory [21], i.e., health may be considered a crucial resource capable of deeply affecting workers' relationship with their job. In particular, the findings suggest that physical well-being helps workers to keep available psychological resources to accomplish relational-type job demands. Therefore, our findings are consistent with the WHO perspective that conceptualizes health as a capital in which it is important to invest to achieve positive future outcomes [45].

Table 1 Multi-sample (MSDs free vs. diagnosed MSDs) confirmatory factor analyses (CFAs) – Test of alternative models – Goodness-of-fit indexes

Model	χ^2(df)	χ^2/df	CFI	TLI	SRMR	RMSEA	Model comparisons	$\Delta\chi^2$(p)
M1 (1 factor)	892.73 (108)	8.26	.50	.49	.13	.18 [.17–.19]	–	–
M2 (2 factors)	538.37 (104)	5.17	.72	.70	.13	.12 [.14–.15]	M2-M1	534.36 (.0001)
M3 (3 factors)	140.10 (98)	2.02	.94	.93	.06	.07 [.05–.08]	M3-M2	398.27 (.0001)

Note: *df* degree of freedom, *CFI* comparative fit index, *TLI* tucker-lewis index, *SRMR* standardized root mean square residual, *RMSEA* root mean square error of approximation

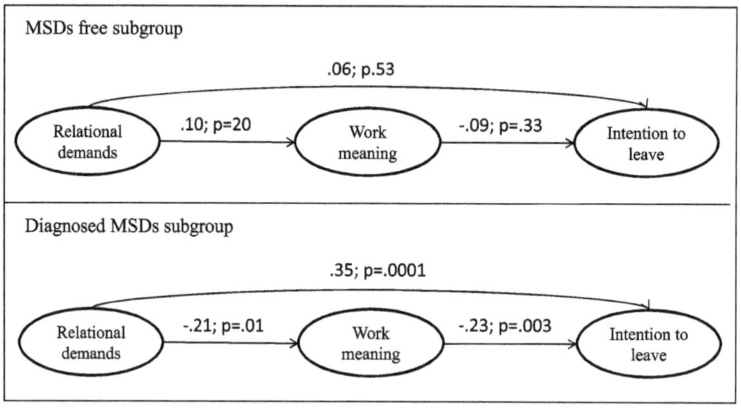

Fig. 1 Multi-sample structural equation models across (MSDs free vs. diagnosed MSDs)

Moreover, the present study has brought to light that the role of relational demands in affecting worker attitudes may change as a function of health conditions. In particular, for the group reporting MSDs, relational demands were found to operate as an initiator of a loss spiral, leading to diminished work meaning, and in turn, to intention to leave. On the other hand, in the subgroup free from MSDs, the loss spiral was not observed, since no significant relationships were found among the variables under study.

Therefore, our findings contain novelty, highlighting that relational demands do not inevitably represent a risk factor. Moreover, they also identified an exacerbating condition (i.e., diagnosed MSDs), never highlighted before, for relational demands. Future studies may be also directed at verifying whether the results found in the present sample, consisted of female preschool teachers, could be applied also to men. Further, to provide evidence for the generalizability of our findings, future studies should investigate whether the same mechanism is also effective in other working populations that have in common with preschool teachers the exposure to relational demands as well as to the risk to develop MSDs (e.g., nurses).

The present study has some limitations. The most relevant is its cross-sectional design. Future researchers should employ a longitudinal design to explore the cross-lagged associations between the constructs examined across various health conditions. Indeed, as suggested by the COR theory [21, 25], the relationship between all these constructs, more than unidirectional, may be cyclic. Longitudinal studies may also be useful to understand whether and how the relationship between these constructs changes over time.

Another limitation is that all of the measures employed were self-reported. Data coming from a single source may introduce the issue of common method variance [46]. Future studies may benefit from the employment of research designs that include a combination of objective and subjective measures or use data from multiple sources (e.g., the inclusion of a medical assessment for the measurement of MSDs would increase the reliability of its measure).

Finally, the representativeness of the results may be a limiting factor. The present study was conducted among a specific professional group, i.e., preschool teachers. Therefore, caution should be exercised when generalizing the results to other working populations employed as well as to other kinds of teachers.

Conclusions

The relevance of the present paper was to demonstrate that suffering from MSDs impairs workers' ability to invest psychological resources at work, thus activating a spiral that may encompass loss not only for such individuals, but also for the recipients of their services and their employer organizations.

From a practical point of view, the present findings suggest that organizations may take advantage of developing actions aimed at protecting and, most of all, promoting physical health. Investing in preventive measures focused on promoting physical health may be ever more important in light of the consideration that one of the most important emerging work-related issues is the aging workforce [47]. In our study, it was found that the incidence of MSDs tends to increase with age ($M_{MSDs\ free} = 47$, $M_{MSDs\ diagnosed} = 52.10$, $F = 40.91$ $p = .0001$). In this view, investing in workers' physical health may represent a measure that contributes to maximizing the likelihood that workers *play as a full resource* (being healthier and more committed in their work) for a longer time during their work life span.

Finally, regarding the preschool context in particular, the present study highlighted that it is necessary to urgently intervene: a relevant segment of the sample reported MSDs and continued working despite the fact that this condition led to the development of the desire to leave their job. In this context, organizations need to develop a set of composite measures aimed to both minimize the risk to develop MSDs among those who have not yet reported them and to contain further secondary losses among who have yet to develop MSDs. First, it might be a crucial health promotion action to re-design kindergarten school facilities to convert them into an ergonomically appropriate environment to minimize the occurrence of movements that place strain on the preschool teachers' bodies and that have potential to cause injuries to the musculoskeletal system. Second, continuing education programs should be implemented, especially if focused on learning techniques that are useful to perform daily work activities without negatively impacting the musculoskeletal system (e.g., how to correctly lift or to prevent injuries due to the assumption of awkward postures). Posture exercise classes aimed at lessening and preventing musculoskeletal pain and diseases may also be beneficial. Health promotion programs may also include informative actions aimed at enabling workers to increase control over their health and at encouraging them to adopt a healthier lifestyle (e.g., diet modification, the introduction of physical activities). Finally, but no less important, it seems necessary to identify specific interventions for those who report MSDs that should be tailored to the specific needs/characteristics of the workers. This may include rehabilitation treatment and, in the case in which MSDs is serious or not reversible, it should be combined with programs that accompany workers to job replacement (e.g., for younger) or early retirement (e.g., for older that have not yet reached the retirement age).

However, considering the relevance of MSDs issue among preschool teachers, in addition to the engagement of the single organization in investing in preventive/protective measures, the development of specific guidelines and recommendations from the international health and safety public agencies may be necessary to help employer organizations and country governments to correctly identify measures to address the problem of MSDs among preschool teachers.

Abbreviations

ANOVA: analysis of variance; CFA: confirmatory factor analysis; CFI: comparative fit index; COR: conservation of resource; df: degrees of freedom; ML: maximum likelihood; MSDs: musculoskeletal disorders; RMSEA: root mean square error of approximation; SEM: structural equation modeling; SRMR: standardized root mean square residual; TLI: Tucker-Lewis index

Funding

The funder for this study is the Municipality of Turin (Italy) through the Department of Psychology of the University of Turin (Italy) within a program aimed at assessing the quality of working life among pre-school teachers. Particularly, this funding body supported the following phase of the research: study design, data collection, and data analysis.

Authors' contributions

Study conception and design: DC, SV, GG, IS, VC. Acquisition of data: DC, SV, GG, IS, VC. Contributions to the analysis and interpretation of data: SV, DC, GG, IS, VC. Drafting the article and revising it critically for important intellectual content: DC, SV (DC and SV equally contributed), GG, IS, VC. Approval of the final version to be submitted for publication: DC, SV, GG, IS, VC.

Competing interests

The authors declared no potential conflicts of interests with respect to the authorship and/or publication of this article.

Author details

[1]Department of Psychology, University of Turin, Via Giuseppe Verdi 8, 10124 Turin, Italy. [2]ASL TO1, Turin, Italy.

References

1. Hall-Kenyon KM, Bullough RV, MacKay KL, Marshall EE. Preschool teacher well-being: a review of the literature. Early Child Educ J. 2014;42(3):153–62.
2. Bloechliger, OR, Bauer GF. Demands and job resources in the child care workforce: Swiss lead teacher and assistant teacher assessments. Early Educ Dev. 2017 (a-head-of-print, DOI: https://doi.org/10.1080/10409289.2016.1154419).
3. Gratz RR, Claffey A, King P, Scheuer G. The physical demands and ergonomics of working with young children. Early Child Dev Care. 2002; 172(6):531–7.
4. Wortman AM. Preventing work-related musculoskeletal injuries. Child Care Information Exchange. 2001; July:50–3.
5. Grant K, Habes D, Tepper A. Work activities and musculoskeletal complaints among preschool workers. Appl Ergon. 1995;26(6):405–511.
6. Gratz R, Claffey A. Adult health in childcare: health status, behaviors, and concerns of teachers, directors, and family child care providers. Early Child Res Q. 1996;11(2):243–67.
7. McGrath B, Huntington AD. The health and wellbeing of adults working in early childhood education. Australian journal early. Childhood. 2007;32:33–8.
8. Converso D, Viotti S, Sottimano I, Cascio V, Guidetti G. Work ability, psycho-physical health, burnout, and age among nursery school and kindergarten teachers: a cross-sectional study. Med Lav. 2015;106(2):91–108.
9. Erick PN, Smith DR. A systematic review of musculoskeletal disorders among school teachers. BMC Musculoskelet Disord. 2011;12:260.
10. Widanarko B, Legg S, Devereux J, Stevenson M. The combined effect of physical, psychosocial/organisational and/or environmental risk factors on the presence of work-related musculoskeletal symptoms and its consequences. Appl Ergon. 2014;45(6):1610–21.
11. Widanarko B, Legg S, Stevenson M, Devereux J, Eng A, Cheng S, Pearce N. Prevalence and work-related risk factors for reduced activities and absenteeism due to low back symptoms. Appl Ergon. 2012;43(4):727–37.
12. D'Errico A, Viotti S, Baratti A, Mottura B, Barocelli AP, Tagna M, [...], Converso D. Low back pain and associated presenteeism among hospital nursing staff. J Occup Health 2013; 55(4):276–283.
13. Miranda H, Kaila-Kangas L, Heliövaara M, PäiLeino-Arjas P, Haukka E, Juha Liira J, Viikari-Juntura E. Musculoskeletal pain at multiple sites and its effects on work ability in a general working population. Occup Environ Med. 2010; 67(7):449–55.
14. Bailey TS, Dollard MF, McLinton SS, Richards PA. Psychosocial safety climate, psychosocial and physical factors in the aetiology of musculoskeletal disorder symptoms and workplace injury compensation claims. Work Stress. 2015;29(2):190–211.
15. Trinkoff AM, Lipscomb JA, Geiger-Brown J, Brady B. Musculoskeletal problems of the neck, shoulder, and back and functional consequences in nurses. Am J Ind Med. 2002;41(3):170–8.
16. Trinkoff AM, Lipscomb JA, Geiger-Brown J, Storr CL, Brady BA. Perceived physical demands and reported musculoskeletal problems in registered nurses. Am J Prev Med. 2003;24(3):270–5.
17. Neupane S, Leino-Arjas P, Nygård CH, Miranda H, Siukola A, Virtanen P. Does the association between musculoskeletal pain and sickness absence due to musculoskeletal diagnoses depend on biomechanical working conditions? Int Arch Occup Environ Health. 2015;88(3):273–9.

18. Kelly AL, Berthelsen DC. Preschool teachers' experiences of stress. Teach Teach Educ. 1995;11(4):345–57.
19. Li-Grining C, Raver CC, Champion K, Sardin L, Metzger M, Jones SM. Understanding and improving classroom emotional climate and behavior management in the "real world": the role of head start teachers' psychosocial stressors. Early Educ Dev. 2010;21(1):65–94.
20. Bakker AB, Demerouti E. The job demands-resources model: state of the art. J Manag Psychol. 2007;22(3):309–28.
21. Hobfoll SE. Conservation of resources: a new attempt at conceptualizing stress. Am Psychol. 1989;44(3):513–24.
22. Kristensen TS, Hannerz H, Høgh A, Borg V. The Copenhagen psychosocial questionnaire-a tool for the assessment and improvement of the psychosocial work environment. Scand J Work Environ Health. 2005;31(6): 438–49.
23. Wright TA, Cropanzano R. Emotional exhaustion as a predictor of job performance and voluntary turnover. J Appl Psychol. 1998;83(3):486–93.
24. Social HSE. Psychological resources and adaptation. Rev Gen Psychol. 2002; 6(4):307–24.
25. Hobfoll SE, Shirom A. Conservation of resources theory: applications to stress and management in the workplace. In: Golembiewski RT, editor. Handbook of Organizational Behavior (2nd ed.). New York, NY, US: Marcel Dekker; 2001. P. 57–80.
26. Leiter MP, Maslach C. The impact of interpersonal environment on burnout and organizational commitment. J Organ Behav. 1988;9(4):297–308.
27. Tham P. Why are they leaving? Factors affecting intention to leave among social workers in child welfare. Br J Soc Work. 2007;37(7):1225–46.
28. Janik M, Rothmann S. (2015). Meaningful work and secondary school teachers' intention to leave. S Afr J Educ. 2015;35(2):1–13.
29. Arnold KA, Turner N, Barling J, Kelloway EK, McKee MC. Transformational leadership and psychological well-being: the mediating role of meaningful work. J Occup Health Psychol. 2007;12(3):193–203.
30. Rosso BD, Dekas KH, Wrzesniewski A. On the meaning of work: a theoretical integration and review. Res Organ Behav. 2010;30:91–127.
31. Dormann C, Zapf D. Customer-related social stressors and burnout. J Occup Health Psychol. 2004;9:61–82.
32. Viotti S, Guidetti G, Loera B, Martini M, Sottimano I, Converso D. Stress, work ability, and an aging workforce: a study among women aged 50 and over. Int J Stress Manag. 2017;24(S1):98–121.
33. Cammann C, Fichman M, Jenkins GD, Klesh JR. Assessing the attitudes and perceptions of organizational members. In: Seashore SE SE, Lawler EE EE, Mirvis PH PH, Cammann C, editors. Assessing organizational change. New York: John Wiley and Sons; 1983. p. 71–138.
34. Kuorinka I, Jonsson B, Kilbom A, Vinterberg H, Biering-Sørensen F, Andersson G, Jørgensen K. Standardised Nordic questionnaires for the analysis of musculoskeletal symptoms. Appl Ergonomics. 1987;18(3):233–7.
35. Spielholz P, Silverstein B, Morgan M, Checkoway H, Kaufman J. Comparison of self-report, video observation and direct measurement methods for upper extremity musculoskeletal disorder physical risk factors. Ergonomics. 2001;44(6):588–613.
36. Kline RB. Principles and Practices of structural equation modelling. 2nd ed. New York: Guilford Press; 2005.
37. Bentler PM. EQS structural equations program manual. Encino, CA: Multivariate Software; 1995.
38. Hoyle RH. Structural equation modeling. Thousand Oaks, CA: Sage Publications Inc; 1995.
39. Hu L, Bentler PM. Cutoff criteria for fit indexes in covariance structure analysis: conventional criteria versus new alternatives. Struct Equ Modeling. 1999;6(1):1–55.
40. Byrne BM. Structural equation modeling with LISREL, PRELIS and SIMPLIS: basic concepts, applications and programming. Mahwah, NJ: Lawrence Erlbaum Associates; 1998.
41. Sottimano I, Viotti S, Guidetti G, Converso D. Protective factors for work ability in preschool teachers. Occup Med. 2017;67(4):301–4.
42. Baron RM, Kenny DA. The moderator–mediator variable distinction in social psychological research: conceptual, strategic, and statistical considerations. J Pers Soc Psychol. 1986;51(6):1173–82.
43. Cheung GW, Lau RS. Testing mediation and suppression effects of latent variables: bootstrapping with structural equation models. Organ Res Methods. 2008;11(2):296–325.
44. MacKinnon DP, Lockwood CM, Hoffman JM, West SG, Sheets V. A comparison of methods to test mediation and other intervening variable effects. Psychol Method. 2002;7(1):83.
45. Williamson DL, Carr J. Health as a resource for everyday life: advancing the conceptualization. Crit Public Health. 2009;19(1):107–22.
46. Podsakoff PM, MacKenzie SB, Lee JY, Podsakoff NP. Common method biases in behavioral research: a critical review of the literature and recommended remedies. J Appl Psychol. 2003;88(5):879–903.
47. Converso D, Sottimano I, Guidetti G, Loera B, Cortini M, Viotti S. Aging and Work Ability: The Moderating Role of Job and Personal Resources. Frontiers in Psychology 8. 2018.

10

Biomechanical effects of metastasis in the osteoporotic lumbar spine: a finite element analysis

Giuseppe Salvatore[1], Alessandra Berton[1], Hugo Giambini[2], Mauro Ciuffreda[1], Pino Florio[1], Umile Giuseppe Longo[1*], Vincenzo Denaro[1], Andrew Thoreson[2] and Kai-Nan An[2]

Abstract

Background: Cancer patients are likely to undergo osteoporosis as consequence of hormone manipulation and/or chemotherapy. Little is known about possible increased risk of fracture in this population. The aim of this study was to describe the biomechanical effect of a metastatic lesion in an osteoporotic lumbar spine model.

Methods: A finite element model of two spinal motion segments (L3-L5) was extracted from a previously developed L3-Sacrum model and used to analyze the effect of metastasis size and bone mineral density (BMD) on Vertebral bulge (VB) and Vertebral height (VH). VB and VH represent respectively radial and axial displacement and they have been correlated to burst fracture. A total of 6 scenarios were evaluated combining three metastasis sizes (no metastasis, 15% and 30% of the vertebral body) and two BMD conditions (normal BMD and osteoporosis).

Results: 15% metastasis increased VB and VH by 178% and 248%, respectively in normal BMD model; while VB and VH increased by 134% and 174% in osteoporotic model. 30% metastasis increased VB and VH by 88% and 109%, respectively, when compared to 15% metastasis in normal BMD model; while VB and VH increased by 59% and 74% in osteoporotic model.

Conclusion: A metastasis in the osteoporotic lumbar spine always leads to a higher risk of vertebral fracture. This risk increases with the size of the metastasis. Unexpectedly, an increment in metastasis size in the normal BMD spine produces a greater impact on vertebral stability compared to the osteoporotic spine.

Keywords: Metastasis, Vertebral fracture, Vertebroplasty, Osteoporosis, Finite element analysis, Lumbar spine

Background

The spine is the most common site for skeletal metastasis, with one third of all cancer patients developing metastases of the spine [1]. Because advancements in oncological treatments have improved patients' survival, the prevalence of spinal metastases is bound to increase [2]. Vertebral fractures caused by spine metastases result in pain, deformity, loss of mobility, and/or neurological complications, significantly affecting quality of life [3–5].

Many patients with metastases of the spine are likely to decrease their bone mineral density (BMD), leading to osteopenia or osteoporosis, as a consequence of hormone manipulation and/or chemotherapy [6], increasing the risk of vertebral fractures. Snyder et al. developed a computed tomography-based structural analysis (CTRA) method to predict fracture risk associated with osteolytic vertebral lesions [7]. Although highly sensitive and more specific than radiographs, validation studies are still ongoing. On the other hand, little is known about the increased risk of fracture in osteoporotic patients with metastatic lesions. Predictive tools, such as dual absorptiometry (DXA), quantitative computed tomography-based finite element analysis (QCT/FEA), biomechanical computed tomography-based FEA (BCT/FEA), have been implemented to improve fracture risk assessment in osteoporotic patients, but they have not been considered for osteoporotic cancer patients [8–11].

* Correspondence: g.longo@unicampus.it
[1]Department of Orthopaedic and Trauma Surgery, Campus Bio-Medico University, Via Alvaro del Portillo, 200, 00128 Trigoria, Rome, Italy

Biomechanical studies investigating the risk of fracture in metastatic spines lack realistic models and are not ideal for parametric analyses [12]. Because cadaveric studies are performed with normal spines, simulated lytic defects are typically developed by removing a core of trabecular bone and penetrating the cortical structure [13–16]. Similarly, clinical studies, including retrospective reviews of patients, can hardly extrapolate the influence of every individual variable as the patients population is generally heterogeneous and uncontrolled multiple factors can influence the results [12]. On the other hand, finite element analysis, successful in predicting failure loads and fracture patterns for bone structures [8, 17–24], allows a parametric representation of complex geometric and material property distributions.

The aim of this study was to evaluate the biomechanical effects of a metastatic lesion in an osteoporotic model of the lumbar spine.

Methods

Finite element model

A finite element model of two spinal motion segments (L3-L5) was extracted from a previously developed and validated three-dimensional, nonlinear, ligamentous L3-Sacrum model [25, 26] (Fig. 1). Development of the model is described in more details in the prior publication [25] and summarized here for convenience. The geometry and dimensions of the model were obtained from a high-resolution computed tomography scan (Siemens Helical CT Scanner, Siemens Corp., Munich, Germany - 0.293 mm in plane pixel size, 0.4 mm slice thickness) of a fresh, frozen human cadaveric spine specimen (male, 52 yrs. old). DICOM images were imported into Mimics image processing and editing software (Materialise US, Plymouth, MI USA) for segmentation. Since soft tissue was poorly visualized on CT scans, the discs were generated using the wrap function in 3-matic 4.2 (Materialise, Ann Arbor, MI, USA). Discs was modeled as a composite of a solid matrix with embedded fibers in concentric rings. The Nucleus pulposum was surrounded by seven annulus fibrosus lamellae, containing two evenly spaced layers of fibers oriented at approximately ±30° to the horizontal plane [27, 28]. The fibers were defined using 3-D two-node truss elements. Collagenous fiber content varies from 23% in the outermost layer to 5% in the innermost layer [29, 30]. Thus, the cross-sectional area of the truss elements was determined based on the annular layer volume and the number of elements to satisfy the fiber content distribution. The fiber thickness and stiffness increased in the radial direction. A "no compression" option was defined for the annulus fibrosus such that the elements resist tension only. The solid matrix of the annulus fibrosus was modeled as a neo-Hookean solid, while the nucleus pulposum was linearly elastic.

The finite element mesh was generated using HyperMesh 10.0 (Altair Engineering, Inc., Troy, MI, USA).

The model included the vertebral bodies consisting of a cortical shell, cancellous centrum, endplates and posterior elements. Intervertebral discs consisted of a nucleus pulposus, annulus ground substances, and annulus fibrosus (seven layers). All major ligaments were represented: (anterior longitudinal, posterior longitudinal, intertransverse, ligamentum flavum, interspinous, supraspinous, and capsular). The ligaments were modeled with 3-D two node truss elements and assigned nonlinear hypoelastic material properties, which allow axial stiffness to be a

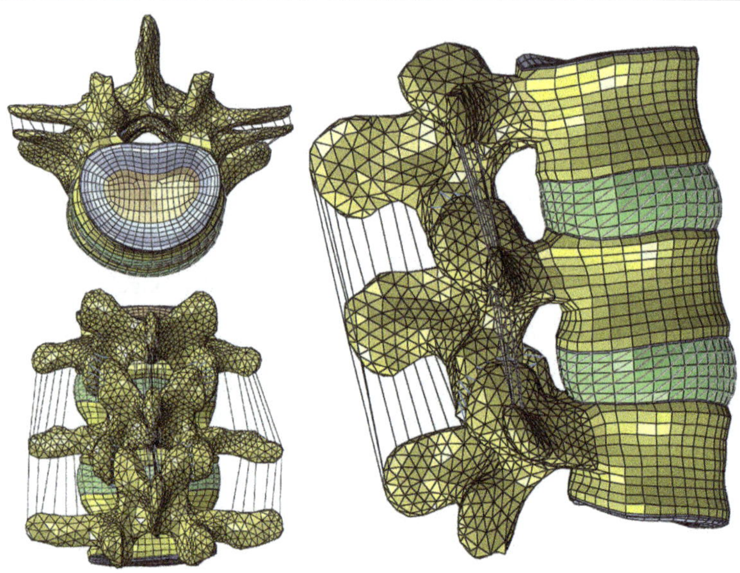

Fig. 1 Finite element model of two spinal motion segments (L3-L5)

function of axial strain. At initially low strains the ligaments exhibit low stiffness, but as the strains increase the ligament stiffness increases. The cross-sectional areas of each ligament were obtained from literature. All elements representing the ligaments were aligned in the anatomical fiber direction and unstressed at the unloaded state [28].

The metastasis was represented as a lytic bone lesion. Material properties for all structures are summarized in Table 1.

Boundary conditions and loads

Nodes at the lower surface of the L5 vertebra, corresponding to the endplate, were encastred and constrained from all three axes of rotation and translations. A reference node was placed 10 mm above the L3 vertebra and surface nodes from the vertebra and the reference node were selected to form rigid bodies and create a kinematic coupling. This constrain limited the motion of aforementioned nodes to the motion applied to the reference node [31]. An axial compressive load of 1200 N was applied to the superior reference node atop the L3 vertebra to represent upper body weight. This load corresponds to a compressive force on the lumbar spine for an individual standing upright holding an 8.3 kg mass with outstretched arms [32].

Table 1 Finite element model material properties

	Elastic Modulus (MPa)	Poisson's Ratio
Vertebra		
Cancellous Bone	100	0.2
Cortical Bone	12,000	0.3
Vertebral Bony Endplate	4000	0.3
Cartilage Endplate	5	0.17
Posterior Bone	3500	0.25
Intervertebral Disc		
Nucleus Polposus	1	0.49
Annular Fibers	Neo-Hooke	
Annular Layers	Neo-Hooke	
Joint		
Facet Joints	3500	
Ligaments		
Anterior Longitudinal	15.6–20.0	0.3
Posterior Longitudinal	10.0–20.0	0.3
Intertransverse	12–58.7	0.3
Ligamentum Flavum	13.0–19.5	0.3
Interspinous	9.8–12.0	0.3
Supraspinous	8.8–15.0	0.3
Capsular	7.5–33.0	0.3
Metastasis		
Lytic Bone Metastasis	0.01	0.4995

Parametric analyses

A parametric analysis was performed varying metastasis size and BMD. Metastatic lesion was varied to represent 15% and 30% of the vertebral body volume by selecting elements at the central core of the L4 vertebral body. (Fig. 2). Osteoporosis was defined by a 66% reduction in the elastic moduli of all bony structures for the cancellous bone, and by 33% for the cortical shell, the endplates, and the posterior elements [33]. Soft tissue structures were left unchanged. A total of 6 scenarios were evaluated, as described in Table 2. Scenario 1 (Normal BMD - Metastasis size 0%) was used as a baseline for comparison with other normal BMD conditions. Scenario 4 (Osteoporotic - Metastasis size 0%) was used as baseline for comparison with other osteoporotic conditions.

Outcomes variables

Vertebral fracture risk was analyzed based on vertebral bulge (VB) and vertebral height (VH) outcomes [13]. Vertebral bulge, representing the maximum radial displacement at the transverse midline of the vertebral body, has been noted to correlate with load-induced spinal canal narrowing, vertebral cortex tensile hoop strains, and bone marrow pressurization [13]. Vertebral

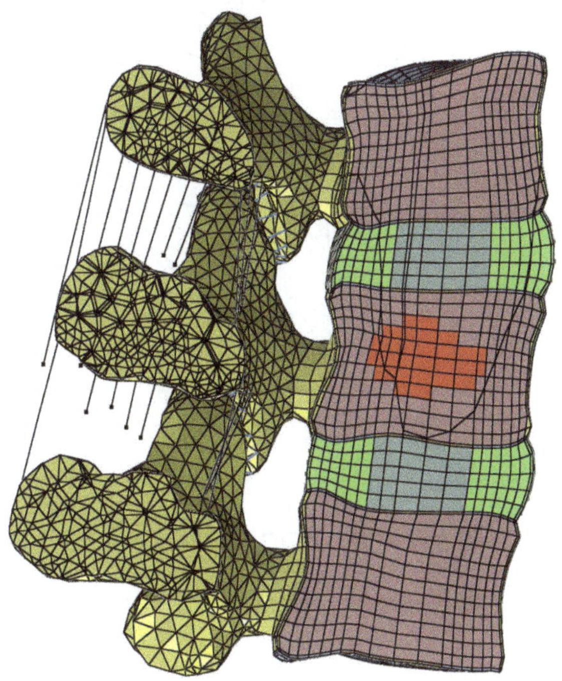

Fig. 2 The metastatic lesion was configured as roughly elliptical mass by selecting a core of elements that covered approximately 15% of the volume of L4 vertebral body

Table 2 Investigated scenarios

Scenario	BMD	Metastasis Size
1	Normal	0%
2	Normal	15%
3	Normal	30%
4	Osteoporotic	0%
5	Osteoporotic	15%
6	Osteoporotic	30%

Scenario 1 (Normal BMD - Metastasis size 0%) and scenario 4 (Osteoporotic - Metastasis size 0%) were used as baseline

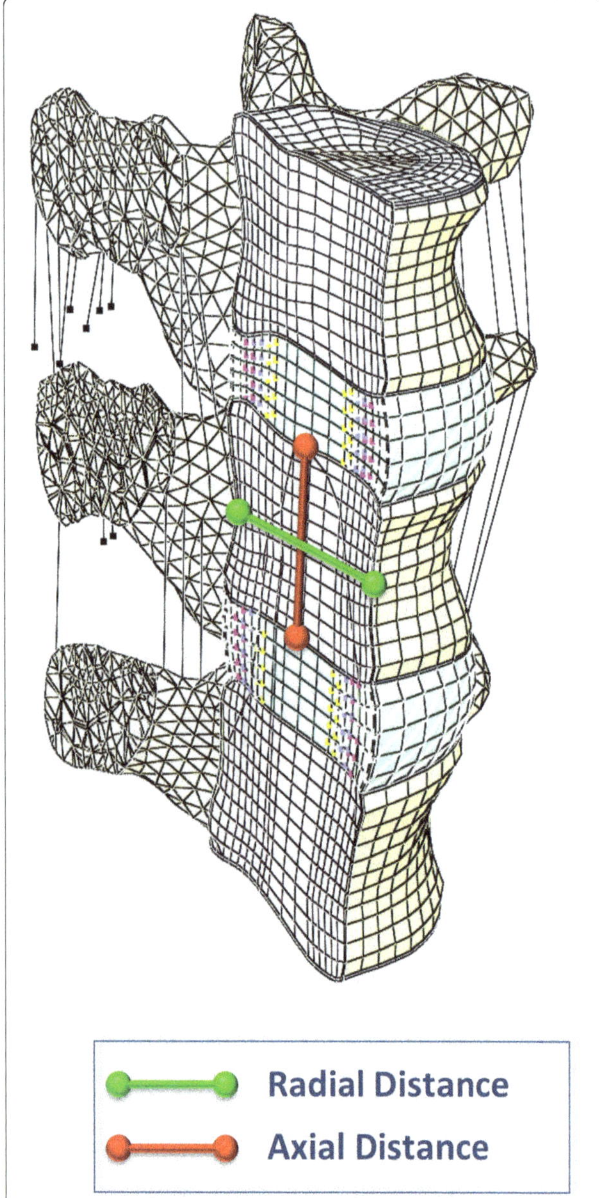

Fig. 3 Radial Distance (green line): distance between two standard nodes at the mid-height of L4 on the sagittal plane. Axial Distance (red line): distance between two standard nodes at the center of the inferior and superior endplates of L4

height, representing the maximum axial displacement of the endplates, characterizes the risk of endplate failure leading to subsequent burst fracture [13].

The distance between two standard nodes at the mid-height of L4 on the sagittal plane was measured (Radial Distance, Fig. 3). VB was calculated as the difference between the Radial Distance before and after the axial compressive load was applied (VB = Radial Distance after load – Radial Distance before load).

The distance between two standard nodes at the center of the inferior and superior endplates of L4 was measured (Axial Distance, Fig. 3). VH was calculated as the difference between the Axial Distance before and after the axial compressive load was applied (VH = Axial Distance before load – Axial Distance after load).

Results

Results for the simulations with metastasis were normalized to relative baseline scenarios of intact vertebra without metastasis (Scenario 1: VB 0.05 mm, VH 0.15 mm and Scenario 4: VB 0.123 mm, VH 0.417 mm). In normal BMD scenarios, 15% metastasis increased VB by 178% (0.139 mm) and VH by 248% (0.522 mm); while a 30% metastasis increased VB by 424% (0.262 mm) and VH by 626% (1.09 mm). A comparison of metastatic lesion size showed a 30% metastasis to increase VB by 88% (0.139 mm vs 0.262 mm) and VH by 109% (0.522 vs 1.09) when compared to a 15% metastasis. In osteoporotic scenarios, a 15% metastasis increased VB by 134% (0.288 mm) and VH by 174% (1.145 mm); while a 30% metastasis increased VB by 272% (0.458 mm) and VH by 479% (1.996 mm). Comparing the two metastatic scenarios (15% and 30%), VB increased by 59% (0.288 vs 0.458) and VH by 74% (1.145 vs 1.996). When same metastasis size scenarios were compared, the osteoporotic spine had larger VB and VH values compared to normal BMD scenario. Results are summarized in Table 3 and Fig. 4.

Discussion

The purpose of this study was to describe the biomechanical effect of a metastatic lesion in an osteoporotic lumbar spine model in order to better understand the risk of vertebral fractures in this population. A finite element model of two spinal motion segments (L3-L5) was used to analyze the effect of metastasis size and osteoporosis on VB and VH. Results from the study showed osteoporosis can represent a risk of fracture

Table 3 VB and VH for each scenario, absolute values

BMD	Normal		Osteoporotic	
Metastasis size	15%	30%	15%	30%
VB	0.133	0.262	0.288	0.458
VH	0.522	1.09	1.145	1.996

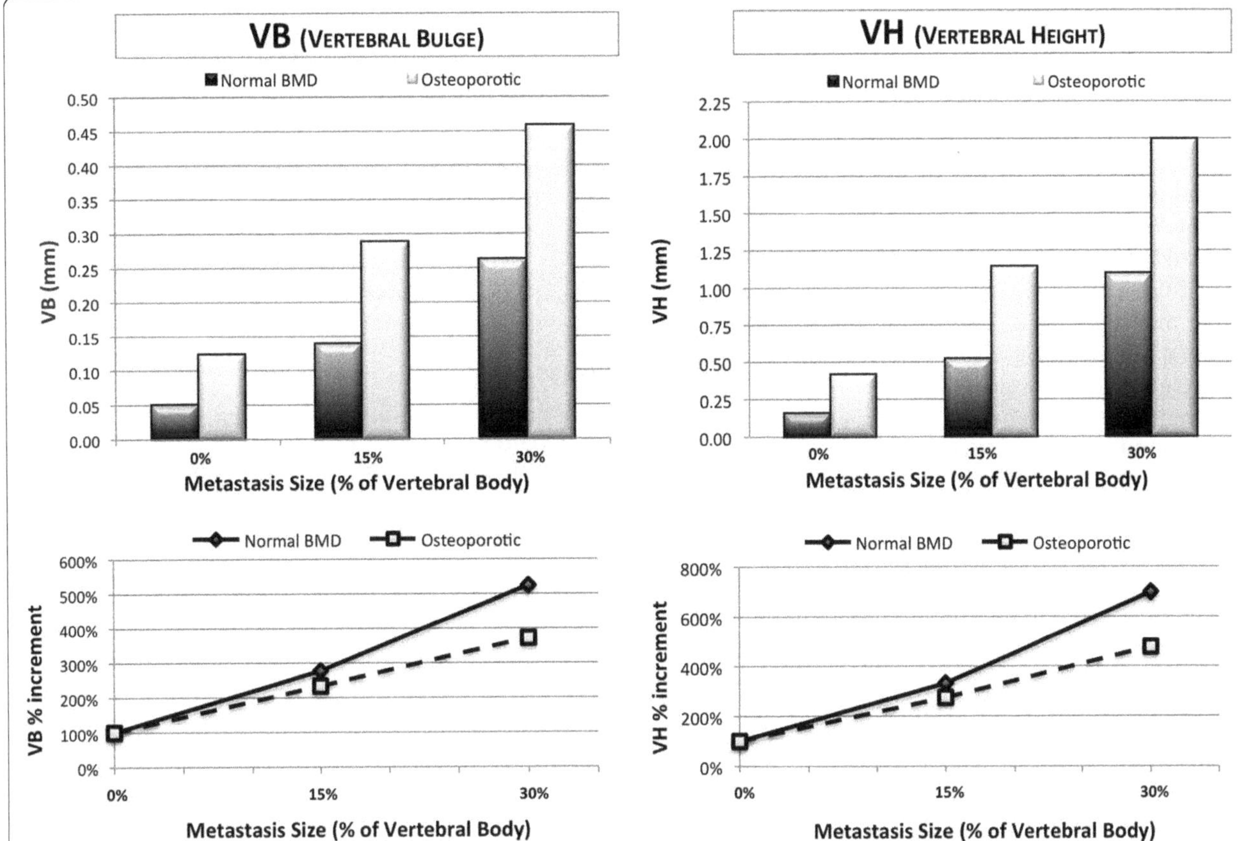

Fig. 4 Histograms show values of VB and VH (in mm) in simulated scenarios. Results show that osteoporotic models are less stable compared to respective normal BMD models. Scatterplots show increments of VB and VH (in percentage) normalized to the respective baseline values, to highlight the trend of increment. Results show that metastasis size greater affects normal BMD models stability compared to osteoporotic ones

regardless of metastasis size compared to patients with normal BMD. Furthermore, an increase in metastasis size has a greater impact on the risk of fracture in patients with normal BMD compared to osteoporotic patients.

A previous study by Taneichi et al. [34] identified the following criteria of impending collapse: 1) 50–60% involvement of the vertebral body with no destruction of other structures, or 25–30% involvement with costovertebral joint destruction in the thoracic spine; and 2) 35–40% involvement of vertebral body, or 20–25% involvement with posterior elements destruction in thoracolumbar and lumbar spine. It is well known that the load bearing capacity of bone is influenced by the geometry, location, biological activity of the tumor, and the geometry and material properties of the host bone [34]. Several studies have investigated the risk of vertebral fracture in osteoporotic bones [35–45]. However, there is still a lack of knowledge relating the interactive and/or cumulative effect of metastatic cancer and osteoporosis [46, 47].

To the best of our knowledge, this is the first three-dimensional, anatomical model of two spinal motion segments (L3-L5) that investigates a metastatic lesion in an osteoporotic spine. A previous study by Whyne et al., investigated the effects of tumor size, material properties and compressive loading rate on vertebral strength, using a two-dimensional, symmetric finite element model of the L1 vertebral body without posterior elements [48]. Two additional studies by Whyne et al. implemented a three-dimensional finite element model of the L1 vertebra including the posterior arch but no additional posterior elements were represented [13, 49]. These studies showed tumor size to be the predominant contributor towards the risk of initiating a burst fracture, followed by the applied load magnitude and bone density. However, the biomechanical response, including stress distribution and geometrical changes, is more complex in a spine segment comprised of the vertebral bodies with posterior elements and soft tissues (intervertebral discs and ligamentous structures). The posterior elements, facet joints and ligaments share a substantial portion of the loads applied to the spine, stabilizing and preventing vertebral bulge [50]. Tschirat et al. developed a geometrical three-dimensional finite element model of a thoracic spine segment to understand the effects of vertebral level, geometry, and metastasis on the cortical shell [51, 52]. The study demonstrated that upper thoracic vertebrae are at greater risk of burst fracture, and that kyphotic segments, ribcage and transcortical tumor provided lower risk of burst fracture initiation [52]. Moreover, the effect of multiple loading conditions on metastatically-involved thoracic spinal motion segment was investigated showing axial loading as the predominant load type leading to increased risk of burst fracture initiation [51]. However, the load distribution in the lumbar spine might differ from that observed in the thoracic spine due to the presence of the ribcage, vertebral size, lordotic angle, and articular facet angles. Our results showed osteoporosis to highly affect vertebral outcomes of the model. Previous studies have only modified trabecular bone material properties based on an assumed apparent density [13, 48, 49]. In order to obtain a reliable representation of an osteoporotic spine, the current model included changes in the material properties of the cortical shell, endplates and posterior elements.

This study has limitations. The L3-L5 finite element model was extracted from a previously developed and validated three-dimensional, nonlinear, ligamentous L3-Sacrum model [25, 26]. Prior validation of the L3-Sacrum model allows considering results derived from the L3-L5 model as reasonable. However, the two spinal motion segment model cannot be considered as properly validated. The metastatic lesion was represented as an ellipsoid, and tumor shape can influence vertebral bulge and vertebral axial displacements [33, 41]. However, the ellipsoidal geometry is frequently used in finite element models of metastasis [13, 41, 49]. Second, only an axial compressive load of 1200 N was studied. However, this represents a compressive force on the lumbar spine for an individual standing upright holding an 8.3 kg mass with outstretched arms [32]. Lower loading regime should be studied in order to simulate daily life tasks of endstage cancer patients that can be translated to clinical practice. Third, additional motions or loads were not simulated. Tschirhart et al. [51] suggested focusing primarily on axial compressive loading rather than complex load/boundary conditions since it is the predominant load type leading to increased risk of burst fracture initiation of the thoracic spine and it is likely to be the same for the lumbar segment. Fourth, it could be argued that metastatic lesions are more common in the thoracic spine rather than in the lumbar spine. However, we aimed to evaluate the effect of axial loading without the influences of the ribs, which can contribute to reduce the effective axial loading applied on the vertebra. Therefore, we decided to study the lumbar spine segment. In future studies, we are planning to study localization of metastasis to the thoracic spine. Fifth, we only simulated a lytic metastasis. Blastic lesions are frequent and should be investigated in future studies. However, it should be taken into account that, both lytic and blastic metastasis lead to a decrease in bone mineralization [46, 53]. Mineral content have been demonstrated to be strongly correlated with strength/stiffness [54–56]. Thus, the reason for fracture of a metastatic vertebra is related to poor bone quality, both in case of lytic and blastic metastasis. Finally, our parametric study was limited to metastasis size and bone mineral density. Future studies should evaluate metastasis location, vertebral level, pedicle involvement, metastasis type, and disc degeneration.

Conclusions

A metastasis in the osteoporotic lumbar spine always leads to a higher risk of vertebral fracture. This risk increases with the size of the metastasis. Unexpectedly, an increment in metastasis size in the normal BMD spine produces a greater impact on vertebral stability compared to the osteoporotic spine.

Abbreviations

BCT/FEA: Biomechanical computed tomography-based FEA; BMD: Bone mineral density; CTRA: Computed tomography-based structural analysis; DXA: Dual absorptiometry; QCT/FEA: Quantitative computed tomography-based finite element analysis; VB: Vertebral bulge; VH: Vertebral height

Acknowledgements

No one else contributed towards the article except for the authors.
None of the authors received funding.
No one else contributed materials essential for the study except for the authors.

Funding

The authors declare that they have no conflict of interest and no funding source.

Authors' contributions

GS and AB wrote the manuscript, optimized the FEA model and performed the FEA simulations. AB, MC and PF performed the data extraction and analysis, and draw figures and Tables. HG contributed to the creation and validation of the FEA model. UGL, VD, AT and KNA contributed to data interpretation and reviewed the manuscript. All authors read and approved the final manuscript.

Consent for publication

Not applicable.

Competing interests

AB, UGL and AT are members of the Editorial Board of BMC Musculoskeletal Disorders. The other authors declare that they have no competing interests.

Author details

[1]Department of Orthopaedic and Trauma Surgery, Campus Bio-Medico University, Via Alvaro del Portillo, 200, 00128 Trigoria, Rome, Italy. [2]Biomechanics Laboratory, Division of Orthopaedic Research, Mayo Clinic, Rochester, MN, USA.

References

1. Aaron AD. The management of cancer metastatic to bone. JAMA : the journal of the American Medical Association. 1994;272(15):1206–9.
2. Ohmori K, Matsui H, Yasuda T, Kanamori M, Yudoh K, Seto H, Tsuji H. Evaluation of the prognosis of cancer patients with metastatic bone tumors based on serial bone scintigrams. Jpn J Clin Oncol. 1997;27(4):263–7.
3. Hortobagyi GN, Theriault RL, Lipton A, Porter L, Blayney D, Sinoff C, Wheeler H, Simeone JF, Seaman JJ, Knight RD, et al. Long-term prevention of skeletal complications of metastatic breast cancer with pamidronate. Protocol 19 Aredia breast cancer study group. J Clin Oncol. 1998;16(6):2038–44.
4. Hortobagyi GN. The status of breast cancer management: challenges and opportunities. Breast Cancer Res Treat. 2002;75(Suppl 1):S61–5. discussion S57–69
5. Hipp JA, Springfield DS, Hayes WC. Predicting pathologic fracture risk in the management of metastatic bone defects. Clin Orthop Relat Res. 1995;312: 120–35.
6. Mincey BA, Moraghan TJ, Perez EA. Prevention and treatment of osteoporosis in women with breast cancer. Mayo Clinic proceedings Mayo Clinic. 2000;75(8): 821–9.
7. Snyder BD, Cordio MA, Nazarian A, Kwak SD, Chang DJ, Entezari V, Zurakowski D, Parker LM. Noninvasive prediction of fracture risk in patients with metastatic cancer to the spine. Clin Cancer Res. 2009;15(24):7676–83.
8. Wang X, Sanyal A, Cawthon PM, Palermo L, Jekir M, Christensen J, Ensrud KE, Cummings SR, Orwoll E, Black DM, et al. Prediction of new clinical vertebral fractures in elderly men using finite element analysis of CT scans. J Bone Miner Res. 2012;27(4):808–16.
9. Morgan SL, Lopez-Ben R, Nunnally N, Burroughs L, Desmond R. Nonprogression of vertebral area or bone mineral content on DXA does not predict compression fractures. J Clin Densitom. 2006;9(3):261–4.
10. Shepherd JA, Schousboe JT, Broy SB, Engelke K, Leslie WD. Executive summary of the 2015 ISCD position development conference on advanced measures from DXA and QCT: fracture prediction beyond BMD. J Clin Densitom. 2015; 18(3):274–86.
11. Zysset P, Qin L, Lang T, Khosla S, Leslie WD, Shepherd JA, Schousboe JT, Engelke K. Clinical use of quantitative computed tomography-based finite element analysis of the hip and spine in the Management of Osteoporosis in adults: the 2015 ISCD official positions-part II. J Clin Densitom. 2015;18(3): 359–92.
12. Whyne CM. Biomechanics of metastatic disease in the vertebral column. Neurol Res. 2014;36(6):493–501.
13. Whyne CM, Hu SS, Lotz JC. Burst fracture in the metastatically involved spine: development, validation, and parametric analysis of a three-dimensional poroelastic finite-element model. Spine. 2003;28(7):652–60.
14. Windhagen HJ, Hipp JA, Silva MJ, Lipson SJ, Hayes WC. Predicting failure of thoracic vertebrae with simulated and actual metastatic defects. Clin Orthop Relat Res. 1997;344:313-319.
15. Dimar JR 2nd, Voor MJ, Zhang YM, Glassman SD. A human cadaver model for determination of pathologic fracture threshold resulting from tumorous destruction of the vertebral body. Spine. 1998;23(11):1209–14.
16. McGowan DP, Hipp JA, Takeuchi T, White AA 3rd, Hayes WC. Strength reductions from trabecular destruction within thoracic vertebrae. J Spinal Disord. 1993;6(2):130-136.
17. Huiskes R, Hollister SJ. From structure to process, from organ to cell: recent developments of FE-analysis in orthopaedic biomechanics. J Biomech Eng. 1993;115(4B):520–7.
18. Lotz JC, Cheal EJ, Hayes WC. Fracture prediction for the proximal femur using finite element models: part I-linear analysis. J Biomech Eng. 1991; 113(4):353–60.
19. Matsuura Y, Giambini H, Ogawa Y, Fang Z, Thoreson AR, Yaszemski MJ, Lu L, An KN. Specimen-specific nonlinear finite element modeling to predict vertebrae fracture loads after vertebroplasty. Spine. 2014;39(22):E1291–6.
20. Morgan EF, Yeh OC, Keaveny TM. Damage in trabecular bone at small strains. Eur J Morphol. 2005;42(1–2):13–21.
21. Morgan EF, Bayraktar HH, Yeh OC, Majumdar S, Burghardt A, Keaveny TM. Contribution of inter-site variations in architecture to trabecular bone apparent yield strains. J Biomech. 2004;37(9):1413–20.
22. Morgan EF, Bayraktar HH, Keaveny TM. Trabecular bone modulus-density relationships depend on anatomic site. J Biomech. 2003;36(7):897–904.
23. Keaveny TM, Morgan EF, Niebur GL, Yeh OC. Biomechanics of trabecular bone. Annu Rev Biomed Eng. 2001;3:307–33.
24. Amin S, Kopperdhal DL, Melton LJ 3rd, Achenbach SJ, Therneau TM, Riggs BL, Keaveny TM, Khosla S. Association of hip strength estimates by finite-element analysis with fractures in women and men. J Bone Miner Res. 2011; 26(7):1593–600.
25. Ellingson AM, Shaw MN, Giambini H, An KN. Comparative role of disc degeneration and ligament failure on functional mechanics of the lumbar spine. Comput Methods Biomech Biomed Engin. 2015:1–10.
26. Viceconti M, Olsen S, Nolte LP, Burton K. Extracting clinically relevant data from finite element simulations. Clin Biomech. 2005;20(5):451–4.
27. Goel VK, Monroe BT, Gilbertson LG, Brinckmann P. Interlaminar shear stresses and laminae separation in a disc. Finite element analysis of the L3-L4 motion segment subjected to axial compressive loads. Spine. 1995;20(6):689–98.
28. White AAPM. Clinical biomechanics of the spine. 2nd ed. Philadelphia: JB Lippincott; 1990.
29. Shirazi-Adl A, Ahmed AM, Shrivastava SC. A finite element study of a lumbar motion segment subjected to pure sagittal plane moments. J Biomech. 1986;19(4):331–50.
30. Schmidt H, Kettler A, Heuer F, Simon U, Claes L, Wilke HJ. Intradiscal pressure, shear strain, and fiber strain in the intervertebral disc under combined loading. Spine. 2007;32(7):748–55.
31. Corp. DSS (ed.): Abaqus Analysis User's Manual. Providence, RI.; 2008 a.
32. Schultz A, Andersson G, Ortengren R, Haderspeck K, Nachemson A. Loads on the lumbar spine. Validation of a biomechanical analysis by measurements of intradiscal pressures and myoelectric signals. J Bone Joint Surg Am. 1982; 64(5):713–20.
33. Polikeit A, Nolte LP, Ferguson SJ. The effect of cement augmentation on the load transfer in an osteoporotic functional spinal unit: finite-element analysis. Spine. 2003;28(10):991–6.
34. Taneichi H, Kaneda K, Takeda N, Abumi K, Satoh S. Risk factors and probability of vertebral body collapse in metastases of the thoracic and lumbar spine. Spine. 1997;22(3):239–45.
35. Longo UG, Loppini M, Denaro L, Maffulli N, Denaro V. Conservative management of patients with an osteoporotic vertebral fracture: a review of the literature. J Bone Joint Surg Br. 2012;94(2):152–7.
36. Longo UG, Loppini M, Denaro L, Maffulli N, Denaro V. Osteoporotic vertebral fractures: current concepts of conservative care. Br Med Bull. 2012;102:171–89.
37. Denaro V, Longo UG, Denaro L. Vertebroplasty versus conservative treatment for vertebral fractures. Lancet. 2010;376(9758):2071. author reply 2071-2072
38. Longo UG, Denaro L, Campi S, Maffulli N, Denaro V. Upper cervical spine injuries: indications and limits of the conservative management in halo vest. A systematic review of efficacy and safety. Injury. 2010;41(11):1127–35.
39. Denaro L, Longo UG, Denaro V. Vertebroplasty and kyphoplasty: reasons for concern? Orthop Clin North Am. 2009;40(4):465–71. viii
40. Denaro V, Longo UG, Maffulli N, Denaro L. Vertebroplasty and kyphoplasty. Clin Cases Miner Bone Metab. 2009;6(2):125–30.
41. Tschirhart CE, Nagpurkar A, Whyne CM. Effects of tumor location, shape and surface serration on burst fracture risk in the metastatic spine. J Biomech. 2004;37(5):653–60.
42. Longo UG, Denaro V. Spinal augmentation: what have we learnt? Lancet. 2009;373(9679):1947. author reply 1947-1948
43. Kopperdahl DL, Aspelund T, Hoffmann PF, Sigurdsson S, Siggeirsdottir K, Harris TB, Gudnason V, Keaveny TM. Assessment of incident spine and hip fractures in women and men using finite element analysis of CT scans. J Bone Miner Res. 2014;29(3):570–80.
44. Anderson DE, Demissie S, Allaire BT, Bruno AG, Kopperdahl DL, Keaveny TM, Kiel DP, Bouxsein ML. The associations between QCT-based vertebral bone measurements and prevalent vertebral fractures depend on the spinal locations of both bone measurement and fracture. Osteoporos Int. 2014; 25(2):559–66.
45. Fields AJ, Keaveny TM. Trabecular architecture and vertebral fragility in osteoporosis. Curr Osteoporos Rep. 2012;10(2):132–40.
46. Nazarian A, von Stechow D, Zurakowski D, Muller R, Snyder BD. Bone volume fraction explains the variation in strength and stiffness of cancellous bone affected by metastatic cancer and osteoporosis. Calcif Tissue Int. 2008;83(6):368–79.
47. Snyder BD, Piazza S, Edwards WT, Hayes WC. Role of trabecular morphology in the etiology of age-related vertebral fractures. Calcif Tissue Int. 1993; 53(Suppl 1):S14–22.

48. Whyne CM, Hu SS, Lotz JC. Parametric finite element analysis of vertebral bodies affected by tumors. J Biomech. 2001;34(10):1317–24.
49. Whyne CM, Hu SS, Lotz JC. Biomechanically derived guideline equations for burst fracture risk prediction in the metastatically involved spine. J Spinal Disord Tech. 2003;16(2):180–5.
50. Whyne CM, Hu SS, Klisch S, Lotz JC. Effect of the pedicle and posterior arch on vertebral body strength predictions in finite element modeling. Spine. 1998;23(8):899–907.
51. Tschirhart CE, Finkelstein JA, Whyne CM. Metastatic burst fracture risk assessment based on complex loading of the thoracic spine. Ann Biomed Eng. 2006;34(3):494–505.
52. Tschirhart CE, Finkelstein JA, Whyne CM. Biomechanics of vertebral level, geometry, and transcortical tumors in the metastatic spine. J Biomech. 2007;40(1):46–54.
53. Sone T, Tamada T, Jo Y, Miyoshi H, Fukunaga M. Analysis of three-dimensional microarchitecture and degree of mineralization in bone metastases from prostate cancer using synchrotron microcomputed tomography. Bone. 2004;35(2):432–8.
54. Burr DB. The contribution of the organic matrix to bone's material properties. Bone. 2002;31(1):8–11.
55. Currey JD. The mechanical consequences of variation in the mineral content of bone. J Biomech. 1969;2(1):1–11.
56. Currey JD. The effect of porosity and mineral content on the Young's modulus of elasticity of compact bone. J Biomech. 1988;21(2):131–9.

11

Posterior decompression and occipitocervical fixation followed by intraoperative vertebroplasty for metastatic involvement of the axis

Xinjie Wu[1,2], Mingsheng Tan[1,2*], Yingna Qi[1,3], Ping Yi[1], Feng Yang[1], Xiangsheng Tang[1] and Qingying Hao[1]

Abstract

Background: Metastases to the upper cervical spine were rarely reported in the literature. However, metastases to this area may cause spinal instability and cord compression, which in turn can result in respiratory failure and neurological dysfunction. The present study investigated the efficacy and safety of posterior decompression and occipitocervical fixation followed by intraoperative vertebroplasty for this disease.

Methods: This was a retrospective study that included 10 patients with metastatic involvement of the axis from March 2002 to May 2014. All cases presented with occipitocervical pain: 5 patients with compressive myelopathy and 6 patients with radiculopathy. Japanese Orthopedic Association (JOA) scores and Visual Analogue Scale (VAS) were used to evaluate the improvement of neurological function and pain intensity, respectively.

Results: All patients underwent posterior decompression and occipitocervical fixation followed by intraoperative vertebroplasty. The VAS scores and JOA scores both improved postoperatively, from 8.2 ± 0.4 to 2.3 ± 0.2 and from 10.1 ± 2.2 to 14.2 ± 2.9, respectively. Additionally, the improvement rate of JOA was $52.4 \pm 1.8\%$. The mean overall survival was 12.8 months. The median survival time was 7 months. The 6-month and 12-month survival rates were 70% and 40%, respectively. The mean duration of operation was 182 min and blood loss was 450 mL. The mean volume of bone cement injected was 4.0 mL. The cement extravasation was observed in only 1 patient without clinical symptoms. One patient developed tumour recurrence and died 1 month later.

Conclusions: Posterior decompression and occipitocervical fixation followed by intraoperative vertebroplasty was a safe and valuable palliative method with relatively less invasion to treat metastatic involvement of the axis.

Keywords: Vertebroplasty, Occipitocervical fixation, Axis, Metastasis

Background

The spine ranks first in the list of cancer metastasis in the skeletal system. Approximately 8-20% of metastases occur in the cervical spine [1–3]. However, metastases to the upper cervical spine were rarely reported in the literature [4, 5]. Due to the importance of this area, metastatic involvement of the axis may cause spinal instability and cord compression, which in turn can result in respiratory failure and neurological dysfunction. For advanced patients, the aim of surgical intervention was not to cure the disease but to relieve the pain and spinal cord compression, reconstruct spinal stability, and improve the quality of remaining life. The treatments included external immobilization, conventional surgical resection and percutaneous cement augmentation. However, conventional surgical treatment itself had risks of mixed infection, speech change, tongue oedema, cerebrospinal fluid leakage, etc., due to poor clinical conditions, comorbidities, and its transoral approach, while percutaneous vertebroplasty in this area was challenging [6, 7].

* Correspondence: doctortan_123@126.com
[1]Department of Spinal Surgery, China-Japan Friendship Hospital, Beijing 100029, People's Republic of China
[2]Graduate School of Peking Union Medical College, Beijing 100730, People's Republic of China

Therefore, combining intraoperative vertebroplasty and posterior decompression and occipitocervical fixation may be advisable, which is less invasive and could provide strong stability. To our knowledge, palliative surgical treatment of such disease has rarely been reported. This palliative method was used to treat 10 patients with metastatic involvement of the axis in our study and produced desirable outcomes.

Methods

Patients

Between March 2002 and May 2014, 10 patients (7 males, 3 females) with metastatic involvement of C2 who underwent surgery were retrospectively analysed. The mean age was 68.9 years, ranging from 49 to 82. In this study, all cases presented with occipitocervical pain: 5 patients with compressive myelopathy, and 6 patients with radiculopathy. The clinical data of the patients are displayed in Table 1.

Surgical indication and contraindication

The indications for surgery were intractable pain resistant to nonsurgical treatment, instability, progressive neurologic dysfunction, and expected survival time>3 months. The contraindication included intolerance to surgery; severe heart, lung, liver or kidney diseases; and extensively widespread metastasis. Four patients were excluded from the study due to short life expectancy or poor conditions. Preoperatively, the Modified Tokuhashi Scoring System [8] was used to predict the survival period for the patients. Four patients had a score of 0-8 (life expectancy<6 months), while 6 patients had a score between 9 and 11 (life expectancy>6 months). Furthermore, the Spinal Instability Neoplastic Score (SINS) [9] was employed to determine spinal instability. Five patients had a SINS of 7-12 (indicating impending instability) and 5 patients had a SINS of 13-18 (indicating an unstable spine).

Table 1 Clinical data of patients

Parameters	n (total 10 patients)
Average age	68.9
Sex ratio (male/female)	7/3
Primary tumor	
Lung	4
Breast	2
Prostate	2
Kidney	1
Unknown	1
Clinical symptom	
Occipitocervical pain	10
Compressive myelopathy	5
Radiculopathy	6
Complication	
Cement extravasation	1
Tumor recurrence	1

Surgery preparation

All 10 patients underwent meticulous oncological examination preoperatively. The radiological data were evaluated using X-ray, CT scans and MRIs. In addition, radionuclide bone scanning was performed to further identify the location of the primary neoplasm and metastases. All procedures were performed by the same surgeon (M.S. Tan).

Procedure

Neurological function was monitored by intraoperative somatosensory-evoked potentials. After endotracheal intubation and general anaesthesia, the patient was placed in the prone position with his or her head immobilized and slightly flexed by a Mayfield head holder. After disinfecting and routine draping, a standard midline incision was made to expose the posterior structure of the occipitocervical area. The laminar ligaments and muscles were dissected. Then, laminectomy and removing the superior and inferior facet joints and pedicle were performed using a high-speed burr and rongeur. The spinal cord, nerve root and vertebral artery were protected carefully during procedures. Transpedicular vertebroplasty with polymethylmethacrylate (PMMA) was performed during surgery using a C-arm image intensifier (Fig. 1). Intraoperative vertebroplasty was accurate and visual to inject bone cement. The leakage of bone cement could be detected and cleared in time. The PMMA was injected at high viscosity. Under C-arm guidance, the occipital plate and lateral mass screws or pedicle screws were placed and connected with a pre-curved rod bilaterally (O-C5) (Fig. 2). After irrigation, the incision was closed in layers and a drainage tube was placed inside.

Postoperatively, all patients were transferred to the oncology department for further treatment, such as radiotherapy or chemotherapy, as decided by the medical oncologists.

Evaluation indexes

Postoperative outcomes were obtained and evaluated both clinically and radiologically. The Japanese Orthopedic Association (JOA) score was used to assess the improvement of neurological function. The formula of improvement rate of JOA was as follows: postoperative improvement rate = (postoperative score − preoperative score) / (17 − preoperative score) × 100%. The pain intensity was compared before and after operation by the VAS score, which had a scale of 0-10. Moreover, the dose of painkillers before and after the intervention was also recorded. For the radiological follow-up, plain X-ray film and CT scans were performed to evaluate the status of internal fixators and cement leakage, and MRIs

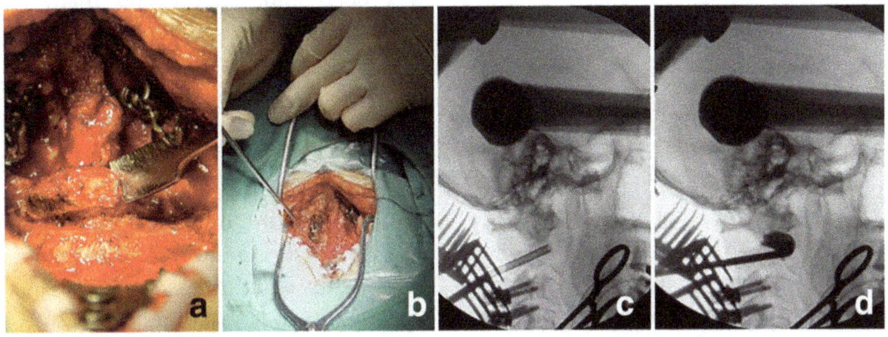

Fig. 1 The surgical process. **a** Posterior decompression. **b** Intraoperative vertebroplasty via the transpedicular approach. **c** and **d** Intraoperative vertebroplasty under C-arm guidance

were used to assess tumour recurrence. In addition, overall patient survival was calculated.

Statistical analysis

Paired *t* test was used to compare changes before and after the operation with parametric values. The t test was considered significant if the *P* value level was less than 0.05. Statistical analyses were performed using SPSS 20.0 software.

Results

Surgical result

The mean duration of operation was 182 min (range 120-255) and intraoperative blood loss ranged from 250 to 850 mL (mean 450). The mean volume of bone cement injected was 4.0 mL, ranging from 3.0 to 5.0 mL. The amount of bone cement injected was calculated by measuring the remaining amount in the syringe. The cement extravasation was observed in only 1 patient according to postoperative CT scans. However, the cement leakage event was not related to clinical symptoms.

None of the significant complications, i.e., vertebral artery (VA) or spinal cord injuries, occurred during the operation or the follow-up period. Surgical site infection was not seen in our study. One patient had a pulmonary infection that resolved with antibiotic therapy. Similarly, no hardware failure or neurological worsening occurred during the whole follow-up period. However, 1 patient developed tumour recurrence and died 1 month later.

Functional result

All patients received various extents of pain relief, which were sustained to the final follow-up period. Symptoms of myelopathy were presented in 5 patients, improved in 4 cases and remained unchanged in only 1 patient. All 6 patients who presented with radiculopathy obtained complete relief. The VAS scores and JOA scores both demonstrated improvement postoperatively (Table 2). In addition, the improvement rate of JOA was 52.4% (range: 49.6% to 57.1%). Due to the advanced stage of the tumours, all patients were prescribed oral morphine to relieve pain. The average preoperative daily dose was 125 mg (range: 80-150 mg), which decreased to an average of 60 mg (range: 50-100 mg) ($P<0.001$). The surgery significantly reduced the daily use of painkillers.

Overall survival

All patients were followed up, until they died, for an average of 12.8 (range: 3 to 29) months. The overall

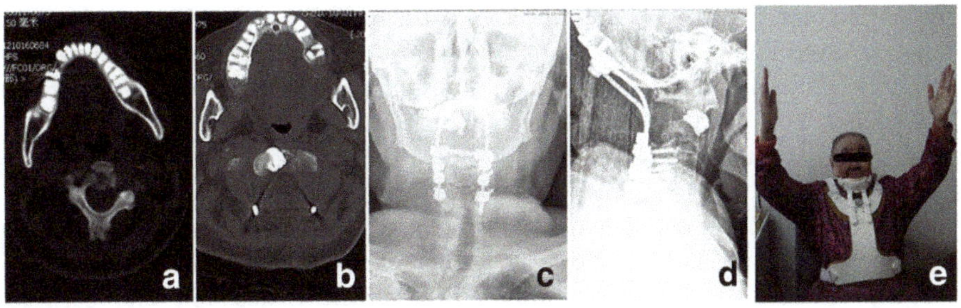

Fig. 2 A 78-year-old female with a C2 metastatic tumour, presenting with occipitocervical pain and quadriplegia, was treated with intraoperative vertebroplasty combined with posterior decompression and occipitocervical fixation in 2012. **a** and **b** Preoperative and postoperative axial CT scans. **c** and **d** Postoperative anterior, posterior and lateral radiographs. **e** The muscle power of the patient returned to normal and pain was completely relieved

Table 2 VAS and JOA outcome

$n = 10$	Pre-op	Final follow-up	P value
VAS	8 (1)	2 (1)	$P < 0.001$
JOA	10 (2)	14 (2)	$P = 0.003$

Note: All data were expressed in median (interquartile range)

median survival time was 7 months. The 6-month and 12-month survival rates were 70% and 40%, respectively. Furthermore, the mean overall survival period was 6.8 months for prostate cancer, followed by lung (7.4 months), kidney (10 months), unknown (10 months), and breast (27.5 months).

Discussion

Metastasis to the spine are commonly spread through the Batson plexus, a valveless vertebral venous complex. Additionally, the vertebral body is the most common site to be affected compared with the posterior elements [10]. In our study, all cases had an affected vertebral body of C2. The clinical picture of metastatic involvement of the upper cervical region ranges from localized pain to a variable extent of the neurological deficits and even death induced by spinal cord compression [11, 12]. Occipitocervical pain occurred in approximately 89% to 100% of patients, was not linked to daily activities and worsened in the night [13–15]. All patients in our study presented with occipitocervical pain. Furthermore, given the relatively larger sagittal diameter of the C1 and C2 level compared to the counterpart of the subaxial cervical spine, the neurological deficit was overt only in the later stages. Hence, the preoperative JOA score was 10.1 ± 2.2 in our study.

With the development of internal fixators and surgical techniques, more invasive approaches were recommended for patients with upper cervical metastases who met strict selective criteria. The aim of the surgery for upper cervical metastases was to decompress the spinal cord, reconstruct spinal stability and obtain pain relief. The main goal was improving the quality of the remaining life rather than cure the disease. Previous studies suggested that metastases to the cervical spine have a worse prognosis than metastases to other sites [16, 17]. However, a recent matched pair analysis showed that metastatic spinal cord compression had similar clinical outcomes to those of thoracic and lumbar spine metastasis in terms of postoperative survival, surgery-related complication, and pain outcome [18].

Total *en bloc* spondylectomy (TES) was widely used to avoid local recurrence of spinal metastases. However, TES also had adverse aspects, such as a longer operation time, massive blood loss and difficulty to perform in the upper cervical spine because of the distinct anatomy of the vertebral arteries and the complex bony architecture. In addition, the transoral approach to the operative field was deep and narrow and many complications may occur, such as mixed infection, speech change, tongue oedema, retropharyngeal haematoma or cerebrospinal fluid leakage [6]. Sakaura et al. [19] described that the recurrence rate was similar for palliative surgery compared with TES. In our study, we only observed one patient with recurrence.

Vertebroplasty or kyphoplasty was widely used on spinal metastases and had gained effective clinical results in patients with osteolytic spinal metastases. Recently, kyphoplasty was even applied in osteoblastic spinal metastases and caused a significant reduction of pain [20]. The mechanism of pain relief was thought to be that bone cement stopped vertebral micro- or macromovement and the destruction of pain receptors through exothermic reactions and chemical and toxic effects [21]. Percutaneous vertebroplasty (PVP) has a shorter operation period, minimal blood loss, rare intra-operative injuries and low cost [22]. The relief of pain was commensurate with an increase in activity, which in turn decreased the risk of concomitant infections and the need for further hospitalization. In our study, all patients experienced a certain extent improvement in occipitocervical pain and a decrease in VAS from 8.2 ± 0.4 to 2.3 ± 0.2. However, this method could not address the problem of spinal cord compression. Interestingly, several studies demonstrated that PMMA had an antitumoural effect, which may be due to the cytotoxicity, thermal effects and ischaemic effects [23, 24]. However, others proposed that the low recurrence rate was attributed to the short survival time rather than the antitumoural effect. Hence, the antitumoural effect needs further study. In addition, transoral PVP also had the demerits itself.

Therefore, posterior surgery combined with intraoperative vertebroplasty may be a feasible and less invasive method. Intraoperative vertebroplasty was accurate and visual to inject bone cement. In our study, cement extravasation was only detected in 1 case, but with no clinical significance (10%).This was overtly lower than PVP (51%) [25]. According to our experience, it was important that the cement injection was under high viscosity, with intraoperative fluoroscopy and preoperative evaluation of the integrity of the vertebral endplates and posterior wall of the vertebrae. Furthermore, laminectomy and removing the pedicles could provide a better way to perform vertebroplasty and the possibility of an immediate clearing of the leaked bone cement.

In our study, our patients had either impending instability or an unstable spine according to SINS, of which sensitivity and specificity was 96% and 80%, respectively [26]. If patients were in good clinical and stable oncological condition, extended posterior fixation (O-C5) was highly recommended [14]. Patients in our study were long-term bedridden and malnourished, with a mean age of 68.9 years.

In addition, the upper cervical spine lacked the support of ribs, which was different from the thoracic spine. Thus, all these factors contributed to the decision to perform an extended posterior fixation. This could achieve the maximum and most long-lasting stability. The shorter posterior fixation might later become insufficient and increases the risk of reoperation. Due to the nature of palliative surgery, we do not ordinarily perform a bone graft. This was consistent with a previous study [27].

Lung, breast and prostate cancer were the 3 main tumours that metastasized to the spine [28, 29], which accounted for 80% in our study. The average survival time of our study was 12.8 months, which was within the range of previous studies, 3-18 months [2, 30]. Patients with primary tumours from lung and prostate had the worst prognosis and a relatively shorter survival time. This was consistent with previous studies [31]. It was worth noting that postoperative radiotherapy and chemotherapy were also important in terms of prolonging life and improving the quality of life. Treatment of spinal metastases is challenging and needs multidisciplinary collaboration.

There were several limitations. First, there was the nature of the retrospective study. Second, the number of patients included was relatively limited due to the rarity of this disease. Third, there was the absence of the control group. A larger controlled study is required to identify the efficacy of this method.

Conclusion

Posterior decompression and occipitocervical fixation followed by intraoperative vertebroplasty was a safe and valuable palliative method with relatively less invasion to treat metastatic involvement of the axis.

Abbreviations

PMMA: Polymethylmethacrylate; PVP: Percutaneous vertebroplasty; SINS: Spinal Instability Neoplastic Score; TES: Total en bloc spondylectomy; VA: Vertebral artery

Acknowledgements

Not applicable.

Funding

Capital Characteristic Clinical project of Beijing Municipal Science & Technology Commission.

Authors' contributions

MS T and XJ W participated in concept development, data generation, quality control of data, data analysis and interpretation, and writing of the manuscript. YN Q, FY and P Y were responsible for data analysis and participated in the interpretation and presentation of the data. XS T and QY H were involved in concept development, quality control of data and data analysis and interpretation. All authors have read and approved the final version of the submitted manuscript.

Consent for publication

The authors have received written consent from participants to publish individual patient data (clinical information and images).

Competing interests

The authors declare that they have no competing interests.

Author details

[1]Department of Spinal Surgery, China-Japan Friendship Hospital, Beijing 100029, People's Republic of China. [2]Graduate School of Peking Union Medical College, Beijing 100730, People's Republic of China. [3]Graduate School of Beijing University of Chinese Medicine, Beijing 100029, People's Republic of China.

References

1. Ibrahim A, Crockard A, Antonietti P, Boriani S, Bunger C, Gasbarrini A, Grejs A, Harms J, Kawahara N, Mazel C, et al. Does spinal surgery improve the quality of life for those with extradural (spinal) osseous metastases? An international multicenter prospective observational study of 223 patients. Invited submission from the joint section meeting on disorders of the spine and peripheral nerves, March 2007. J Neurosurg Spine. 2008;8(3):271–8.
2. Tokuhashi Y, Matsuzaki H, Oda H, Oshima M, Ryu J. A revised scoring system for preoperative evaluation of metastatic spine tumor prognosis. Spine. 2005;30(19):2186–91.
3. Fehlings MG, David KS, Vialle L, Vialle E, Setzer M, Vrionis FD. Decision making in the surgical treatment of cervical spine metastases. Spine. 2009; 34(22 Suppl):S108–17.
4. Fourney DR, York JE, Cohen ZR, Suki D, Rhines LD, Gokaslan ZL. Management of atlantoaxial metastases with posterior occipitocervical stabilization. J Neurosurg. 2003;98(2 Suppl):165–70.
5. Fung KY, Law SW. Management of malignant atlanto-axial tumours. J Orthop Surg. 2005;13(3):232–9.
6. Frempong-Boadu AK, Faunce WA, Fessler RG. Endoscopically assisted transoral-transpharyngeal approach to the craniovertebral junction. Neurosurgery. 2002;51(5 Suppl):S60–6.
7. Mont'Alverne F, Vallee JN, Cormier E, Guillevin R, Barragan H, Jean B, Rose M, Chiras J. Percutaneous vertebroplasty for metastatic involvement of the axis. AJNR Am J Neuroradiol. 2005;26(7):1641–5.
8. Rimondi E, Rossi G, Bartalena T, Ciminari R, Alberghini M, Ruggieri P, Errani C, Angelini A, Calabro T, Abati CN, et al. Percutaneous CT-guided biopsy of the musculoskeletal system: results of 2027 cases. Eur J Radiol. 2011;77(1):34–42.
9. Kawahara N, Tomita K, Murakami H, Demura S. Total en bloc spondylectomy for spinal tumors: surgical techniques and related basic background. Orthop Clin North Am. 2009;40(1):47–63. vi
10. Eleraky M, Setzer M, Vrionis FD. Posterior transpedicular corpectomy for malignant cervical spine tumors. Eur Spine J. 2010;19(2):257–62.
11. Sciubba DM, Petteys RJ, Dekutoski MB, Fisher CG, Fehlings MG, Ondra SL, Rhines LD, Gokaslan ZL. Diagnosis and management of metastatic spine disease. A review. J Neurosurg Spine. 2010;13(1):94–108.
12. Phillips E, Levine AM. Metastatic lesions of the upper cervical spine. Spine. 1989;14(10):1071–7.
13. Mazel C, Balabaud L, Bennis S, Hansen S. Cervical and thoracic spine tumor management: surgical indications, techniques, and outcomes. Orthop Clin North Am. 2009;40(1):75–92. vi-vii
14. Papp Z, Marosfoi M, Szikora I, Banczerowski P. Treatment of C-2 metastatic tumors with intraoperative transoral or transpedicular vertebroplasty and occipitocervical posterior fixation. J Neurosurg Spine. 2014;21(6):886–91.

15. Wu X, Ye Z, Pu F, Chen S, Wang B, Zhang Z, Yang C, Yang S, Shao Z. Palliative surgery in treating painful metastases of the upper cervical spine: case report and review of the literature. Medicine. 2016;95(18):e3558.
16. Bartels RH, Feuth T, van der Maazen R, Verbeek AL, Kappelle AC, Andre Grotenhuis J, Leer JW. Development of a model with which to predict the life expectancy of patients with spinal epidural metastasis. Cancer. 2007;110(9):2042–9.
17. Sciubba DM, Gokaslan ZL, Suk I, Suki D, Maldaun MV, McCutcheon IE, Nader R, Theriault R, Rhines LD, Shehadi JA. Positive and negative prognostic variables for patients undergoing spine surgery for metastatic breast disease. Eur Spine J. 2007;16(10):1659–67.
18. Lei M, Liu Y, Yan L, Tang C, Liu S, Zhou S. Posterior decompression and spine stabilization for metastatic spinal cord compression in the cervical spine. A matched pair analysis. Eur J Surg Oncol. 2015;41(12):1691–8.
19. Sakaura H, Hosono N, Mukai Y, Ishii T, Yonenobu K, Yoshikawa H. Outcome of total en bloc spondylectomy for solitary metastasis of the thoracolumbar spine. J Spinal Disord Tech. 2004;17(4):297–300.
20. Zhang HT, Chen GD, Yang HL, Luo ZP. Percutaneous Kyphoplasty in the Treatment of Osteoblastic-related Spinal Metastases. Clin spine Surg. 2017; 30:80–4.
21. Muijs SP, van Erkel AR, Dijkstra PD. Treatment of painful osteoporotic vertebral compression fractures: a brief review of the evidence for percutaneous vertebroplasty. J Bone Joint Surg Br. 2011;93(9):1149–53.
22. Quraishi NA, Arealis G, Salem KM, Purushothamdas S, Edwards KL, Boszczyk BM. The surgical management of metastatic spinal tumors based on an Epidural Spinal Cord Compression (ESCC) scale. Spine J. 2015;15(8):1738–43.
23. San Millan Ruiz D, Burkhardt K, Jean B, Muster M, Martin JB, Bouvier J, Fasel JH, Rufenacht DA, Kurt AM. Pathology findings with acrylic implants. Bone. 1999;25(2 Suppl):85S–90S.
24. Brahimi Y, Antoni D, Buy X, Gangi A, Noel G. Bone metastases relapse after cementoplasty: case report and discussion about the combination of radiotherapy and cementoplasty. Cancer Radiother. 2016;20(2):109–14.
25. Potet J, Weber-Donat G, Curis E, Arnaud FX, Thome A, Valbousquet L, Peroux E, Geffroy Y, Bouzad C, Kervella Y, et al. Incidence of pulmonary cement embolism after real-time CT fluoroscopy-guided vertebroplasty. J Vasc Interv Radiol. 2013;24(12):1853–60.
26. Fourney DR, Frangou EM, Ryken TC, Dipaola CP, Shaffrey CI, Berven SH, Bilsky MH, Harrop JS, Fehlings MG, Boriani S, et al. Spinal instability neoplastic score: an analysis of reliability and validity from the spine oncology study group. J Clin Oncol. 2011;29(22):3072–7.
27. Quan GM, Vital JM, Pointillart V. Outcomes of palliative surgery in metastatic disease of the cervical and cervicothoracic spine. J Neurosurg Spine. 2011;14(5):612–8.
28. Sundaresan N, Boriani S, Rothman A, Holtzman R. Tumors of the osseous spine. J Neuro-Oncol. 2004;69(1-3):273–90.
29. Mesfin A, Buchowski JM, Gokaslan ZL, Bird JE. Management of metastatic cervical spine tumors. J Am Acad Orthop Surg. 2015;23(1):38–46.
30. Perrin RG, Laxton AW. Metastatic spine disease: epidemiology, pathophysiology, and evaluation of patients. Neurosurg Clin N Am. 2004;15(4):365–73.
31. Leithner A, Radl R, Gruber G, Hochegger M, Leithner K, Welkerling H, Rehak P, Windhager R. Predictive value of seven preoperative prognostic scoring systems for spinal metastases. Eur Spine J. 2008;17(11):1488–95.

Introduction of a guide based on a femoral neck section for fixation with multiple screws

Qiuliang Zhu*, Bin Xu, Jinzhu Lv and Maohua Yan

Abstract

Background: The design and application of assisted instrumentation for internal fixation of femoral neck fractures with multiple screws are still evolving. A novel guide based on a femoral neck section was designed to improve the accuracy of screw placement, and its efficacy was evaluated.

Methods: A guide based on a femoral neck section was designed for assisted fixation of femoral neck fractures with multiple screws. Femoral specimens from 10 adults (20 femurs) underwent assisted internal fixation for a femoral neck fracture with 3 cannulated screws using the new guide technique or conventional technique. The accuracy of screw orientation and entry point, the accuracy of optimal screw positioning, and drilling attempts, operative time, and fluoroscopy time were recorded.

Results: Among all 20 specimens, 60 screws were inserted successfully. Screw parallelism, operative time, and fluoroscopy time showed no statistical difference between the new guide technique and conventional technique ($P > 0.05$). The accuracy of optimal screw positioning was determined by the contained screw area ratio, distance between screws, distance from the centre of the femoral neck section, distance between screws and the femoral neck cortex, and Drilling attempts were statistical significantly better (data in the first three were larger and in the latter two was smaller) with the new guide technique, than with conventional technique ($P < 0.05$).

Conclusions: This new, two-dimensional, fluoroscopy-assisted, percutaneous guide technique enables accurate and optimal screw positioning in internal fixation of femoral neck fractures, compared with conventional technique.

Keywords: Femoral neck fracture, Internal fixation, Guide, Multiple screws, Femoral neck section

Background

Use of 3 cannulated screws has been the standard method for internal fixation of femoral neck fractures in young patients and elder adults with nondisplaced fractures. Bhandari et al. [1] queried 442 surgeons and found that 82.8% preferred cannulated screws for nondisplaced fractures, with a 17% preference for displaced fractures. Luttrell et al. [2] surveyed 272 Orthopaedic Trauma Association members regarding treatment of high-angle "vertical" femoral neck fractures, and found that 43.1% preferred cannulated screws, with or without off-axis screw placement. Some thought that optimal biomechanical stability and minimally-invasive technique could be achieved if accuracy of optimal screw placement could be maintained.

For accuracy of optimal screw placement, two-dimensional, fluoroscopy-assisted commercial guides and improved versions have focused on screw orientation and entry point. The advantage was reflected in reduction of operative and fluoroscopy time [3–5]. Three-dimensional, computer-assisted navigation systems generated more discussion on the accuracy of optimal screw positioning. Related studies showed that navigation systems were superior for parallel screw placement, had greater spread, and distributed cortical support using a femoral neck section (FNS), but the complex equipment, complicated surgical procedure, and prolonged operative time limited clinical use [6–9]. Therefore, the design and application of assisted instrumentation for internal

* Correspondence: zhuqiuliang666@163.com
Department of Orthopedics, People's Hospital of Anji, Zhejiang 313000, China

fixation of femoral neck fractures with multiple screws are still evolving.

We designed a novel instrument based on the specific anatomy of the FNS for internal fixation of femoral neck fractures, and called it "the guide of femoral neck section (GFNS)." The present study demonstrated that simulated surgery using GFNS for internal fixation of femoral neck fractures enhanced accuracy of screw position in 10 dry cadaveric femurs under two-dimensional fluoroscopic (C-arm) control, compared with conventional technique.

Methods

The shape of FNS (Fig. 1): FNS was roughly elliptical. The long axis of the ellipse rotated forward formed an angle with the coronal plane of the proximal femur called the femoral neck torsion angle (FNTA), with a value of approximately 20° [10–12]. Thus, iatrogenic perforation could occur in the posterosuperior and anterorinferior quadrants of the lateral femoral wall during internal fixation of the femoral neck with multiple screw insertions [13].

GFNS (Fig. 2): GFNS is made of titanium, making it lighter (about 220 g) and easier to fix, and consists of a carrier with angle logo and a cuboid. The cuboid is 6-cm long, with 8 rows and 11 columns of parallel guide holes, each with diameter of 2.6 mm, with 2.4-mm hole spacing. The bottom row includes a centre hole and adjustment holes, for connection with the single hole at the inner surface of the cuboid, with hole spacing of 2. 1 mm. At the top of the lateral aspect of the cuboid, the angle logo carrier is set on an angle with the bottom row centre hole at the centre of acircle 0 °- 40 ° to the left and right, matching the FNTA. Anon-parallel mounting hole with 2 mm diameter is below the logo. The elevation angle of the inner surface of the cuboid is 130°, matching the surface soft tissue of the thigh.

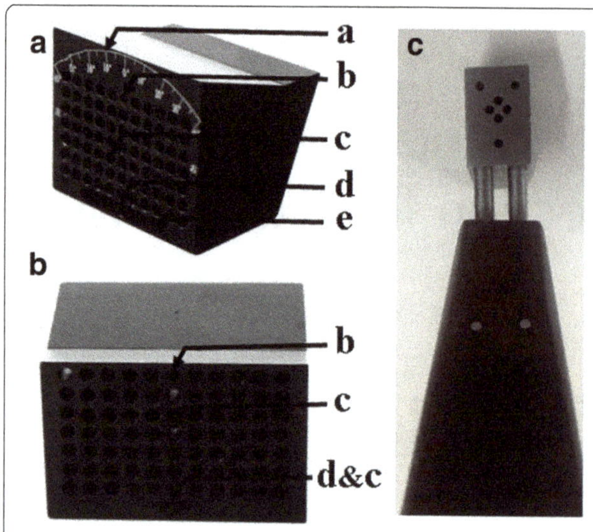

Fig. 2 Overall view (A) and medial surface (B) of the guide of femoral neck section (GFNS) and the conventional guide (C) supplied by manufacturer for internal fixation of femoral neck fracture: a angle logo; b mounting hole; c parallel guide hole; d centre hole; e adjust hole

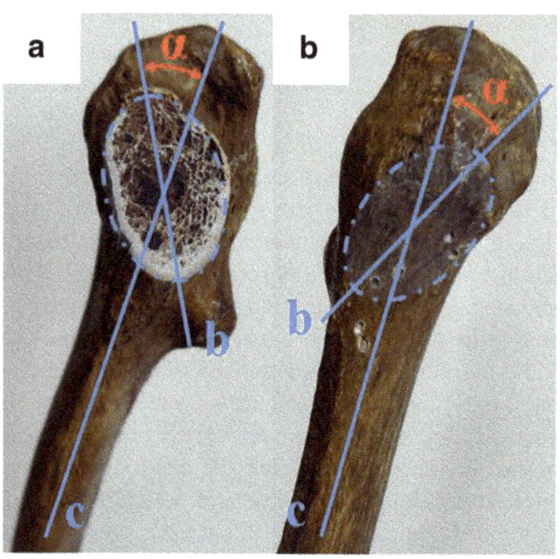

Fig. 1 Picture showed that the shape of femoral neck section (FNS) related with the medial aspect (A) and lateral surface (B) of proximal femur: The ellipse represented FNS; ∠α Femoral neck torsion angle; b Long axis of FNS; c Coronal axis of proximal femur

Specimens: 20 dry, intact femoral specimens from 10 adults (7 men and 3 women; average age 47.5 years, range, 37 to 58y) were obtained from the Department of Anatomy, Zhejiang University School of Medicine. No visible deformity and no defects on distal and proximal femurs were observed. Two different operating techniques were used in the right or left femur of one adult, and were grouped using random numbers. The long and short axis of the femoral neck and the FNTA were calculated (Table 1). All femurs were mounted on an operating table and covered with a surgical drape to imitate soft tissue for percutaneous screw placement.

Technique description

Conventional AO technique: First, the guide wire was freehand inserted from the trochanteric lateral wall to the femoral head under image intensification, to ensure

Table 1 The general data of 20 femurs

Group	Number	Femoral neck section (mm)		Femoral neck torsion angle (deg.)
		Long axis	Short axis	
DFNS	10	36.67 ± 3.62*	25.57 ± 2.44*	19.30 ± 3.01*
Conventional	10	37.08 ± 2.74	24.98 ± 2.95	20.12 ± 2.36

*$P > 0.05$ Comparing with Conventional Group

that the guide wire was located on the central axis of the femoral neck in anteroposterior (AP) and lateral views. Second, a manufacturing guide (Chuangsheng, Jiangsu, China. Figure 2C) was placed over the wire through its central hole, with selection of 3 appropriate outer holes for greater spread close to the femoral neck cortex, and an inverted triangle was constructed, followed by insertion of 3 guide-wires. The manufacturing guide and the central wire were removed, with verification of the correct placement of wires using C-arm fluoroscopy in AP and lateral views. Finally, 7.3-mm cannulated screws were inserted over the guide wires.

GFNS technique (Fig. 3): With C-arm fluoroscopy guidance, the first wire (inferior wire) was placed freehand in the middle or slightly posterior region of the femoral neck on the lateral view, parallel to the femoral neck axis and attached to the femoral calcar on AP projection. GFNS was placed over the wire through the central hole on the bottom (wire anteversion could be adjusted using the adjustment holes on the bottom, if needed). A 2-mm Kirschner wire was inserted along the fixing hole to the greater trochanter to fix the GFNS. Assuming 20°placement relative to the pre-measured long axis of the femoral neck, 2-4 guide wires inserted into GFNS but outside the femoral cortex were adjusted using AP and lateral images. The edge of FNS was confirmed and the projection of FNS (red line) on GFNS was drawn. The screw positions were located such that hole placement was within 3 mm of the femoral neck cortex (considered excellent, red spot); location in the middle of the FNS is considered good (blue spot) and location outside the red line is poor (white spot). Using the "excellent" guide-holes, 3 were selected for maximum distance from each other. The second wire (anterosuperior) was inserted and placed near the anterosuperior cortex. The third guide wire (medial and posterior wire) was placed close to the medial and posterior cortex. After making sure the guide wires were in ideal positions using lateral and AP images, appropriate length screws were used for fixation.

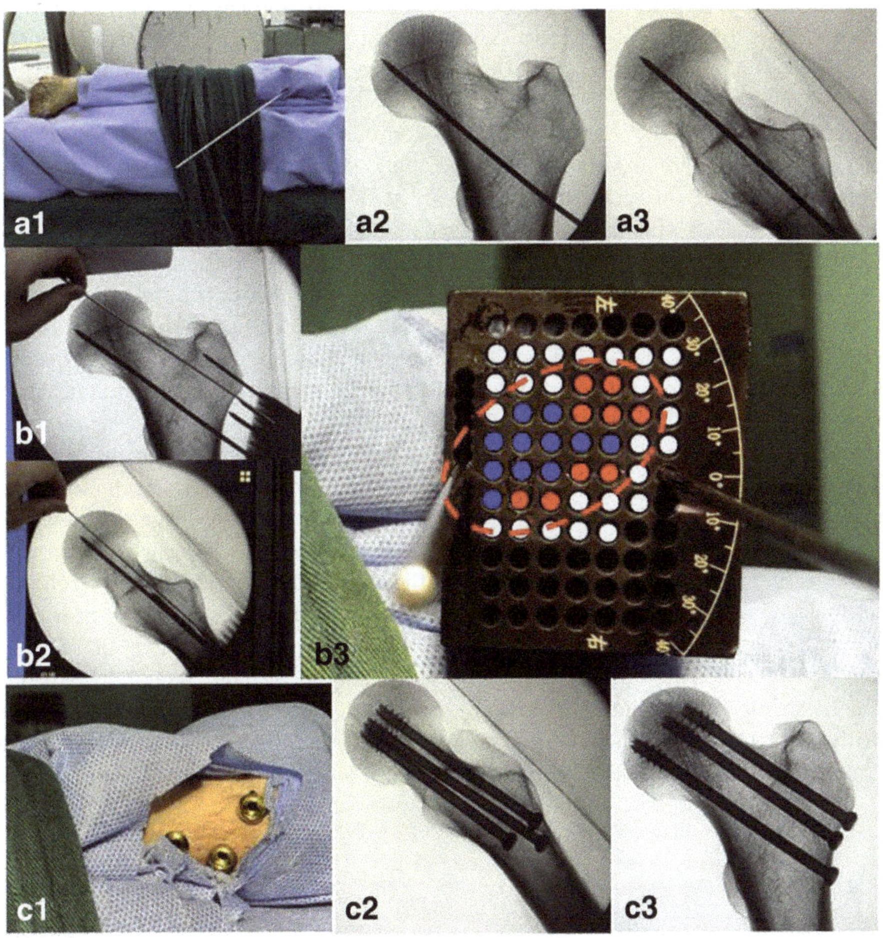

Fig. 3 The operative process with GFNS: Inserted the first guide-wire into appropriate place with freehand under AP and lateral views (A). Fixed and draw FNS on GFNS (red ellipse) by related data, identify the excellent hole (red point), good hole (blue point) and bad hole (white hole). After making sure the guide wires were in ideal positions by lateral and AP image, fixed with appropriate length screws

Measurement parameters

Screw accuracy of orientation and placement: Screw parallelism, distance between screws (defined as total length of connecting lines between 3screw centres), screw area ratio (consisting of the triangle screw area and the FNS area), distance from the centre of FNS to the screws, and distance from the screws to the femoral neck cortex were measured by a resident who was blinded to the surgical procedure.

Operative time was measured from the moment of initial wire placement to the point when the 3screws were finally fixed. Fluoroscopy time was determined by the number of fluoroscopic single shots during the operation. Perforation for insertion of a guide wire into the femoral trochanteric wall, including drill reversal, was counted as a drilling attempt.

Statistical methods

Analyses were performed using SPSS version 16.0 statistical software (SPSS Inc., Chicago, IL, USA). Values are presented as mean ± SD. The paired Student's t-test was used to compare the measured parameters between 2groups, and p values ≤0.05 were considered statistically significant.

Results

Among all 20 cases, 60 screws were inserted successfully. The results of measurements of screw placement accuracy are presented in Table 2 and the parameters measured during surgery are shown in Table 3.

Screw parallelism on AP and lateral imaging showed no statistical difference between the 2 groups. Screw area ratio, distance between screws, distance from the centre of FNS, and distance from screws to femoral neck cortex in GFNS group were statistical significantly better (data in the first three were larger and in the latter was smaller) than those in the conventional group ($P < 0.05$). The operative and fluoroscopy times showed no statistical difference between the 2 groups. Drilling attempts with GFNS were significantly fewer than with use of the conventional guide.

Discussion

Despite superior biomechanical properties and greater fracture stability with sliding hip screws in internal fixation of femoral neck fractures, use of 3 cannulated screw has been the most popular technique, as superior torsion stability, minimally-invasive insertion, and limited disruption of femoral head blood supply may be lead to better postoperative function [1, 2, 14–16]. Greater screw spread, screw placement close to the cortex for cortical support, and parallel screw placement reflect screw placement accuracy, and are thought to achieve greater stability and decreased risk of nonunion of the fracture [17–20]. For accuracy of screw placement, a series of guides and instruments have been developed to assist the surgical procedure. However, there is no consensus regarding the optimal instrument or guide for both screw precision and minimum invasion.

Two-dimensional, fluoroscopy (C-arm)-assisted guides have been used to improve the technique of femoral neck fracture repair, with improved versions reported by Xia et al. and Yuenyongviwat et al. in synthetic femurs [3, 5]. These studies showed the benefits of reduced operative time and radiation exposure but did not consider screw position accuracy. Yin et al. and Tai et al. described a novel guide/screw (as a sleeve) that was simple in structure and easy to apply, and that facilitated accuracy of guide wire orientation and entry point. However, the accuracy of optimal screw distribution in FNS has not been considered [4, 21]. Three-dimensional, computer-assisted navigation systems have been increasingly studied [6–9]. Previous literature demonstrated that the accuracy of screw placement distribution, which included the guide wire entry point, orientation, and optimal screw distribution, was improved with use of navigation systems, but the radiation exposure and operative time were increased. In addition, the complex equipment and complicated surgical procedure (scanning, registering, planning, etc.) limited the use in clinical practice.

The advantage of the accuracy associated with screw placement distribution in femoral neck fixation was demonstrated in the present study. This is because the projection of FNS is clearly drawn on the GFNS using the following process: with reference to the first guide wire placement, based on previous measured data (FNTA, long and short axis of FNS) or historical information, the AP and lateral intraoperative images were integrated to form the real-time shape of FNS. Therefore, according to the requirement of optimal screw position for greater spread and cortical support, the

Table 2 Comparative analysis of screw placement accuracy in 2 groups

group	Screw parallelism (deg.)		Screw area ratio	DS (mm)	DC (mm)	DSC (mm)
	AP	Lateral				
conventional	1.73 ± 0.62	1.52 ± 0.60	0.16 ± 0.02	10.38 ± 3.91	8.02 ± 1.51	4.21 ± 1.31
GFNS	1.68 ± 0.83#	1.61 ± 0.57#	0.29 ± 0.02*	16.87 ± 4.12*	11.05 ± 1.94*	2.40 ± 1.24*

GFNS guide of femoral neck section, *DS* distance between screws, *DC* distance between the centre of FNS, *DSC* distance between screw to femoral neck cortex
*$P < 0.05$; #$p > 0.05$ Comparing with Conventional group

Table 3 comparative analysis of parameters during surgical procedure in 2 groups

Group	Operation time (min)	Fluoroscopic time (no.)	Drilling attempt (no.)
conventional	24.80 ± 9.12	8.89 ± 2.17	7.97 ± 3.60
GFNS	27.33 ± 7.61#	9.51 ± 1.72#	4.81 ± 1.27*

*$P < 0.05$; #$p > 0.05$ Comparing with Conventional group

"excellent" guide-holes were easily confirmed on visible projection (Fig. 3B3). In this study, the screw area ratio, distance between screws, and distance from the centre of FNS were greater in GFNS compared with those in the conventional group, and the distance from the screws to the femoral neck cortex was smaller. The results were better than with use of two-dimensional, fluoroscopy-assisted guide technique and similar three-dimensional, computer-assisted systems described in previous literature [7, 8]. The improvement in accuracy of screw orientation and entry point were not considered in the design of GFNS; as a result, the screw parallelism showed no significant difference between the 2 groups in this study.

This study used fewer drilling attempts with GFNS technique than with conventional technique. Multiple drilling attempts might weaken the bone and lead to unsuccessful adjustment, as the guide wire may slide along the initial drilling track. With GFNS technique, before guide wire insertion, a virtual extended drilling track from the "excellent" hole was confirmed on fluoroscopy (Fig. 3), limiting the need for further drilling attempts. The results are analogous to those in previous reports with computer-assisted navigation technique [7, 8]. The reduction in drilling attempts shortened the operative and fluoroscopy time, but the time needed to verify the "excellent" drilling holes on GFNS was prolonged; therefore, the operative and fluoroscopy times were similar in the GFNS group and conventional groups.

The limitation of this study is the inadequacy of soft tissue coverage and femoral neck fracture simulation models. In clinical practice, thicker soft tissue coverage may interfere with the accuracy of screw orientation and entry point. Use of a surgical drape to simulate thin soft tissue probably oversimplified the complexity of the surgical procedure, suggesting that the percutaneous GFNS technique should not be used in obese patients. To simplify the trial process, we used the intact proximal femur to simulate anatomic reduction of a femoral neck fracture. This may have decreased the difficulty of the surgical procedure, but had little influence on the trial results.

Conclusion

Two-dimensional, fluoroscopy-assisted, percutaneous GFNS technique can increase the accuracy of optimal screw positioning and can decrease drilling attempts in internal fixation of femoral neck fractures. There was no difference in accuracy of screw orientation and entry point or operative and fluoroscopy time compared with conventional technique. The percutaneous GFNS technique should be considered for use in clinical practice, as three-dimensional, computer-assisted navigation systems have not been widely employed.

Abbreviations

AP: Anteroposterior view; DC: Distance between the centre of FNS; DS: Distance between screws; DSC: Distance between screw to femoral neck cortex; FNS: Femoral neck section; FNTA: Femoral neck torsion angle; GFNS: Guide of femoral neck section

Acknowledgements

There have no acknowledgements.

Funding

This subject have received funding from the Science Technology Department of Zhejiang Province (government).

Authors' contributions

ZQL made the conception and design, and was a major contributor in writing the manuscript. XB performed the operation and completed the acquisition of data. LJZ and YMH analyzed and interpreted the data. All authors stated that the manuscript had been read and approved.

Consent for publication

Not applicable.

Competing interests

The authors declare that they have no competing interests.

References

1. Bhandari M, Tornetta P, Hanson B, Swiontkowski MF. Optimal internal fixation for femoral neck fractures: multiple screws or sliding hip screws? J Orthop Trauma. 2009;23:403–9.
2. Luttrell K, Beltran M, Collinge CA. Preoperative decision making in the treatment of high-angle "vertical" femoral neck fractures in young adult patients. An expert opinion survey of the Orthopaedic Trauma Association's (OTA) menbership. J Orthop Trauma. 2014;28(9):e221–5.
3. Yuenyongviwat V, Tuntarattanapong P, Tangtrakulwanich B. A new adjustable parallel drill guide for internal fixation of femoral neck fracture: adevelopmental and experimental study. BMC Musculoskelet Disord. 2016; 17:8. https://doi.org/10.1186/s12891-015-0845-2.
4. Yin WJ, Xu HT, Xu PJ, Hu T, An ZQ, Zhang CQ, Sheng JG. A novel guidewire aiming device to improve the accuracy of guidewire insertion in femoral neck fracture surgery using cannulated screw fixation. Med Sci Monit. 2016; 22:2893–9. https://doi.org/10.12659/MSM.897120

5. Xia SL, Wang ZP, Wang MH, et al. Self-designed femoral neck guide pin locator for femoral neck fractures. Orthopedics. 2014;37(1):19–23.
6. Kendoff D, Hüener T, Citak M, Geerling J, Maier C, Wesemeier F, Krettek C. Implementation of a new navigated parallel drill guide for femoral neck fractures. Comput Aided Surg. 2006;11(6):317–21.
7. Müller MC, Belei P, Pennekamp PG, Kabir K, Wirtz DC, Burger C, Weber O. Three- dimensional computer-assisted navigation for the placement of cannulated hip screws. A pilot study. Int Orthop. 2012;36(7):1463–149. https://doi.org/10.1007/s00264-012-1496-7.
8. Hamelinck HKM, Haagmans M, Snoeren MM, Biert J, Vugt ABV, Frolke PM. Safety of computer-assisted surgery for cannulated hip screws. Clin Orthop Relat Res. 2006;455:241–5.
9. Wang JQ, Zhao CP, Su YG, Zhou L, Hu L, Wang TM, Wang MY. Computer-assisted navigation systems for insertion of cannulated screws in femoral neck fractures: a comparison of bi-planar robot navigation with optoelectronic navigation in a Synbone hip model trial. Chin Med J. 2011; 124(23):3906–11.
10. Kate BR. Anteversion versus torsion of the femoral neck. Acta Anat (Basel). 1976;94(3):457–63.
11. Maximilian JH, Andreas P, Anne S, et al. Determination of femoral neck angle and torsion angle utilizing a novel three-dimensional modeling and analytical technology based on CT datasets. PLoS One. 2016;11(3):e0149480.
12. Zhu QL, Yuan JF, Zhao LL, et al. Discerning the femoral neck anteversion (FNA) from the torsion angle on 3D CT. China J Orthop Traumatol. 2012; 25(10):831–3.
13. Zhang YQ, Chang SM, Huang YG, et al. The femoral neck safe zone: a radiographic simulation study to prevent cortical perforation with multiple screw insertion. J Orthop Trauma. 2015;29(5):178–82.
14. Gupta M, Arya RK, Kumar S, Jain VK, Sinha S, Naik AK. Comparative study of multiple cancellous screws versus sliding hip screws in femoral neck fractures of young adults. Chin J Traumatol. 2016;19(4):209–12.
15. The FAITH Investigators. Fixation using alternative implants for the treatment of hip fracture (FANTH): design andrationale fora multi-centre randomized trial comparing sliding hip screws and cancellous screws on revision surgery rates and quality of life in the treatment of femoral neck fractures. BMC Musculoskelet Disord. 2014;15:219. https://doi.org/10.1186/1471-2474-15-219.
16. Mosseri J, Trinquart L, Nizard R, Ravaud P. Meta-analysis of a complex network of non-pharmacological interventions: the example of femoral neck fracture. PLoS One. 2016;11(1):e0146336. https://doi.org/10.1371/journal.pone.0146336.
17. Ye Y, Hao J, Mauffrey C, et al. Optimizing stability in femoral neck fracture fixation. Orthopedics. 2015;38(10):625–30.
18. Gurusamy K, Parker MJ, Rowlands TK. The complications of displaced intracapsular fractures of the hip: the effect of screw positioning and angulation on fracture healing. J Bone Joint Surg Br. 2005;87(5):632–4.
19. Tan V, Wong KL, Born CT, Harten R, DeLong WG Jr. Two-screw femoral neck fracture fixation: a biomechanical analysis of 2 different configurations. Am J Orthop (Belle Mead NJ). 2007;36(9):481–5.
20. Zdero R, Keast-Butler O, Schemitsch EH. A biomechanical comparison of two triple-screw methods for femoral neck fracture fixation in a synthetic bone model. J Trauma. 2010;69(6):1537–44. https://doi.org/10.1097/TA.0b013e3181efb1d1.
21. Tai TW, Lien FC, Lee PY, Jou IM, Lin CJ, Huang YH. Using a cannulated screw as a drill guide and sleeve: a simple technique for multiple-screw fixation for intracapsular femoral neck fracture. Orthopedics. 2010;33(8). https://doi.org/10.3928/01477447-20100625-05.

Vertebral column decancellation in Pott's deformity: use of Surgimap Spine for preoperative surgical planning, retrospective review of 18 patients

Wenhao Hu[1†], Xuesong Zhang[1†], Jiayi Yu[2], Fanqi Hu[1], Hao Zhang[1] and Yan Wang[1*]

Abstract

Background: In the late stage of Spinal tuberculosis, the bony destruction and vertebral collapse often leads to significant kyphosis, presenting clinically as a painful gibbus deformity, with increased instability, vertebral body translations and increased risk of neurologic involvement. Vertebral column decancellation is thought to be suitable for most patients with severe rigid kyphosis. Surgimap Spine, could offer a pragmatic graphical method for the surgical planning of osteotomies. The aim of this study was to evaluate the efficacy of Vertebral column decancellation planned preoperatively with the computer software-assistance in the patients with Pott's kyphosis.

Methods: Between May 2012 and May 2015, 18 patients with Pott's kyphosis underwent the Vertebral column decancellation using Surgimap Spine for preoperative surgical planning. Preoperative and postoperative Konstam's angle, sagittal vertical angle, lumbar lordosis, thoracic kyphosis, pelvic tilt and pelvic incidence were measured. Visual analog scale and American Spinal Injury Association were documented.

Results: The Konstam's angles decreased from 88.1° (range, 70–105°) preoperatively to 18.5° (range, 7–31°) ($P < 0.01$). All patients reached the physiological limits at the final follow-up. The mean VAS score was reduced from preoperative 7.1 (range, 6–8) to 1.8 (range, 1–3, $P < 0.01$) and the ODI improved from 65.8% (range, 58–74%) to 20.2% (range, 12–38%, $P < 0.01$). At final follow-up, there was radiographic evidence of solid fusion at the osteotomy site and fixed segments in all patients. Neurological function improved from ASIA scale D to E in 5 patients. The patients were followed up for 30.4 months on average.

Conclusion: Vertebral column decancellation is an effective treatment option for severe Pott's kyphosis. The surgical planning software Surgimap Spine can be a reliable and helpful tool that provides a simplified method to evaluate and analyze the spino-pelvic parameters and simulate the osteotomy procedure. According to individual character, the appropriate surgery strategy should be selected.

Keywords: Pott's deformity, Vertebral column decancellation, Surgimap Spine, Vertebral column resection, Pedicle subtraction osteotomy, Sagittal vertical angle, Visual analog scale, American spinal injury association

* Correspondence: yanwang301spine1@sina.com
†Equal contributors
[1]The Department of Orthopedics, Chinese PLA General Hospital, Fuxing Rd. 28, Haidian District, Beijing, China
Full list of author information is available at the end of the article

Background

Tuberculosis (TB) is an important cause of morbidity and mortality and The People's Republic of China has the second highest incidence of TB worldwide [1]. Spinal TB is the most common form of extra-pulmonary TB, and accounts for nearly half of all musculoskeletal TB cases [2]. Delayed diagnosis is common and patients treated with anti-TB chemotherapy alone or with simple surgical debridement without fusion may develop disease reactivation [3]. In the late stage, bony destruction and vertebral collapse often leads to significant kyphosis, presenting clinically as a painful gibbus deformity, with increased instability, vertebral body translations and increased risk of neurologic involvement [4].

Anterior, posterior, and combined anterior and posterior (AP) procedures show various degrees of success for correcting kyphosis in TB [5–7]. The late correction of stiff and sharp angular deformities (more than 60°) is only feasible with three-column osteotomy or vertebral column resection (VCR) [8]. Pedicle subtraction osteotomy (PSO), 30–40°recommended as a safe range [9], is usually insufficient to correct severe kyphosis. Despite VCR is considered as the most powerful tool for correction of spinal deformity, this technique is a formidable last resort technique for severe fixed sagittal and coronal deformity due to its technical difficulty and potential for complications [10]. Vertebral column decancellation (VCD), a combination of the eggshell technique, Smith-Petersen osteotomy (SPO), PSO and VCR, is thought to be suitable for most patients with severe rigid kyphosis. VCD technique is a simpler and safer osteotomy procedure, while VCR provides the greatest amount of correction with higher risk of complications.

To obtain satisfactory outcomes, preoperative surgical planning must be performed carefully [11]. Several mathematical formulas [12–16] and graphical methods [17–20] for preoperative planning have been described. For most methods, however, global sagittal balance was not accurately evaluated and the effect of spinopelvic parameters, especially pelvic incidence (PI) and pelvic tilt (PT), were neglected, leading to postoperative undercorrection. Moreover, these are relatively complex for routine clinical use. An optimal approach to quantifying sagittal parameters and planning precise correction is lacking [21]. It is important to select the best surgery strategy in accordance with the characteristics of individuals. Surgimap Spine, a free computer program (Nemaris Inc., New York, NY, USA) that integrates spine-related measurement and tools for surgical planning in combination with knowledge gained from the published literature, offers a pragmatic graphical method for the surgical planning of osteotomies [21]. Surgimap Spine has been used in the surgical treatment of kyphosis deformity secondary to ankylosing spondylitis, [22] osteomalacia, or inappropriate past fusion procedures [23]. The software not only provides a practical and convenient method to analyze preoperative sagittal parameters and predict proper postoperative alignment, but also simulates the procedure of osteotomy to help surgeons select appropriate surgical methods.

In the current study, we evaluate the efficacy of VCD technique planned preoperatively with computer software-assistance, in the patients with Pott's kyphosis.

Methods

Twenty six patients diagnosed with Pott's kyphosis were admitted to our department from May 2012 to May 2015. Diagnosis was based on radiographic examination, laboratory tests and histopathology. This study was conducted with approval from the Ethics Committee of Chinese PLA General Hospital and was performed in accordance with the Declaration of Helsinki. Written informed consent was obtained from all participants. The indications for surgery were as follows: (1) healed tubercular kyphosis; (2) low back pain refractory to conservative treatment; (3) inability to lie down in dorsal position; (4) increasing neurological deficit. Patients with active infection and who cannot tolerate surgery due to poor cardiopulmonary function were excluded. Surgical planning was performed using Surgimap Spine, development of an accurate plan required determination of parameters such as thoracic kyphosis (TK) and lumbar lordosis (LL). Patients whose fused vertebrae involved both T12 and L1, in which TK and LL cannot be measured, were also excluded.

Anteroposterior and lateral spine radiographs, 3-dimensional computed tomography (3-D CT) reconstruction, and magnetic resonance imaging (MRI) were available for all patients (Fig. 1). The plain radiographs were taken in the standing position for all patients. One American Spinal Injury Association (ASIA) C patient (Case 7) had standing radiographs 2 weeks prior to admission. At that time, he had ASIA grade D and could stand unsupported. However, he declined surgery because of financial issues. However, his neurological deficits rapidly progressed and his ASIA grade deteriorated to C before surgery. Lateral radiography was processed with Surgimap Spine. Local and global sagittal parameters were measured and analyzed including Konstam's angle [24], sagittal vertical angle (SVA),lumbar lordosis (LL), thoracic kyphosis(TK), pelvic tilt (PT), pelvic incidence (PI). Preoperative planning was executed in 3 phases [22]: 1. Spino- pelvic parameters were measured and analyzed (Fig. 2a). 2. Identification of the site of osteotomy and the location of wedge-shaped resection (Fig. 2b). The level of osteotomy wasselected with these fused vertebrae treated as one targeted vertebra. 3. Simulation of the osteotomy and evaluation of

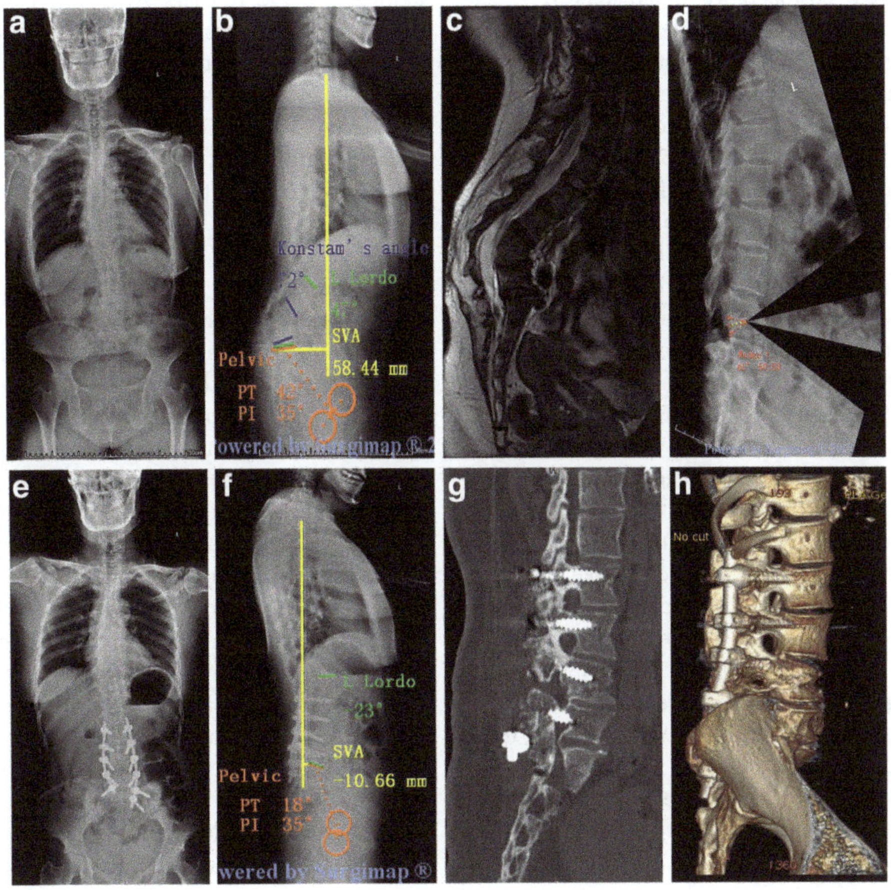

Fig. 1 A 38-year-old man with Kyphotic deformity secondary to spinal Tuberculosis suffers from severe back pain and numbness in the left lower extremity. Pre-operative radiographs (**a**, **b**) and MRI (**c**) show that the apex of kyphosis is located at L3. L4, The Konstam's angle was 72°, PI-LL: 82°, PT: 42°, The simulation of VCD osteotomy in Surgimap (**d**). The kyphosis was corrected to only 11° immediately after the surgery,PI-LL: 8°, PT: 18° (**e**, **f**, **g**). Three-dimensional reconstruction demonstrated that solid fusion of resection site was achieved 3.5 years postoperatively (**f**)

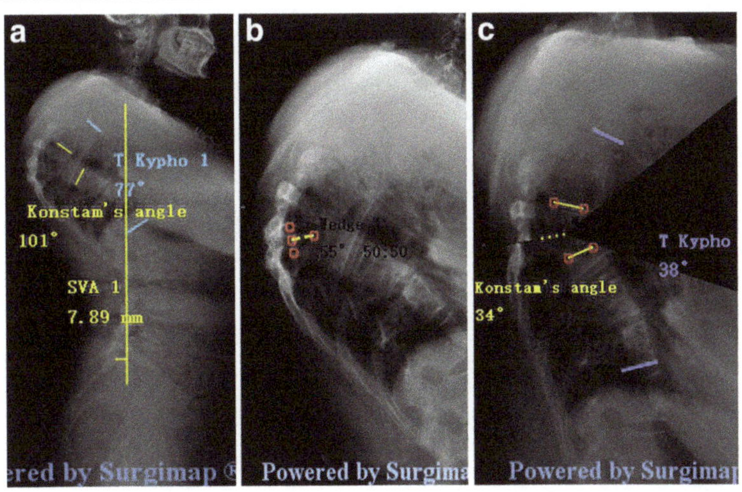

Fig. 2 The process of Surgimap Spine for surgical planning. **a** Measurement the preoperative sagittal parameters: Konstam's angle, SVA,TK; **b** Identification the site of osteotomy and the location of wedge-shaped resection. **c** Simulation of the osteotomy and evaluate the Surgimap-predicted postoperative parameters to check if VCD is sufficient for the correction

Surgimap-predicted postoperative parameters (Fig. 2c). This phase consists in applying a resection angle at the posterior column using the "Wedge Osteotomy" tool and graphically tracing the osteotomy directly on the radiographic image. The success of correction according to physiological limits was set at: SVA < 5 cm, TK < 50° (the apical vertebra was located at the thoracic level), PI-LL < 10° and PT < 20° [25] (the apical vertebra was located at the lumbar level). It was checked if VCD was sufficient for the correction. If not, VCR was applied. Of note, VCR, as the most aggressive method, allows a greater correction angle. However, it is a technically demanding and exhausting procedure with higher risk of major complications. It is generally the last-resort technique for severe spinal deformity [10].

Of 26 patients, 2 were excluded because of poor cardiopulmonary function and inability to tolerate surgery; 3 only had mild back pain without a neurological deficit, and refused surgery; and 3 were advised to have VCR surgery because their severe kyphosis was found to be inappropriate for VCD, based on osteotomy simulation using Surgimap. In all, 18 patients of whom (8males, 10 females; mean age 37.7 years) underwent the VCD technique. The mean Konstam's angle was 88.1° (ranging from 70° to 105°). Among the 18 patients, 5 patients had previously underwent an initial debridement without fusion. Neurologic deficits were assessed according to the American Spinal Injury Association (ASIA) grading system as follows: ASIA E, 10 cases; ASIA D, 7 cases; and ASIA C, 1 case. Pain was assessed using the visual analogue scale (VAS). Disability status was assessed using the Oswestry Disability Index (ODI). All patients' radiological and clinical records were recorded preoperatively, postoperatively and during the last follow-up period. Operation time, blood loss, and osteotomy levels were noted (Table 1).

Operative technique

All surgeries were performed under monitoring of somatosensory-evoked potentials, transcranial motor-evoked potentials, and free-running electromyography. Under general anesthesia, the patient was placed prone on the operating table, and a standard posterior middle incision was made at the predetermined level. The spine was exposed by dissection lateral to the costotransverse joint at the thoracic level and the lumbar transverse process. The segmental vessels were coagulated using electric cauterization and hemostatic gauze. Pedicle screws (Weigao Orthopedic,Shandong, China) were then placed three levels above and below the damaged vertebral body by freehand technique. C-arm fluoroscopy was used to confirm the appropriate insertions.

Then, VCD was performed (Fig. 3). A pedicle probe and drill were used to create and enlarge relatively normal pedicle holes in the target vertebra on both sides of the pedicles. Cancellous bone of the posterior half of the osteotomy column was adequately removed through the

Table 1 Demographic and clinical data

Patient	Age/Sex	ASIA	Osteotomy level	Instrumented levels	Operative time (min)	Blood loss (ml)	Follow-up (mon)
1	32/M	E	T8-T9	T6-T8,T10-T12	230	450	28
2	41/M	D	T9-T11	T7-T9,T12-L2	260	600	34
3	28/F	E	L2-L3	T12-L2,L4-S1	210	430	30
4	35/M	D	T9-T10	T7-T9,T11-L1	200	450	32
5	37/F	D	L1-L2	T11-L1,L3-L5	220	500	29
6	33/F	E	L1-L2	T11-L1,L3-L5	230	400	31
7	39/M	C	T8-T9	T6-T8,T10-T12	230	420	27
8	44/F	D	T10-T12	T8-T10,L1-L3	220	480	26
9	29/M	E	L1-L2	T11-L1,L3-L5	240	500	29
10	40/F	D	T10-T12	T8-T10,L1-L3	260	550	30
11	36/M	E	L2-L3	T12-L2,L4-S1	200	430	35
12	44/F	D	T10-T12	T8-T10,L1-L3	220	500	31
13	43/F	E	T11-T12	T8-T11,L1-L3	240	580	36
14	35/F	E	T9-T10	T6-T9,T11-L1	210	460	29
15	46/F	D	T11-T12	T9-T11,L1-L3	220	420	28
16	38/M	E	L3-L4	L1-L3,L5-S1	240	500	34
17	42/M	E	L1-L2	T11-L1,L2-L4	200	430	31
18	36/F	E	T8-T9	T6-T8,T10-T12	220	450	28

ASIA indicates American Spinal Injury Association

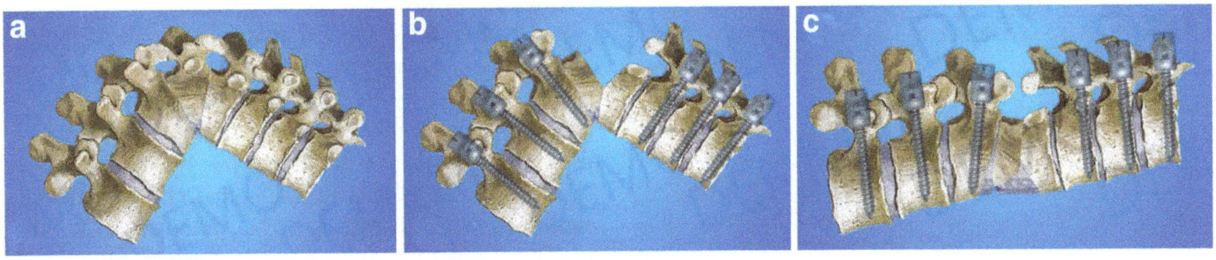

Fig. 3 VCD osteotomy for Pott's deformity. **a** Pott's Kyphotic deformity **b** A wedge-shaped posterior column was removed **c** The anterior column was opening when the posterior wedge space was closed

pedicle holes, using a rongeur and curette. A high-speed drill was used to thin the anterior cortex and lateral walls of the vertebral body and linear fractures of the anterior cortex were created using an osteotome. Then the spinal canal was opened laterally, and the posterior elements including the spinous process, bilateral lamina, transverse process, and the adjacent facet joints were removed. After removing the posterior cortical bone of the osteotomized vertebra, the kyphotic spine was corrected using gentle manual force,and was stabilized with a temporary rod. The operating table and position of the patient were adjusted for correction.

During the correction procedure, an anterior opening wedge was created and the hinge was located at the border of the anterior and medial column. VCD technique is a "Y" type osteotomy rather than a "V" type osteotomy (PSO) (Fig. 4). The posterior interlaminar fusion was completed over the fixed segments with residual autogenous bone. After confirmation of absent soft or bony compression, a drainage tube was placed in the surgical field, and the wound was closed in layers.

Statistical analysis

All statistical analysis was performed with SPSS v19.0 software (SPSS Inc., Chicago, Illinois). Paired t tests were used to determine significant changes between data that were collected preoperatively and postoperatively; the Wilcoxon signed rank test was used as a nonparametric alternative for which the required conditions were not satisfied, and the one-way ANOVA test was performed to compare mean values of three samples. p-value < 0.05 was considered statistically significant.

Result

VCD osteotomy was performed in all patients according to preoperative surgical planning. All patients completed follow-up of 30.4 months on average, ranging from 26 to 36 months. The average operation time was 225 min (range, 200–260 min) with a mean intraoperative blood loss of 475 mL (range, 400–600 mL). The Konstam's angles decreased from 88.1° (range, 70–105°) preoperatively to 18.5° (range, 7–31°) at the final follow-up ($P < 0.01$). All patients reached the physiological limits and the preoperative and last follow-up data for the 18 patients are shown in Table 2.

The mean VAS score decreased from a preoperative 7.1 (range, 6–8) to 1.8 (range, 1–3, $P < 0.01$) and the ODI improved from 65.8% (range, 58–74%) to 20.2% (range, 12–38%, $P < 0.01$). At final follow-up, there was radiographic evidence of solid fusion at the osteotomy site and fixed segments in all patients. Neurological function improved from ASIA scale D to E in 5 patients.

Dural tears were encountered in two cases that underwent an initial debridement, and were successfully repaired with 6–0 Prolene suture. No deep wound infection was identified. One patient had transient partial neurological deficit post-operatively and recovered completely within 3 months. To make a comprehensive comparison between VCD and VCR and PSO, we retrospectively reviewed 51 patients with Pott's kyphosis who

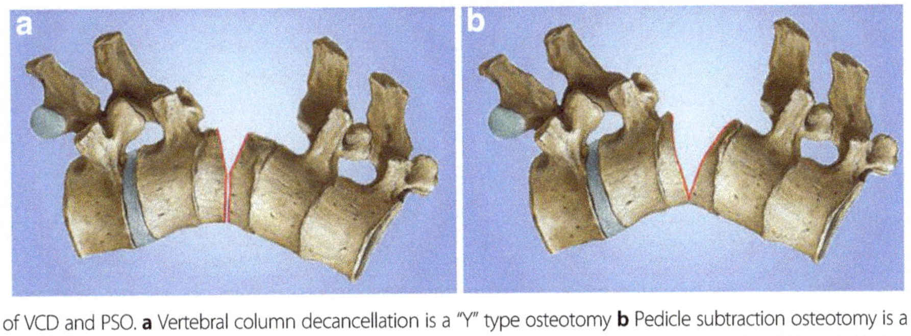

Fig. 4 Comparison of VCD and PSO. **a** Vertebral column decancellation is a "Y" type osteotomy **b** Pedicle subtraction osteotomy is a "V" type osteotomy

Table 2 The preoperative and last follow-up data

Parameters	Pre-operative	Post-operative	*p*-value
Konstam's angle(°)	88.1	18.5	<0.001
TK(°)[a]	76.9	31.1	<0.001
PI-LL(°)[b]	78.7	5.7	<0.001
PT(°)[b]	43	14.3	<0.001
SVA(cm)	5.3	2.4	<0.001
VAS	7.1	1.8	<0.001
ODI(%)	65.8	20.2	<0.001

TK thoracic kyphosis, *PI* pelvic incidence, *LL* lumbar lordosis, *PT* pelvic tilt, *SVA* sagittal vertical angle, *VAS* visual analogue score, *ODI* oswestry disability index
[a]$n = 11$, measured when the apical vertebra was located at the thoracic level;
[b]$n = 7$, measured when the apical vertebra was located at the lumbar level

underwent three-column osteotomies (PSO, $n = 23$; VCD, $n = 18$, VCR, $n = 10$) between May 2010 and May 2015 in our department by 2 spinal deformity surgeons. All the patients completed a minimum of 2 years of follow-up. The data comparing radiological and clinical outcomes in the PSO, VCD, and VCR groups are shown in Table 3.

Discussion

TB spondylitis can lead to significant osteolysis and collapse of the vertebral bodies, resulting in hyperkyphosis and tethering of the spinal cord [26]. Late stages of rigid hyperkyphosis are difficult to treat [8]. The sharp angular hyperkyphosis often requires complex three-column osteotomies. Currently, the one-stage posterior approach is most often used for minimizing the risk of injury to anterior vascular and visceral structures. PSO, the most popular osteotomy technique, has been applied for progressive TB thoracic and thoracolumbar kyphosis. The osteotomy should be limited to 30–40° as a safe single segment range; otherwise, the spinal cord is excessively shortened and distorted [27]. Although VCR or its variation, posterior-only VCR, can provide the greatest amount of surgical correction when compared to all other spinal osteotomy types [28], its use is limited due to its high inherent neurological risk related to instability induced during correction of the malformation [29, 30]. The complication rate has been estimated as high as 59% for posterior VCR [31].

Therefore, we prefer the VCD technique. This technique allows greater correction angles than PSO, and is a simpler and safer procedure with lower risk of complications compared with VCR. The main challenge for VCD is in determining the exact location of the hinge intraoperatively. The location of the hinge differs and the postoperative correction angle is variable. Until now, the surgeon's experience was the determinant. To solve this challenge, Surgimap was used for preoperative planning and C-arm technique was used to confirm the appropriate position. VCD is a newer technique, with insufficient data on long-term outcomes for assessment

Table 3 Comparison of the PSO, VCD, VCR group in radiological and clinical outcomes

	VCD	PSO	VCR	*p*-value
Patients	18(8 M,13F)	23(12 M,11F)	10(6 M, 4F)	
Mean age (yrs) (range)	37.7(29 to 46)	35.6(25 to 43)	41.2(31 to 48)	0.23
Preoperative Konstam's angle(°)	88.1(70–105)	63.5(52–81)	96.4(82–131)	0.04
Follow-up Konstam's angle(°)	18.5(7–31)[&]	16.3(8–29)[&]	32.1(18–42)[&]	0.02
Preoperative SVA(cm)	5.3(3.6–5.9))	4.5(2.2–5.1)	5.7(3.3–6.2)	0.31
Follow-up SVA(cm)	2.4(1.2–4.1)[&]	1.5(1.2–4.1)[&]	3.4(2.2–5.1)[&]	0.27
Preoperative TK(°)*	76.9(53–96)	65.2(51–85)	84.8(73–113)	0.03
Follow-up TK(°)*	14.3(10–23)[&]	16.3(12–32)[&]	32.5(24–62)[&]	0.02
Preoperative PI-LL(°)[#]	78.7(53–89)	62.3(42–74)	83.5(65–96)	0.01
Follow-up PI-LL(°)[#]	5.7(3–9)[&]	6.1(2–10)[&]	9.4(5–17)[&]	0.01
Operating time (mins)	225(200–260)	237(200–280)	370(320–400)	0.03
Loss of blood (ml)	475(400–600)	420(380–600)	625(500–980)	0.02
Complications (n)(%)	3(16.7)	4(17.4)	3(30)	0.03
Time of hospitalization(d)	11.3(7–17)	10.5(7–15)	15.2(10–21)	0.43
Preoperative VAS	7.1(6–9)	7.3(6–9)	8.4(7–9)	0.12
Follow-up VAS	1.8(1–3)[&]	1.5(1–4)[&]	4.1(3–7)[&]	0.02
Preoperative ODI(%)	65.8(59–84)	63.6(57–81)	74.8(65–89)	0.24
Follow-up ODI(%)	20.2(15–41)[&]	21.1(16–38)[&]	35.6(25–51)[&]	0.03

VCD vertebral column decancellation, *PSO* pedicle subtraction osteotomy, *VCR* vertebral column resection, *TK* thoracic kyphosis, *PI* pelvic incidence, *LL* lumbar lordosis, *SVA* sagittal vertical angle, *VAS* visual analogue score, *ODI* oswestry disability index. [&]< 0.05 vs. preoperative data; *$n = 11$, measured when the apical vertebra was located at the thoracic level ; [#]$n = 7$,measured when the apical vertebra was located at the lumbar level.

of effectiveness. As our medical team follows up all patients, more long-term outcomes of VCD technique for spinal deformity will be reported.

Of note, no way is perfect. VCD is not suitable for all deformities. Our maximum preoperative Konstam's angle was 105°. VCR, as the most aggressive method, is still recommended for some severe kyphosis despite of the high risk of complications. Thus, it is important to select the appropriate individual treatment. The surgeon-developed surgical planning software, Surgimap Spine, is increasingly popular among spine surgeons. It offers a pragmatic and systematic approach involving evaluation of important spinopelvic parameters and simulation of spinal osteotomy with the goal of optimal treatment. As VCD technique is a "Y" type osteotomy, the Wedge Osteotomy tool was used in surgical planning using Surgimap. The portion of the wedge-shaped resection was determined by two lines consisting of three points. The anterior point was located at the border of the anterior and medial column. The cephalad and caudad junction points of the pedicle and vertebral body were selected as the posterior points of the upper and lower resection line. The wedge shape was set to a 50:50 angle bisector. Upon application of the osteotomy, the image was modified directly: the wedge shape portion was removed, the posterior column closed, and the anterior column opened (Fig. 1d and Fig. 5d). Then, the key parameters were measured to determine whether sagittal alignment was restored to the normal physiological limits. Subsequently, the optimal surgical strategy was decided. Intraoperatively, it was essential to determine the anterior point of the wedge-shaped resection. Generally, the length between the anterior point and the pedicle is measured in Surgimap; after placing the pedicle screw above and below the damaged vertebral body, a pedicle probe with appropriate depth was inserted into the targeted vertebral body through the pedicle hole. C-arm fluoroscopy confirmed the exact location of the probe and the anterior point was determined. A high-speed drill was used to enlarge the pedicle hole both cephalad and caudad, until the corresponding walls

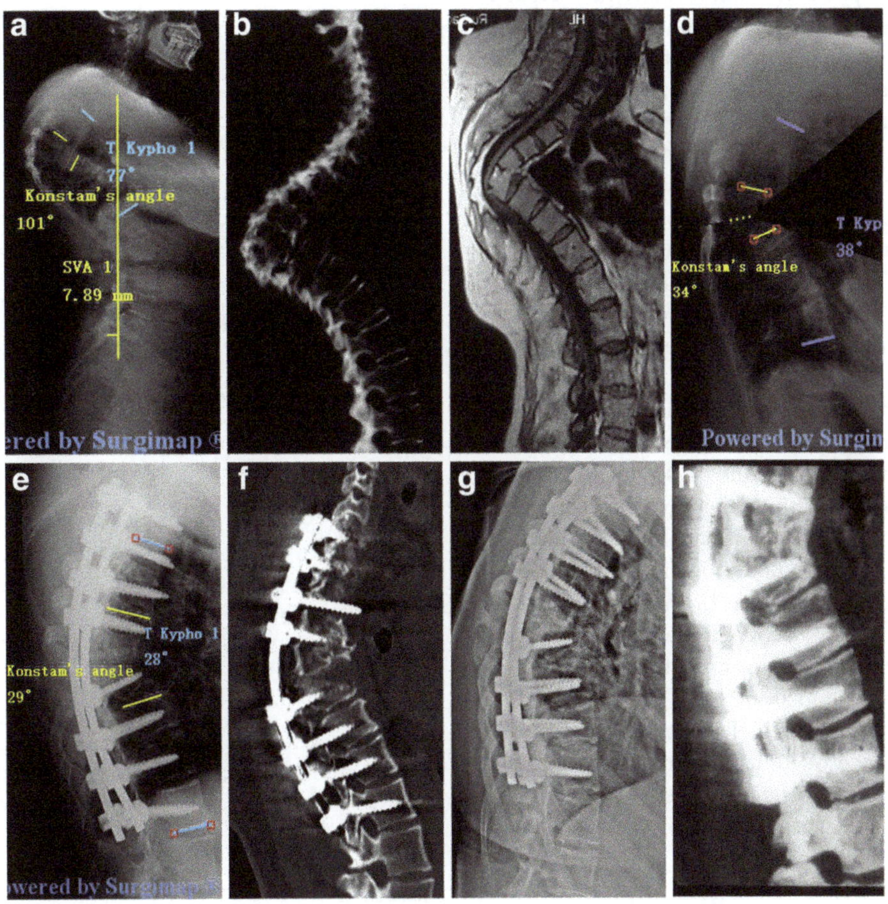

Fig. 5 A 36-year-old patient with Pott's deformity. The patient's main complaints were increasing neurological deficit and cosmetic issues. Pre-operative radiographs (**a**), CT (**b**) and MRI (**c**) show that the apex of kyphosis is located at T6-T9, The Konstam's angle was 101° and the TK was 77°. The simulation of VCD osteotomy in Surgimap (**d**). The Konstam's angle was corrected to 29° and the TK was 28° immediately after the surgery (**e**, **f**). 28 months follow-up X-ray (**g**) and CT (**h**) scan show a solid fusion

were penetrated. The three points of the wedge-shaped resection were determined intraoperatively. Good surgical planning requires exact and full evaluation of sagittal alignment. Surgimap not only measures global and local key parameters, but also takes compensatory mechanisms used in an effort to maintain the trunk and the effect of spinopelvic parameters into account. As a geometrical method, Surgimap allows the surgeon to introduce given angular corrections at any given point of the spine and mimic the surgical maneuvers on preoperative X-rays, thus providing an estimate of the postoperative results. Its novel approach provides a virtual preview of the result of a surgical procedure, and allows the surgeon to evaluate the amount of correction needed and to determine its potential effect. Moreover, Surgimap, an open source archive system and software, is very easy to learn and convenient to use. It is an effective and practical tool for spine surgeons. In 2014, Yunus Atici et al. [23] used Surgimap Spine to evaluate the efficacy of two-level PSO osteotomy, and concluded that computer software (Surgimap) seems to fail as an assisting method in the preoperative surgical planning of sagittal plane deformities, since its incapability of estimation the amount of bleeding and the possible buckling of the spinal cord. In my opinion, however, The main purpose of surgical planning for a spine deformity is to analyze the coronal and sagittal alignment and evaluate the effects of predicted surgical technique in order to choose the best procedure for a given patient. In the current study, Surgimap was used to measure pre- and postoperative spinal parameters and to simulate an osteotomy procedure. The geometrical changes of spinopelvic parameters help surgeons select the optimal osteotomy. It's very helpful and useful method regarding the aspect. The amount of bleeding and spinal cord buckling are influenced by a number of factors, including patient coagulation function, duration of the operation, and the surgeon's experience and skill. Thus, it is difficult to predict outcomes with any existing method and further research is needed. The other weak point of the software is that it is not possible to consider the reciprocal changes that may occur in the unfused segment [21]. In the current study, we found that all patients achieved the satisfactory photographic clinical outcomes as planned before surgery. The reason may be that the main problem in patients with TB kyphosis is the imbalance in local parameters and the compensatory change of unfused segments in the direction of global sagittal balance. When using Surgimap Spine, surgeons should be aware of the following points: first, all angle and length parameters must be measured precisely, because a small error has a large effect on the outcome. Second, before measuring any length, image calibration must be performed. The surgeon draws a line on the image and then defines the realistic length of the line. Third, it is important to make sure that preoperative planning is consistent with surgery, so X-ray or CT should be performed intraoperatively to verify that the location of osteotomy is as planed with Surgimap.

Conclusion

VCD is an effective treatment option for severe Pott's kyphosis. The Surgimap Spine surgical planning software can be a reliable and helpful tool that provides a simplified method to evaluate and analyze the spino-pelvic parameters and simulate the osteotomy procedure. The appropriate surgical strategy should be selected according to individual findings.

Abbreviations

AP: Anterior and posterior; LL: Lumbar lordosis; MRI: Magnetic Resonance Imaging; ODI: Oswestry Disability Index; PI: Pelvic incidence; PSO: Pedicle subtraction osteotomy; PT: Pelvic tilt; SPO: Smith-Petersen osteotomy; SVA: Sagittal vertical angle; TK: Thoracic kyphosis; VAS: Visual analogue score; VCD: Vertebral column decancellation; VCR: Vertebral column resection

Acknowledgements

The authors thank the medical team and all the Participants for their support in this study.

Funding

None.

Authors' contributions

All authors have read and approved the final manuscript. WHH was involved in the study design, data collection, drafting and revising of the manuscript. XSZ was involved in the study design, analysis and interpretation of the data, drafting and revising of the manuscript. JYY was involved in the study design, data collection. FQH was involved in the data collection. HZ was involved in the analysis and interpretation of data. YW was involved in the study design, drafting and revising of the manuscript and has given final approval.

Consent for publication

Not applicable.

Competing interests

The authors declare that they have no competing interests.

Author details

[1]The Department of Orthopedics, Chinese PLA General Hospital, Fuxing Rd. 28, Haidian District, Beijing, China. [2]Department of Renal cancer and Melanoma, Peking University Cancer Hospital, Fucheng Rd. 28, Haidian District, Beijing, China.

References

1. Wang HT, Zhang J, Ji LC, You SH, Bai Y, Dai W, Wang ZY. Frequency of tuberculosis among diabetic patients in the People's Republic of China. Ther Clin Risk Manag. 2014;10:45–9.
2. Yao DC, Sartoris DJ. Musculoskeletal tuberculosis. Radiol Clin N Am. 1995;33(4):679–89.

3. Cheung WY, Luk KD. Clinical and radiological outcomes after conservative treatment of TB spondylitis: is the 15 years' follow-up in the MRC study long enough? European Spine J. 2013;22(Suppl 4):594–602.
4. Jain AK, Aggarwal PK, Arora A, Singh S. Behaviour of the kyphotic angle in spinal tuberculosis. Int Orthop. 2004;28(2):110–4.
5. Song JF, Jing ZZ, Chen B, Ai ZS, Hu W. One-stage anterolateral surgical treatment for lumbosacral segment tuberculosis. Int Orthop. 2012;36(2):339–44.
6. Pang X, Wu P, Shen X, Li D, Luo C, Wang X. One-stage posterior transforaminal lumbar debridement, 360 degrees interbody fusion, and posterior instrumentation in treating lumbosacral spinal tuberculosis. Arch Orthop Trauma Surg. 2013;133(8):1033–9.
7. He Q, Xu J. Comparison between the antero-posterior and anterior approaches for treating L5-S1 vertebral tuberculosis. Int Orthop. 2012;36(2):345–51.
8. Boachie-Adjei O, Papadopoulos EC, Pellise F, Cunningham ME, Perez-Grueso FS, Gupta M, Lonner B, Paonessa K, King A, Sacramento C, et al. Late treatment of tuberculosis-associated kyphosis: literature review and experience from a SRS-GOP site. European Spine J. 2013;22(Suppl 4):641–6.
9. Kawahara N, Tomita K, Kobayashi T, Abdel-Wanis ME, Murakami H, Akamaru T. Influence of acute shortening on the spinal cord: an experimental study. Spine. 2005;30(6):613–20.
10. Suk SI, Kim JH, Kim WJ, Lee SM, Chung ER, Nah KH. Posterior vertebral column resection for severe spinal deformities. Spine. 2002;27(21):2374–82.
11. Schwab FJ, Patel A, Shaffrey CI, Smith JS, Farcy JP, Boachie-Adjei O, Hostin RA, Hart RA, Akbarnia BA, Burton DC, et al. Sagittal realignment failures following pedicle subtraction osteotomy surgery: are we doing enough?: clinical article. J Neurosurg Spine. 2012;16(6):539–46.
12. Boulay C, Tardieu C, Hecquet J, Benaim C, Mouilleseaux B, Marty C, Prat-Pradal D, Legaye J, Duval-Beaupere G, Pelissier J. Sagittal alignment of spine and pelvis regulated by pelvic incidence: standard values and prediction of lordosis. European Spine J. 2006;15(4):415–22.
13. Kim YJ, Bridwell KH, Lenke LG, Rhim S, Cheh G. An analysis of sagittal spinal alignment following long adult lumbar instrumentation and fusion to L5 or S1: can we predict ideal lumbar lordosis? Spine. 2006;31(20):2343–52.
14. Schwab F, Lafage V, Patel A, Farcy JP. Sagittal plane considerations and the pelvis in the adult patient. Spine. 2009;34(17):1828–33.
15. Lafage V, Schwab F, Vira S, Patel A, Ungar B, Farcy JP. Spino-pelvic parameters after surgery can be predicted: a preliminary formula and validation of standing alignment. Spine. 2011;36(13):1037–45.
16. Berjano P, Langella F, Ismael MF, Damilano M, Scopetta S, Lamartina C. Successful correction of sagittal imbalance can be calculated on the basis of pelvic incidence and age. European Spine J. 2014;23(Suppl 6):587–96.
17. Pigge RR, Scheerder FJ, Smit TH, Mullender MG, van Royen BJ. Effectiveness of preoperative planning in the restoration of balance and view in ankylosing spondylitis. Neurosurg Focus. 2008;24(1):E7.
18. Ondra SL, Marzouk S, Koski T, Silva F, Salehi S. Mathematical calculation of pedicle subtraction osteotomy size to allow precision correction of fixed sagittal deformity. Spine. 2006;31(25):E973–9.
19. Van Royen BJ, De Gast A, Smit TH. Deformity planning for sagittal plane corrective osteotomies of the spine in ankylosing spondylitis. European Spine J. 2000;9(6):492–8.
20. Le Huec JC, Leijssen P, Duarte M, Aunoble S. Thoracolumbar imbalance analysis for osteotomy planification using a new method: FBI technique. European Spine J. 2011;20(Suppl 5):669–80.
21. Akbar M, Terran J, Ames CP, Lafage V, Schwab F. Use of Surgimap spine in sagittal plane analysis, osteotomy planning, and correction calculation. Neurosurg Clin N Am. 2013;24(2):163–72.
22. Hu W, Yu J, Liu H, Zhang X, Wang Y. Y shape Osteotomy in Ankylosing Spondylitis, a prospective case series with minimum 2 year follow-up. PLoS One. 2016;11(12):e0167792.
23. Atici Y, Akman YE, Balioglu MB, Kargin D, Kaygusuz MA. Two level pedicle substraction osteotomies for the treatment of severe fixed sagittal plane deformity: computer software-assisted preoperative planning and assessing. European Spine J. 2016;25(8):2461–70.
24. Konstam PG, Blesovsky A. The ambulant treatment of spinal tuberculosis. Br J Surg. 1962;50:26–38.
25. Legaye J, Duval-Beaupere G, Hecquet J, Marty C. Pelvic incidence: a fundamental pelvic parameter for three-dimensional regulation of spinal sagittal curves. European Spine J. 1998;7(2):99–103.
26. Charles YP, Schuller S, Sfeir G, Steib JP. Vertebral column resection for thoracic hyperkyphosis in Pott's disease. European Spine J. 2014;23(3):708–10.
27. Gertzbein SD. Scoliosis Research Society. Multicenter spine fracture study. Spine. 1992;17(5):528–40.
28. Enercan M, Ozturk C, Kahraman S, Sarier M, Hamzaoglu A, Alanay A. Osteotomies/spinal column resections in adult deformity. European Spine J. 2013;22(Suppl 2):S254–64.
29. Liu S, Zhang N, Song Y, Song Z, Zhang L, Liu J, Xie E, Wu Q, Hao D. Radiologic comparison of posterior release, internal distraction, final PSO and spinal fusion with one-stage posterior vertebral column resection for multi-level severe congenital scoliosis. BMC Musculoskelet Disord. 2017;18(1):270.
30. Leatherman KD, Dickson RA. Two-stage corrective surgery for congenital deformities of the spine. J Bone Joint Surg Br Vol. 1979;61-B(3):324–8.
31. Lenke LG, Newton PO, Sucato DJ, Shufflebarger HL, Emans JB, Sponseller PD, Shah SA, Sides BA, Blanke KM. Complications after 147 consecutive vertebral column resections for severe pediatric spinal deformity: a multicenter analysis. Spine. 2013;38(2):119–32.

14

Does Hallux valgus impair physical function?

Akinobu Nishimura[1,2*], Naoya Ito[1], Shigeto Nakazora[3], Ko Kato[3], Toru Ogura[4] and Akihiro Sudo[1]

Abstract

Background: The relationships between radiographic hallux valgus (HV) and various physical functions independent of knee osteoarthritis (KOA) were examined among residents of a mountain village in Japan.

Methods: Study participants were recruited from mountain village residents aged ≥50 years. Participants' height, weight, and body mass index (BMI) were measured, and baseline data, including age, sex, and foot pain, were obtained using interviews and questionnaires. Radiography of the feet and knees was performed to assess the presence of HV (HV angle ≥20°) and KOA (Kellgren-Lawrence grade ≥ II). Grip strength, 6-m walk at usual and maximum speeds, single-leg stance time, and stand up from a chair time were evaluated as physical function performance tests. Plantar pressure patterns were also examined.

Results: Moderate-severe HV (HV angle ≥30 degrees), impaired grip strength and maximum walking speed, and painful HV reduced usual and maximum walking speeds independent of KOA. Hallux plantar pressure decreased according to the HV angle. Hallux plantar pressure was significantly lower in painful HV than in the no HV feet or painless HV.

Conclusions: Moderate-severe HV deformity and HV-related pain impaired physical function independent of KOA. By controlling the pain and severe deformity of HV by treatments such as surgery, the physical function of HV patients might be improved.

Keywords: Hallux valgus, Physical function, Knee osteoarthritis, Epidemiology elderly

Background

Hallux valgus (HV) is one of the most common foot deformities in adults; it is characterized by abnormal angulation, rotation, and lateral deviation of the hallux at the first metatarsophalangeal joint [1]. The prevalence of HV has been reported as 58% in adult women and 25% in adult men (HV angle ≥15°) in the USA [2], 28.4% in adults (self-reported hallux valgus) in the UK [3], 64.7% (HV angle ≥15°) in a Korean population aged between 40 and 69 years [4], and 29.8% (HV angle > 20°) in a Japanese population aged over 65 years [5]. While HV is basically regarded as a structural deformity, there is debate surrounding the association between abnormal foot structure and related disability. Several studies have found no association between HV and disability, such as the Timed Up & Go test [6], walking speed [6–8], and balance tests [8]. On the other hand, increasing HV severity has been shown to negatively impact health-related quality of life and self-reported function [4, 9, 10], and HV has been linked to balance function [11] and increased fall risk in older adults [12, 13].

Our cohort study started in 1997 to investigate the epidemiology of knee osteoarthritis (KOA) [14, 15] and osteoporosis [16]. The study of HV started from 2009, and we reported the prevalence and risk factors for HV [5]. In our study [5], HV showed a significant relationship with KOA. In general, KOA is associated with lower physical extremity function [17]. However, no report has shown a relationship between HV and physical function after taking into account the existence of KOA.

The purpose of this cross-sectional study was to investigate whether HV affects physical function after taking into account KOA among elderly persons.

* Correspondence: meiten@clin.medic.mie-u.ac.jp
[1]Departments of Orthopaedic Surgery, Mie University Graduate School of Medicine, 2-174 Edobashi, Tsu City, Mie 514-8507, Japan
[2]Departments of Orthopaedic and Sports Medicine, Mie University Graduate School of Medicine, Tsu City 514-8507, Mie, Japan

Methods

Individuals aged ≥50 years were recruited from among the inhabitants of a mountain village in Japan. The main industry is the forest industry. The study was started in 1997, with follow-up every two years. All studies were held at the local hospital. This present study analyzed data from the seventh to tenth biennial examinations in 2009, 2011, 2013, and 2015, respectively. The number of participants in 2009, 2011, 2013, and 2015 was 314, 221, 223, and 204, respectively. For individuals who participated in two or more iterations of these four examinations, only the data from the earliest examination were included. For example, if an individual participated in 2009, 2011 and 2015, the data in 2009 were included in this study. Exclusion criteria were rheumatoid arthritis and past history of surgery for hallux valgus. A total of 562 participants (194 male, 368 female) were part of this study.

Before direct examination, a baseline questionnaire including name, age, sex, medical history, and pain was sent to the participants. Direct examination consisted of physical measurement, medical interview, physical examination, X-rays, blood tests, and physical function tests. We measured participants' height and body weight, and the body mass index (BMI) was calculated as weight (kg) divided by height squared (m^2). Medical interviews and physical examinations were performed one-on-one by orthopedic surgeons. Bunions were detected by inspection and palpation. Painful bunions were determined by applying pressure to the bunion. Knee X-rays were taken with the knee in a fully extended standing position. KOA was scored according to the Kellgren-Lawrence grading system [18]. Radiographic KOA was defined as grade ≥ 2. We took foot X-rays with participants standing upright with both feet on the cassette, as described by Saltzman [19]. The HV angle, which is formed by the bone axes of the first metatarsal and the first proximal phalanx, was consistently measured by the same examiner [20]. These imaging data were analyzed using Image J version 1.37 software (National Institutes of Health, Bethesda, MD, USA). Hallux valgus was deemed to be present if the HV angle was ≥20°, according to the Japanese Orthopaedic Society criteria. HV severity was classified as mild (≥20° and < 30°), moderate (≥30° and < 40°), or severe (≥40°). Participants reporting pain in the right or left hallux on most days of a month for at least 1 month in the previous year were classified as having right or left hallux pain. Participants with radiographic HV and self-reported hallux pain or a painful bunion checked by orthopedic surgeons were defined as having painful HV. If a participant had left hallux pain and right radiographic HV, that participant was not included in the painful HV group.

The physical function tests consisted of grip strength, 6-meter (m) walk at usual and maximum speeds, single-leg stance time with eyes open, and stand up from a chair time. Grip strength was measured using a Takei 5401 handgrip dynamometer (Takei Scientific Instruments Co., Niigata, Japan). The participants stood and held the dynamometer with the arm at right angles and the elbow by the side of the body. Two measurements were done for each hand. We used the average of the highest measurement of each hand. Participants were instructed to walk at their usual and maximum speeds. We measured the time was with a stopwatch. The data for plantar pressure patterns were taken using a gait analyzer (Walk Way MW 1000; Anima, Tokyo, Japan). This analyzer has a sheet length of 2.4 m, and this sheet was set in the middle of the 6-m walkway. In order to investigate how strongly participants pushed the ground with the great toe, the percentage of the hallux footprint in the whole footprint was examined. Each footprint was picked up using the gait analyzer (Fig. 1), and the hallux

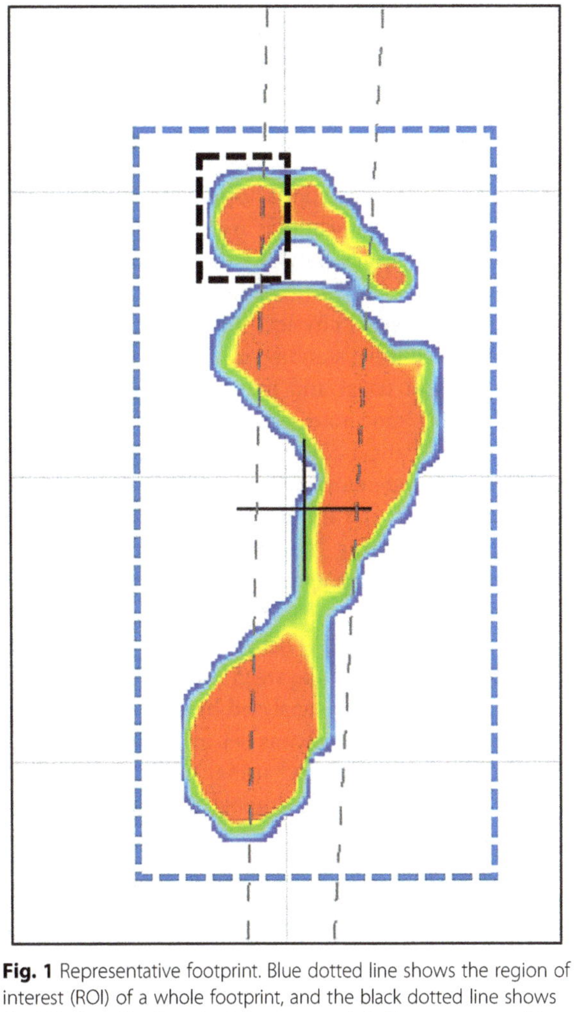

Fig. 1 Representative footprint. Blue dotted line shows the region of interest (ROI) of a whole footprint, and the black dotted line shows the ROI of a hallux footprint for pressure analysis. The percentage of the hallux footprint is calculated as the hallux footprint pressure divided by the whole footprint

footprint and the whole footprint were enclosed, and the pressure was analyzed with analysis software (PREDAS MD-1000; Anima, Tokyo, Japan). The percentage of the hallux footprint was defined as [hallux footprint]/[whole footprint]. Examining the foot pressure patterns, the percentage of hallux footprint was checked, from which was calculated hallux pressure/whole foot pressure. We measured single-leg stance time with eyes open for both legs, and we calculated the average time. Participants were instructed to stand on one leg while elevating the contralateral limb. The time until the raised leg was touched on the floor was measured. The maximum time was 60 seconds (s). The stand up from a chair time was the time taken to stand from a chair five times with hands folded in front of the chest and feet flat on the floor.

Based on the worse HV angle in their feet, the participants were classified into a no HV group (HV angle < 20°) and an HV group (HV angle ≥20°). They were then classified into a no HV-mild HV group (HV angle < 30°) and a moderate-severe HV group (HV angle ≥30°). Finally, they were classified into a painful HV group and a no HV or painless HV group.

Statistical analysis

Means ± standard deviations were calculated for variables unless otherwise noted. Associations among the physical characteristics between the groups were determined by the unpaired *t*-test or Fisher's exact test. The relationships between physical functions (grip strength, single-leg stance time, standing up from a chair, and 6-m walking times at usual and maximum speeds) and HV (HV angle ≥20°), moderate-severe HV (HV angle ≥30°), or painful HV (HV angle ≥20° with pain) were evaluated by multiple linear regression analysis both after adjusting for age, sex, and BMI, and for age, sex, BMI, and KOA. The correlation between the HV angle and the percentage of the hallux footprint was analyzed by Pearson's correlation coefficient. Percentages of the hallux footprint between no HV foot and HV, between no HV-mild HV and moderate-severe HV, and between no HV foot or painless HV and painful HV were analyzed by the Mann-Whitney test. The significance level was set at 5% in a two-tailed test. All data were analyzed using PASW Statistics for Windows version 22 (IBM, Armonk, NY, USA).

Results

The overall prevalence of definite radiographic HV was 28.4% (160/562); it was 13.4% (26/194) in males and 36.4% (134/368) in females. The rates of mild, moderate, and severe HV in the 562 participants were 16.5% (93/562), 9.3% (52/562), and 2.7% (15/562), respectively.

Table 1 shows the physical characteristics of the participants who fulfilled the criteria. The HV group had 160 participants (26 male, 134 female), whereas the no HV group had 402 participants (168 male, 234 female). Participants in the HV group were significantly shorter and older than those in the no HV group, and the percentages of female and KOA were significantly higher in the HV group than in the no HV group. When participants were classified into a no HV-mild HV group and a moderate-severe HV group, participants in the moderate-severe HV group were significantly shorter and lighter than those in the no HV-mild HV group, and the percentages of female and KOA were significantly higher in the moderate-severe HV group than in the no HV-mild HV group. When participants were classified into a no HV or painless HV group and a painful HV group, the participants in the painful HV group were significantly shorter than those in the no HV or painless HV group, and the percentages of female and KOA were significantly higher in the painful HV group than in the no HV or painless HV group.

The relationships between HV and physical functions are shown in Tables 2 and 3. Table 2 shows the results after adjustment for age, sex, and BMI, and Table 3 shows the results after adjustment for age, sex, BMI, and KOA. There was no significant difference between the HV group and the no HV group in physical functions. On the other hand, grip strength and maximal 6-m walking time were significantly stronger and faster in the no HV-mild HV group than in the moderate-severe HV group, respectively. In terms of HV-related pain, both usual and maximum walking speeds were significantly slower in the painful HV group than in the no HV or painless HV group. During 6-m walking, a significant negative correlation was observed between the HV angle and the percentage of hallux footprint (Fig. 2). Pearson's correlation coefficient (r) and the corresponding p value were $r = -0.44$ and $p < 0.01$. The percentage of hallux footprint was significantly higher in no HV feet than in HV feet (Fig. 3a). The percentage of hallux footprint was significantly higher in no HV or mild HV feet than in moderate-severe HV feet (Fig. 3b). Moreover, the percentage of hallux footprint was significantly higher in no HV or painless HV feet than in painful HV feet (Fig. 3c).

Discussion

The results of this cross-sectional study indicated that participants with moderate-severe HV or painful HV had impaired physical functions compared to participants with no HV-mild HV or painless HV after taking into account age, sex, BMI, and radiographic KOA. Hallux loading was reduced with increasing HV severity or HV-related pain.

With regard to standing balance, Menz et al. [21], Spink et al. [22], and Nix et al. [11] reported that poorer lateral stability, poorer coordinate stability, and increased

Table 1 Comparison of participants' basic data between the no HV group and the HV group, between the no HV -mild HV group and the moderate-severe HV group, and between the no HV or painless HV group and the painful HV group

	No HV group ($n = 402$)	HV group ($n = 160$)	No HV-mild HV group ($n = 495$)	Moderate-severe HV group ($n = 67$)	No HV or painless HV group ($n = 529$)	Painful HV group ($n = 33$)
Age (years)	**71.1 ± 8.8	73.3 ± 8.7	71.5 ± 8.9	73.4 ± 8.3	71.6 ± 8.8	74.0 ± 9.1
Sex (% female)	**58.2	83.8	**62.2	89.6	*64.1	87.9
Height (cm)	**154.6 ± 8.9	151.1 ± 7.8	**154.2 ± 8.7	149.7 ± 7.5	*153.9 ± 8.6	148.9 ± 9.0
Weight (kg)	**55.8 ± 10.3	53.5 ± 9.4	*55.5 ± 10.2	52.4 ± 9.5	55.4 ± 10.1	51.9 ± 10.0
BMI (kg/m^2)	23.3 ± 3.2	23.4 ± 3.6	23.3 ± 3.3	23.4 ± 3.5	23.3 ± 3.3	23.4 ± 3.7
KOA (%)	**33.8	55.0	**37.2	59.7	*40.0	42.4

HV hallux valgus, *BMI* body mass index, *KOA* knee osteoarthritis
**$p < 0.01$, *$p < 0.05$

postural sway were associated with HV in elderly populations. On the other hand, Mickle et al. [23] and Menz and Lord [24] showed no relationship between HV and standing balance. These previous reports included much finer analyses, with evaluation of the center of pressure (COP) using a force plate, and/or more severe conditions, such as eyes closed, than the present study. The data of the present study were only for standing time with eyes open to examine standing balance, but there was no relationship between HV and standing balance. If finer evaluations, such as analyzing COP, and/or more severe conditions, such as eyes closed, were performed, some differences might be detected.

To the best of our knowledge, there have been no reports of the relationship between HV and hand grip strength. The present study showed that moderate-severe HV deformity (HV angle ≥30°) was associated with impaired hand grip strength. It is easy to imagine that patients with moderate-severe HV have smaller grip strength of the foot because of poor alignment of the 1st MTP joint. Grip strength of the hallux might be correlated with hand grip strength. Thus, patients with poor grip strength in the moderate-severe HV group may show poor grip strength of the hallux. However, this is just a hypothesis, and further studies are needed.

No significant between-group differences were found in walking performance in some studies [11, 22]. The present data for the no HV group and the HV group are consistent with these previous studies. However, the definitions used in the various studies differed, since the data were self-reported (such as the Manchester scale) or HV < 20° was used, so that the HV groups had many mild HV participants. In the present study, maximum walking speed was faster in the no HV-mild HV group than in the moderate-severe HV group. Cho et al. [4] showed that participants with moderate or greater HV (HV angle > 25°) had significantly worse functional status, foot health function status, and self-assessment of their foot condition. These data support the present data. There were no data about maximum walking speed in previous studies, but maximum walking requires a higher level of physical function than usual walking. Thus, moderate-severe HV appeared to be associated with maximum walking speed in the present study.

Previous studies reported that foot pain was associated with poor physical function. Some studies [24–26] reported that participants with foot pain had more difficulty walking than participants without foot pain. In addition, some reports [1, 4] showed that HV was associated with more self-reported foot pain and poorer self-reported physical function. Abhishek et al. [10] further highlighted the importance of hallux pain with HV, reporting that health-related quality of life was progressively impaired in participants with HV alone, hallux pain alone, and HV with hallux pain. In the present study, walking speeds of participants with painful HV were slower than those of participants with no HV or mild HV.

Previous reports [27–29] showed an inverse relationship between HV severity and reduced hallux loading. Nix et al. [11] and Mickle et al. [13] showed that participants with HV had decreased hallux plantar flexion strength. Sanders et al. [30] reported an inverse relationship between HV angle and hallux plantar flexion strength, as well as lower mean hallux plantar flexion strength in those with painful HV than in those with HV without complaints. Moreover, Mickle et al. [23] reported less hallux loading in HV patients than controls. Hurn et al. [29] reported that participants with moderate (average HV angle = 30.8°) and severe HV (average HV angle = 39.9°) showed significantly reduced hallux plantar pressure-time compared to controls. These reports are consistent with the results of the present study. These reduced hallux plantar pressures might reflect impaired physical function, such as slower walking speed.

Caution must be applied when comparing reports from different studies [1]. Some studies have used self-report information, such as the Manchester scale [21–23, 31], and others have used X-ray definitions. In terms of X-ray examinations, studies have used a range of definitions, such as HV angle > 15° or 20° and so

Table 2 Comparison of physical functions between the no HV group and the HV group, between the no HV-mild HV group and the moderate-severe HV group, and between the no HV or painless HV group and the painful HV group after adjusted for age, sex, and body mass index

		No HV ($n = 402$)	HV ($n = 160$)	Standard partial regression coefficient	*p* Value	No HV-mild HV ($n = 495$)	Moderate-severe HV ($n = 67$)	Standard partial regression coefficient	*p* Value	No HV or painless HV ($n = 529$)	Painful HV ($n = 33$)	Standard partial regression coefficient	*p* Value
Grip strength, kg	Crude	28.6 ± 8.5	25.1 ± 6.2			28.2 ± 8.2	23.1 ± 6.0			27.9 ± 8.1	23.2 ± 7.0		
	Adjusted	27.6 ± 5.2	27.6 ± 5.2	0.007	0.910	27.8 ± 5.1	26.3 ± 5.2	−0.140	*0.034	27.7 ± 5.1	26.4 ± 5.1	−0.088	0.189
Single-leg stance time, s	Crude	31.2 ± 22.8	24.8 ± 22.1			30.0 ± 22.7	24.3 ± 22.7			29.8 ± 22.7	22.5 ± 22.9		
	Adjusted	30.1 ± 18.3	27.4 ± 18.6	−0.079	0.125	29.6 ± 18.2	27.3 ± 18.5	− 0.051	0.332	29.5 ± 18.2	26.3 ± 18.3	− 0.052	0.323
Stand up from a chair time, s	Crude	10.1 ± 3.6	11.1 ± 4.5			10.2 ± 3.6	11.5 ± 5.5			10.3 ± 3.8	11.8 ± 4.3		
	Adjusted	10.3 ± 3.4	10.7 ± 3.5	0.063	0.175	10.3 ± 3.4	11.2 ± 3.5	0.089	0.056	10.3 ± 3.4	11.3 ± 3.4	0.077	0.106
Usual gait speed, m/s	Crude	1.01 ± 0.21	1.01 ± 0.24			1.02 ± 0.21	1.00 ± 0.26			1.02 ± 0.22	0.92 ± 0.25		
	Adjusted	1.01 ± 0.20	1.03 ± 0.20	0.039	0.376	1.02 ± 0.20	1.01 ± 0.20	−0.003	0.949	1.02 ± 0.21	0.93 ± 0.20	− 0.108	*0.017
Maximum gait speed, m/s	Crude	1.33 ± 0.27	1.28 ± 0.31			1.33 ± 0.27	1.22 ± 0.33			1.33 ± 0.27	1.17 ± 0.37		
	Adjusted	1.32 ± 0.24	1.32 ± 0.24	0.002	0.968	1.33 ± 0.24	1.26 ± 0.24	−0.103	*0.037	1.33 ± 0.23	1.22 ± 0.24	−0.120	*0.016

***HV* hallux valgus, *M* male, *F* female, *s* second, *m/s* meters per second**

$^*p < 0.05$

Table 3 Comparison of physical functions between the no HV group and the HV group, between the no HV-mild HV group and the moderate-severe HV group, and between the no HV or painless HV group and the painful HV group after adjustment for age, sex, body mass index, and knee osteoarthritis

		No HV	HV	Standard partial regression coefficient	*p* Value	No HV-mild HV	Moderate-severe HV	Standard partial regression coefficient	*p* Value	No HV or painless HV	Painful HV	Standard partial regression coefficient	*p* Value
		($n = 402$)	($n = 160$)			($n = 495$)	($n = 67$)			($n = 529$)	($n = 33$)		
Grip strength, kg	Crude	28.6 ± 8.5	25.1 ± 6.2			28.2 ± 8.2	23.1 ± 6.0			27.9 ± 8.1	23.2 ± 7.0		
	Adjusted	27.6 ± 5.2	27.7 ± 5.3	0.007	0.813	27.7 ± 5.1	26.4 ± 5.2	−0.055	*0.043	27.7 ± 5.1	26.5 ± 5.1	−0.035	0.206
Single-leg stance time, s	Crude	31.2 ± 22.8	24.8 ± 22.1			30.0 ± 22.7	24.3 ± 22.7			29.8 ± 22.7	22.5 ± 22.9		
	Adjusted	30.1 ± 18.4	27.6 ± 18.7	−0.049	0.162	29.6 ± 18.2	27.5 ± 18.6	− 0.03	0.391	29.5 ± 18.2	26.5 ± 18.3	−0.032	0.351
Stand up from a chair time, s	Crude	10.1 ± 3.6	11.1 ± 4.5			10.2 ± 3.6	11.5 ± 5.5			10.3 ± 3.8	11.3 ± 4.3		
	Adjusted	10.3 ± 3.5	10.7 ± 3.5	0.048	0.222	10.3 ± 3.4	11.1 ± 3.5	0.069	0.072	10.3 ± 3.4	11.8 ± 3.4	0.059	0.118
Usual gait speed, m/s	Crude	1.01 ± 0.21	1.01 ± 0.24			1.02 ± 0.21	1.00 ± 0.26			1.02 ± 0.22	0.92 ± 0.25		
	Adjusted	1.01 ± 0.20	1.03 ± 0.21	0.044	0.279	1.01 ± 0.20	1.02 ± 0.20	0.003	0.931	1.02 ± 0.20	0.94 ± 0.20	−0.091	*0.021
Maximum gait speed, m/s	Crude	1.33 ± 0.27	1.28 ± 0.31			1.33 ± 0.27	1.22 ± 0.33			1.33 ± 0.27	1.17 ± 0.37		
	Adjusted	1.32 ± 0.24	1.32 ± 0.24	0.007	0.849	1.33 ± 0.24	1.27 ± 0.24	−0.072	*0.048	1.33 ± 0.23	1.23 ± 0.24	−0.084	*0.018

HV hallux valgus, *M* male, *F* female, *s* second, *m/s* meters per second

*$p < 0.05$

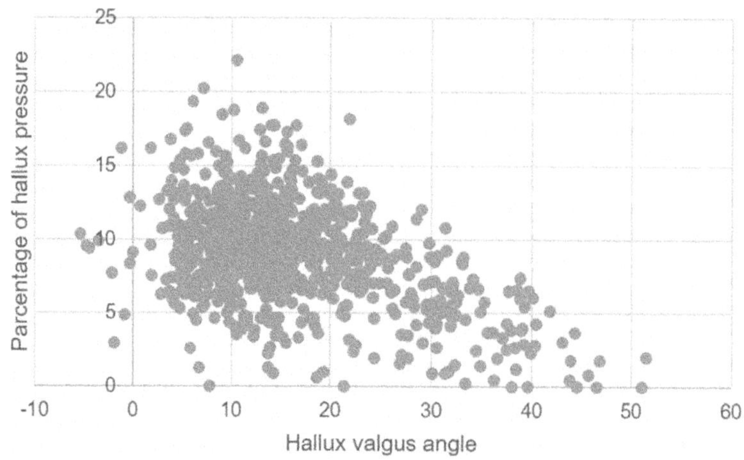

Fig. 2 Relationship between the percentage of hallux footprint and the hallux valgus angle

on. The present study used standardized weight-bearing radiographs, and the definition of HV was an HV angle > 20° according to the definition of the Japanese Foot and Ankle Society.

The present study has several limitations. First, since it was a cross-sectional study, causal relationships cannot be determined. Second, participants could walk to the survey site and could understand and sign an informed consent form. Thus, elderly participants in this study were relatively healthier and had no dementia. Furthermore, since workers in Japan usually retire between 63 and 65 years old, male participants in their 50s usually have health examinations at their work place. Thus, male participants in their 50s who worried about their health

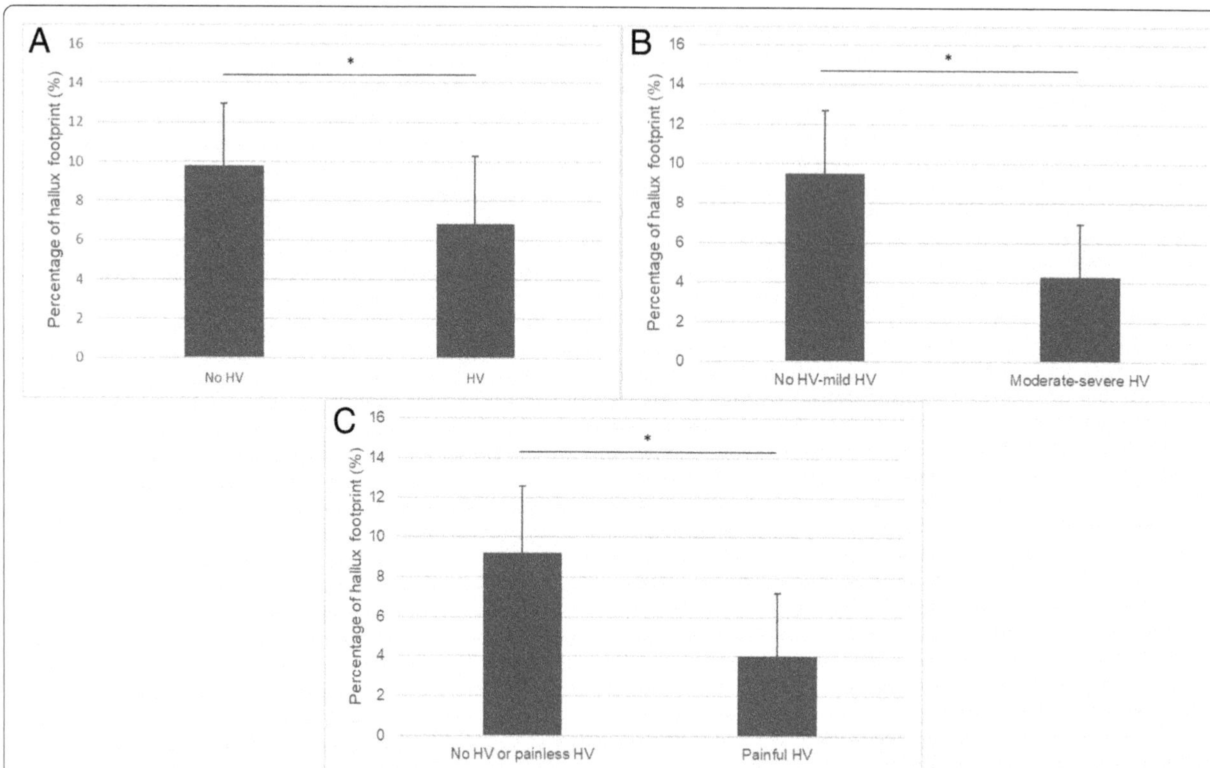

Fig. 3 Comparison of the percentage of the hallux footprint between the no HV group and the HV group (**a**), between the no HV-mild HV group and the moderate-severe HV group (**b**), and between the no HV or painless HV group and the painful HV group (**c**). HV hallux valgus. $^{*}p < 0.01$. Mann-Whitney test

tended to attend our exam. Due to this healthy user bias, the participants in this study do not truly represent the general population. The percentage of men in this study was 34.5%, but the percentage of men over 65 years old in this village was 39.2% in 2009. Further, the percentage of men over 65 years old in Japan was 42.8% in 2009. This sex mismatch is also one of the limitations. Third, the examinations were held in a specific mountain village, so that this study is not necessarily representative of all of Japan. Fourth, the balance test was simply single-leg standing time with eyes open. If a standing test with eyes closed and/or postural sway using a force plate were used, significant differences might be detected in the balance tests. Fifth, hallux pain is not always due to HV. Thus, painful HV does not necessarily mean pain related to HV.

Conclusions

This cross-sectional epidemiological study showed that moderate-severe HV impaired some physical functions (grip strength and maximum walking speed), and painful HV slowed walking speed regardless of radiographic KOA. Hallux plantar pressure decreased according to HV angle and pain. We suspect this reduced hallux pressure is one of the reasons for the functional impairments in participants with moderate-severe HV or painful HV. By controlling pain and treating severe HV deformity with treatments such as surgery, the physical functions of HV patients might be improved.

Abbreviations

BMI: body mass index; HV: hallux valgus; KOA: knee osteoarthritis

Acknowledgements

The authors would like to thank the staff of Houtoku Hospital for their invaluable assistance.

Funding

This study was supported by JSPS KAKENHI Grant Number JP15K08732 and Grants-in-Aid for H25-Choujyu-007 (Director, Noriko Yoshimura) from the Ministry of Health, Labour and Welfare of Japan.

Authors' contributions

AN conceived of this study and participated in the study design, and performed data acquisition, analysis and interpretation, and drafted the manuscript. NI and SN participated in the interpretation of data and performed statistical analyses. KK and AS contributed to the study design and coordination, and helped to draft the manuscript. TO helped to perform statistical analysis and interpretation of data. All authors read and approved the final manuscript.

Competing interests

The authors declare that they have no competing interests.

Author details

[1]Departments of Orthopaedic Surgery, Mie University Graduate School of Medicine, 2-174 Edobashi, Tsu City, Mie 514-8507, Japan. [2]Departments of Orthopaedic and Sports Medicine, Mie University Graduate School of Medicine, Tsu City 514-8507, Mie, Japan. [3]Department of Orthopaedic Surgery, Suzuka Kaisei Hospital, Suzuka City 513-8505, Mie, Japan. [4]Clinical Research Support Center, Mie University Hospital, 2-174 Edobashi, Tsu City, Mie 514-8507, Japan.

References

1. Nix S, Smith M, Vicenzino B. Prevalence of hallux valgus in the general population: a systematic review and meta-analysis. J Foot Ankle Res. 2010;3:21.
2. Nguyen US, Hillstrom HJ, Li W, Dufour AB, Kiel DP, Procter-Gray E, Gagnon MM, Hannan MT. Factors associated with hallux valgus in a population-based study of older women and men: the MOBILIZE Boston study. Osteoarthr Cartil. 2010;18(1):41–6.
3. Roddy E, Zhang W, Doherty M. Prevalence and associations of hallux valgus in a primary care population. Arthritis Rheum. 2008;59(6):857–62.
4. Cho NH, Kim S, Kwon DJ, Kim HA. The prevalence of hallux valgus and its association with foot pain and function in a rural Korean community. J Bone Joint Surg Br. 2009;91(4):494–8.
5. Nishimura A, Kato K, Fukuda A, Nakazora S, Yamada T, Uchida A, Sudo A. Prevalence of hallux valgus and risk factors among Japanese community dwellers. J Orthop Sci. 2014;19(2):257–62.
6. Chaiwanichsiri D, Janchai S, Tantisiriwat N. Foot disorders and falls in older persons. Gerontology. 2009;55(3):296–302.
7. Badlissi F, Dunn JE, Link CL, Keysor JJ, McKinlay JB, Felson DT. Foot musculoskeletal disorders, pain, and foot-related functional limitation in older persons. J Am Geriatr Soc. 2005;53(6):1029–33.
8. Keysor JJ, Dunn JE, Link CL, Badlissi F, Felson DT. Are foot disorders associated with functional limitation and disability among community-dwelling older adults? J Aging Health. 2005;17(6):734–52.
9. Menz HB, Roddy E, Thomas E, Croft PR. Impact of hallux valgus severity on general and foot-specific health-related quality of life. Arthritis Care Res (Hoboken). 2011;63(3):396–404.
10. Abhishek A, Roddy E, Zhang W, Doherty M. Are hallux valgus and big toe pain associated with impaired quality of life? A cross-sectional study. Osteoarthr Cartil. 2010;18(7):923–6.
11. Nix SE, Vicenzino BT, Smith MD. Foot pain and functional limitation in healthy adults with hallux valgus: a cross-sectional study. BMC Musculoskelet Disord. 2012;13:197.
12. Menz HB, Morris ME, Lord SR. Foot and ankle risk factors for falls in older people: a prospective study. J Gerontol A Biol Sci Med Sci. 2006; 61(8):866–70.
13. Mickle KJ, Munro BJ, Lord SR, Menz HB, Steele JR. ISB clinical biomechanics award 2009: toe weakness and deformity increase the risk of falls in older people. Clin Biomech (Bristol, Avon). 2009;24(10):787–91.
14. Nishimura A, Hasegawa M, Kato K, Yamada T, Uchida A, Sudo A. Risk factors for the incidence and progression of radiographic osteoarthritis of the knee among Japanese. Int Orthop. 2011;35(6):839–43.
15. Nishimura A, Hasegawa M, Wakabayashi H, Yoshida K, Kato K, Yamada T, Uchida A, Sudo A. Prevalence and characteristics of unilateral knee osteoarthritis in a community sample of elderly Japanese: do fractures around the knee affect the pathogenesis of unilateral knee osteoarthritis? J Orthop Sci. 2012;17(5):556–61.
16. Nishimura A, Akeda K, Kato K, Asanuma K, Yamada T, Uchida A, Sudo A. Osteoporosis, vertebral fractures and mortality in a Japanese rural community. Mod Rheumatol. 2014;24(5):840–3.
17. Iversen MD, Price LL, von Heideken J, Harvey WF, Wang C. Physical examination findings and their relationship with performance-based function in adults with knee osteoarthritis. BMC Musculoskelet Disord. 2016;17:273.
18. Kellgren JH, Lawrence JS. Radiological assessment of osteo-arthrosis. Ann Rheum Dis. 1957;16(4):494–502.
19. Saltzman CL, Brandser EA, Berbaum KS, DeGnore L, Holmes JR, Katcherian DA, Teasdall RD, Alexander IJ. Reliability of standard foot radiographic measurements. Foot Ankle Int. 1994;15(12):661–5.
20. Helal B, Gupta SK, Gojaseni P. Surgery for adolescent hallux valgus. Acta Orthop Scand. 1974;45(2):271–95.

21. Menz HB, Morris ME, Lord SR. Foot and ankle characteristics associated with impaired balance and functional ability in older people. J Gerontol A Biol Sci Med Sci. 2005;60(12):1546–52.
22. Spink MJ, Fotoohabadi MR, Wee E, Hill KD, Lord SR, Menz HB. Foot and ankle strength, range of motion, posture, and deformity are associated with balance and functional ability in older adults. Arch Phys Med Rehabil. 2011;92(1):68–75.
23. Mickle KJ, Munro BJ, Lord SR, Menz HB, Steele JR. Gait, balance and plantar pressures in older people with toe deformities. Gait Posture. 2011;34(3):347–51.
24. Menz HB, Lord SR. Foot pain impairs balance and functional ability in community-dwelling older people. J Am Podiatr Med Assoc. 2001;91(5):222–9.
25. Leveille SG, Guralnik JM, Ferrucci L, Hirsch R, Simonsick E, Hochberg MC. Foot pain and disability in older women. Am J Epidemiol. 1998;148(7):657–65.
26. Benvenuti F, Ferrucci L, Guralnik JM, Gangemi S, Baroni A. Foot pain and disability in older persons: an epidemiologic survey. J Am Geriatr Soc. 1995;43(5):479–84.
27. Menz HB, Morris ME. Clinical determinants of plantar forces and pressures during walking in older people. Gait Posture. 2006;24(2):229–36.
28. Mueller MJ, Hastings M, Commean PK, Smith KE, Pilgram TK, Robertson D, Johnson J. Forefoot structural predictors of plantar pressures during walking in people with diabetes and peripheral neuropathy. J Biomech. 2003;36(7):1009–17.
29. Hurn SE, Vicenzino B, Smith MD. Functional impairments characterizing mild, moderate, and severe hallux valgus. Arthritis Care Res (Hoboken). 2015;67(1):80–8.
30. Sanders AP, Snijders CJ, van Linge B. Medial deviation of the first metatarsal head as a result of flexion forces in hallux valgus. Foot & ankle. 1992;13(9):515–22.
31. Menz HB, Morris ME. Determinants of disabling foot pain in retirement village residents. J Am Podiatr Med Assoc. 2005;95(6):573–9.

15

Relationships between paraspinal muscle morphology and neurocompressive conditions of the lumbar spine

Jeffrey R. Cooley[1*], Bruce F. Walker[1], Emad M. Ardakani [1], Per Kjaer [2], Tue S. Jensen[3,4,5] and Jeffrey J. Hebert[6,7]

Abstract

Background: Individual study results have demonstrated unclear relationships between neurocompressive disorders and paraspinal muscle morphology. This systematic review aimed to synthesize current evidence regarding the relationship lumbar neurocompressive disorders may have with lumbar paraspinal muscle morphology.

Methods: Searches were conducted in seven databases from inception through October 2017. Observational studies with control or comparison groups comparing herniations, facet degeneration, or canal stenosis to changes in imaging or biopsy-identified lumbar paraspinal muscle morphology were included. Data extraction and risk of bias assessment were performed by review author pairs independent of one another. Morphological differences between individuals with and without neurocompressive disorders were compared qualitatively, and where possible, standardised mean differences were obtained.

Results: Twenty-eight studies were included. Lumbar multifidus fiber diameter was smaller on the side of and below herniation for type I [SMD: −0.40 (95% CI = −0.70, −0.09) and type II fibers [SMD: −0.38 (95% CI = −0.69, −0.06)] compared to the unaffected side. The distribution of type I fibers was greater on the herniation side [SMD: 0.43 (95% CI = 0.03, 0.82)]. Qualitatively, two studies assessing small angular fiber frequency and fiber type groupings demonstrated increases in these parameters below the herniation level. For diagnostic imaging meta-analyses, there were no consistent differences across the various assessment types for any paraspinal muscle groups when patients with herniation served as their own control. However, qualitative synthesis of between-group comparisons reported greater multifidus and erector spinae muscle atrophy or fat infiltration among patients with disc herniation and radiculopathy in four of six studies, and increased fatty infiltration in paraspinal muscles with higher grades of facet joint degeneration in four of five studies. Conflicting outcomes and variations in study methodology precluded a clear conclusion for canal stenosis.

Conclusions: Based on mixed levels of risk of bias data, in patients with chronic radiculopathy, disc herniation and severe facet degeneration were associated with altered paraspinal muscle morphology at or below the pathology level. As the variability of study quality and heterogeneous approaches utilized to assess muscle morphology challenged comparison across studies, we provide recommendations to promote uniform measurement techniques for future studies.

Keywords: Lumbar spine, paraspinal muscle, disc herniation, radiculopathy, fat infiltration, canal stenosis, facet arthrosis

* Correspondence: J.Cooley@murdoch.edu.au
[1]School of Health Professions, Murdoch University, 90 South Street, Murdoch, Western Australia 6150, Australia
Full list of author information is available at the end of the article

Background

Globally, low-back pain (LBP) ranks first in years lived with disability [1]. The lifetime prevalence of LBP is estimated to be as high as 84% [2], with a mean of 38.9% [3]. In Australia, 2001 estimates revealed a direct and indirect cost of LBP of AUD$9.17 billion [4]. In 2014, the estimated annual cost of chronic LBP-related lost productivity in Japan was ¥1.2 trillion (equivalent to AUD$12.6 billion) [5]. It should be noted that these estimated prevalence rates and costs are inclusive of all types of LBP; however, approximately 90% of LBP is non-specific in nature, while specific LBP resulting from an identifiable disorder (e.g., tumor, fracture, stenosis) can only be classified in a small percentage of patients [6]. Although there is very limited data available to quantify the prevalence of neuro-compressive disorders such as lumbar disc herniation, facet joint hypertrophy and lumbar spinal stenosis, these can only make up a portion of the 10% of specific LBP cases.

Despite intensive research efforts aimed at enhancing our understanding of both specific and non-specific LBP, these disorders continues to present diagnostic and therapeutic challenges. In an attempt to identify discrete pain generating tissues or clinically relevant structural changes related to LBP, recent studies have focused on the relationships between morphological changes to the lumbar paraspinal musculature (e.g., atrophy, fat replacement) and both specific and non-specific causes of chronic low back or radicular pain [7–11]. Systematic reviews have assessed the relationship of paraspinal muscle morphology with LBP, the impact of paraspinal muscle atrophy and/or fatty replacement on clinical outcomes, and the predictive value of paraspinal muscle morphology with clinical outcomes [12–14].

Of particular interest to this review is the growing body of research attempting to identify the relationships between spinal pathologies and paraspinal muscle morphology, and their impact on specific LBP and clinical outcomes [15–21]. One specific area of interest focuses on localized injuries or pathologies resulting in nerve root or central neurological compression (neurocompressive disorders), as it is understood that the biological effects of short and long-term skeletal muscle denervation can result in muscle fiber atrophy and adipose tissue replacement [22–24]. However, no prior systematic reviews of these relationships have been identified by the authors. A 2014 review by Steffens et al. [25], explored the ability of MRI-identified pathologies to predict future LBP, concluding that no definitive associations between imaging findings and clinical outcomes could be confirmed due to limited research in this area. However, these authors did not include altered muscle morphology in their pathology criteria, nor did they look at the relationship of paraspinal muscle morphology to regional pathology.

Therefore, the objective of this study was to systematically review the literature to investigate for relationships between lumbosacral neurocompressive disorders and measures of lumbar paraspinal muscle morphology in patients with specific LBP.

Methods

Protocol and registration

This review followed the reporting guidelines and methodologies proposed in *Preferred reporting items of systematic reviews and meta-analysis: the PRISMA statement* [26] and *Meta-analysis of observational studies in epidemiology* (MOOSE) [27]. The initial review protocol was registered with Prospero, 13 February 2015 (PROSPERO 2015 :CRD42015012985), available from: http://www.crd.york.ac.uk/PROSPERO/display_record.asp?ID=CRD42015012985. The original search strategy was applied following the registered protocol; however, due to the large and diverse number of articles meeting the eligibility criteria, a post-hoc decision was made to the original protocol to limit this review to patients with radicular pain or reduced muscle strength in the lower extremities due to neurocompression.

Information sources

With the assistance of specialist librarians, we developed a search strategy using medical subject headings (MeSH) and keywords that encompassed muscle type and morphology; pathology and related clinical syndromes; imaging types, biopsy analyses, and muscle measurement parameters; and, the lumbar spinal region. No language restrictions were applied.

We searched the following databases from inception through October 2017 in PEDro, PubMed (Medline), Web of Science (Core Collection), Web of Science (Medline Advanced), SPORTDiscus, Cumulative Index to Nursing and Allied Health Literature (CINAHL), and EMBASE. The reference lists of included studies from the title/abstract screening, as well as all systematic reviews related to the topic, were also reviewed. Where only an abstract was published as part of a poster or conference proceedings, the authors were contacted via email to determine if the full studies had since been published. The search protocols for each database can be found in Additional file 1.

Eligibility and study selection criteria

The eligibility and selection criteria are provided in Table 1. The outcomes of interest included measures of lumbar paraspinal muscle morphology, such as muscle cross-sectional area, fat infiltration area, and type I and II muscle fiber distribution.

Table 1 Study eligibility and selection criteria

Inclusion criteria
Articles published (including those accepted for publication) in an indexed, peer reviewed journal, or a published[a] thesis
Studies including patients with: disc herniation, facet arthrosis, and/or spinal canal stenosis identified via imaging; specific LBP with confirmed radicular leg pain or muscle weakness on clinical examination
Regional paraspinal muscle morphology assessed with imaging or biopsy for either the lumbar multifidus muscles (LMM), erector spinae muscles (ESM) (including subcomponents), psoas major muscles (PMM), or "paraspinal / paravertebral" muscles (PVM)
Observational human studies with a control or comparison analyses (controls included: "normal" or "non-diseased"; comparisons between different severities of conditions; participants serving as own control when there was a normal and an abnormal side to compare)
Clinical / surgical trials containing baseline data with relevant "pathology to muscle" or "clinical to muscle" comparisons
Exclusion criteria
History of previous lumbar spine surgery
Analysis was solely post-interventional (i.e., no pre-surgical, pre-treatment, or pre-activity/functional muscle measurement data analysed)
Case reports, editorials/letters, literature reviews, guidelines, and abstract-only publications
Patients with primary muscular disease (e.g., muscular dystrophy, parkinsonism)

[a]If archived in an international research database (e.g., ProQuest, EBSCO*host*)

Study selection and data extraction

Selection process

One reviewer (JC) conducted all database searches based on the previously defined strategies and removed all duplicates (Figure 1). Two review authors (JC/EA) independently screened all included titles & abstracts according to the eligibility criteria, and articles denoted as potentially eligible by *either* reviewer (i.e., "yes" or "maybe") were included for the full-text screening stage. Articles were excluded if both reviewers indicated "no". As there were no language restrictions applied to the search, all non-English articles selected for full-text review were professionally translated [Straker Translations (Melbourne, Victoria; Australia)].

Four reviewers participated in the full-text screening phase (JC reviewed all articles in conjunction with either EA, BW, or JH to ensure each article was initially independently assessed by two reviewers). A selection form (developed using EpiData Manager v2.0.4.43 [EpiData Association, Denmark]) was developed and piloted on ten citations, then modified for clarity (Additional File 2). Once trained, viewers assessed full-text copies of the selected articles according to the selection criteria. For full article inclusion, both reviewers of an article had to note "yes". For exclusion, both reviewers had to indicate "no" and the recorded reason(s) agreed. Any disagreement or uncertainty regarding a decision at this stage of the process which could not be resolved by the two reviewers was presented to a third review author (i.e., an author not involved in the initial full-text review of the article) for final determination.

Extraction process

A data extraction form was developed using EpiData Manager (v2.0.4.43 – EpiData Association, Denmark) and pre-tested by the lead reviewer. All reviewers underwent training in the use of the form, which resulted in minor modifications to enhance clarity. Pairs of review authors independently extracted the data. Additional file 2 provides specific details regarding the type of data extracted. When extracting data, if details were not specified in the methods or results sections, "not included" was input by the reviewers.

Following extraction, a consensus meeting was held with each pair of reviewers to ensure accuracy and agreement between reviewers. Where differences were identified, disagreements were resolved via discussion or upon consultation with a third reviewer. Additionally, to identify studies potentially reporting duplicate data once the extracted data was tabulated, the lead reviewer cross-checked the study authors, year of publication, dates of data acquisition (if provided), study aims, participant demographics, methods for assessing muscle changes, and outcomes being analysed. Inter-reviewer agreement was examined by percentage agreement and Kappa coefficients, using IBM SPSS Statistics v24.0 [Armonk, NY: IBM Corp.].

Risk of bias assessment

At the time this review was initiated, no established or validated risk of bias (ROB) tool appropriate for the types of studies predominately being assessed in this review was available. As such, we developed a modified version of the ROB tool developed by Downs and Black [28]. With one exception, the modifications applied were limited to removal of questions relating to interventions (following the approach used by Mills et al. [29], and Munn et al. [30]), and the replacement of guidance scenarios to better match the focus of our review. One reporting criterion assessing for clear descriptions of *interventions* was replaced with a criterion assessing for clear descriptions of *assessment parameters*, to include an otherwise absent key component of this review.

The three overarching criteria for assessing studies included: 1) reporting characteristics (e.g., aims, methods, participant characteristics, confounders, probability values); 2) external validity (e.g., population representation, blinding, appropriateness of analysis); and, 3) internal validity (e.g., recruitment, adjusting for confounders). Additional file 3 details the ROB tool, including more detailed explanations of the modifications applied.

The modified ROB tool for this review was piloted with each review author using three articles. Five authors independently assessed study quality (JC assessed all selected studies; EA, BW, JH, and PK assessed one or more subcomponents ensuring two independent quality assessments

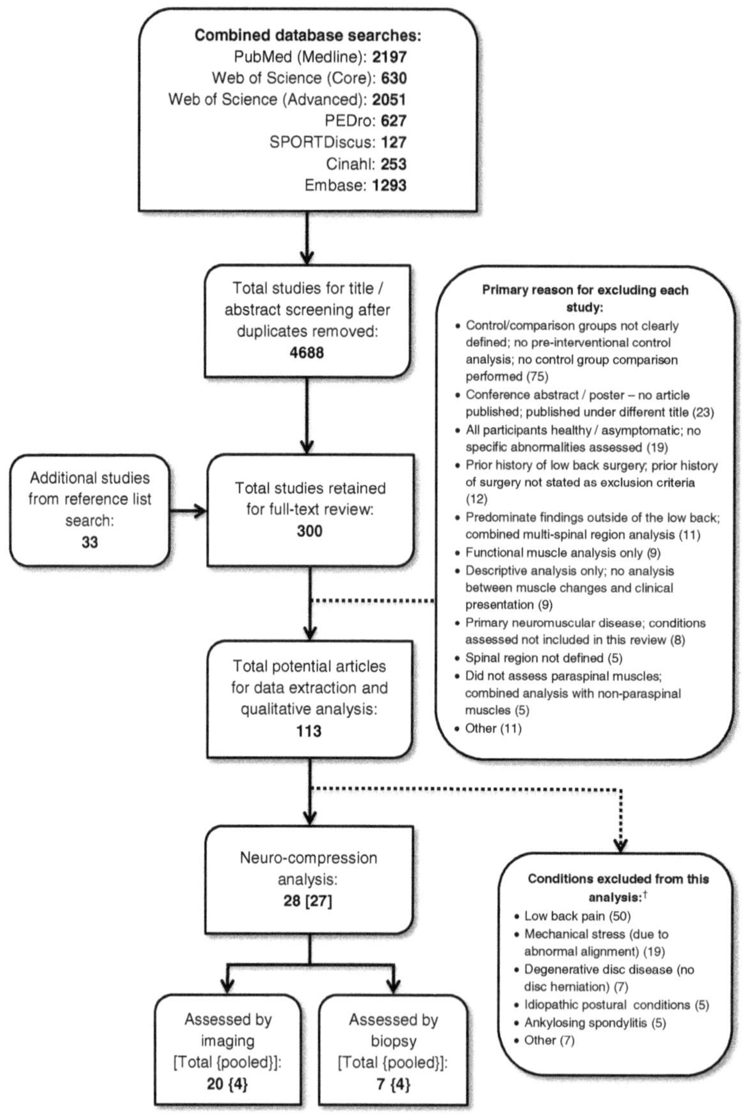

Fig. 1 Flow diagram for search strategy. †Some articles included conditions assessable in more than one subcategory

of each study). Disagreements within each reviewer pairing were discussed and resolved by consensus. A third reviewer was available to resolve irreconcilable differences, but this was not required. When analysing the quality of data, one assumption was made regarding the reporting of blinding: if no indication was discernible from a study's methodology that the investigator(s) extracting clinical data were different from those assessing the imaging, it was considered that no blinding occurred between the clinical and imaging data acquisitions.

Due to the inherent issue of variable item weighting when using scaled/score-based ROB tools, an *a priori* decision was made to apply the study quality criteria used by Munn et al. [30], of <60% (low quality / high risk), 60-74% (moderate quality / moderate risk), and ≥75% (high quality / low risk) for determining overall study quality. While other studies have set a score of 50% as a quality exclusion criteria (e.g., Mills et al. [29]), we agreed with Munn that 60% was fair in our context; studies of low quality were not excluded from analysis, but their potential for increased risk of bias was considered and discussed where applicable. Inter-reviewer reliability of risk of bias was examined by percentage agreement and Kappa coefficients.

Summary measures

For data where meta-analysis was possible, the reported means and standard deviations were used to calculate standardised mean differences (SMD). The SMD was used to allow for direct comparison of pooled results between the different continuous measurement metrics reported in our included studies, as well as to compare different constructs between analyses (e.g., measured area versus ratios or percentages). For non-pooled data, the reported measures were retained and analysed descriptively.

Methods of analysis

For this review we undertook qualitative and quantitative analysis. For quantitative analysis, after evaluating the study outcomes for clinical homogeneity, we performed a random-effects meta-analysis on the included studies, assessing for statistical heterogeneity using both χ^2 and I^2 statistics. The SMD (95% CI), calculated with Hedges' *g*, was used to report parameter estimates.

Criteria to assess clinical homogeneity between studies included patient source, sex, age, chronicity of symptoms related to neurocompression, type of comparison, imaging or biopsy method, muscle parameters assessed, and outcome scales. Meta-analyses were undertaken when three or more homogeneous studies were available. As the study effect sizes were collected from a distribution of variable effect sizes, the random-effects model was applied. Statistical analyses were conducted using Review Manager (RevMan) v5.3 [Copenhagen: The Nordic Cochrane Centre, The Cochrane Collaboration, 2014.].

Additional analyses

Pre-specified subgroup analyses comprised disc herniations and studies with low risk of bias. A post-hoc decision was made to assess for differences in outcomes between muscle biopsy sites located at and below the level of disc herniation.

The percentage difference in muscle fiber diameter between the affected and unaffected sides of patients with LDH was calculated as the average mean diameter on the affected side / average mean diameter on the unaffected side x 100. The "average mean diameter" (AMD) per side was determined by the formula: AMD = [(m*N (S1)) + (m*N (S2)) + (m*N (S3)) + (m*N (S4))] / Total N [*S* = *study*].

Results

Study selection

The database searches identified 7178 studies, with 2490 being duplicates (Figure 1). A total of 267 studies were selected from the title/abstract search, and an additional 33 studies were identified from the reference list search of all selected articles and relevant reviews. Nine non-English language articles were included (Chinese (5), Turkish, Portuguese, Japanese, and German), of which eight met the requirements for full-text review and were fully translated. The number of studies excluded (with primary reasons indicated) at the full-text screening stage is noted in Figure 1. A list of excluded studies from the full-text phase is provided in Additional file 4.

Twenty-three potential studies for inclusion were initially identified as abstracts-only from conference proceedings or poster presentations. Upon further investigation, four of these were published under a different title and were already included for review. Authors of 15 additional abstracts were contacted with a request to confirm if their study had proceeded to full publication. Eight authors replied to either an initial or follow-up request; of these, seven indicated no publication had occurred and one provided publication details under a different title already included. No contact details for any of the authors listed for four of the abstracts could be identified. No additional studies were added from this process.

There were 113 studies initially identified for potential data extraction, of which 28 focussed on conditions relating to neurocompression. The remaining studies were excluded from this report (Figure 1), but will be considered for future systematic reviews. Of the studies identified for extraction, two [31, 32] were noted to provide different analyses of the same data set and were combined, reducing the number of distinct studies to 27. Two additional studies were published by the same lead author drawing patients from the same facility [22, 33]; however, there were sufficient differences in the methodology and patient demographics to consider these as distinct studies.

For the full-text screening phase, we achieved moderate inter-rater agreement (κ ≥ 0.68) [34] (Table 2). A third reviewer was only required on one occasion to clarify the presence of a control group.

Study characteristics

Additional file 5 provides specific extracted participant characteristics and study details. Patients with lumbar disc herniation (LDH) were assessed via imaging in 12 studies [15, 16, 18, 35–43] and via biopsy in six studies [22, 33, 44–47], with one additional study [48] assessing subjects en bloc via biopsy across multiple pathologies

Table 2 Full text screening and risk of bias agreement

Agreement for full text screening				
	Examiners 1 & 2	Examiners 1 & 3	Examiners 1 & 4	Overall
N (articles)	126	65	88	279
% agreement	83%	88%	86%	86%
κ [CI (95%)]	0.68 [0.53-0.80]	0.75 [0.58-0.91]	0.73 [0.57-0.86]	0.71 [0.63-0.80]
Agreement for risk of bias analysis				
ROB section	Reporting	External Validity	Internal Validity	Overall
N (questions)[a]	224	168	84	476
% agreement	83%	81%	73%	81%
κ [CI (95%)]	0.51 [0.38-0.63]	0.63 [0.52-0.74]	0.43 [0.28-0.62]	0.58 [0.51-0.65]

κ Kappa coefficient, *CI* confidence intervals, *N* number of questions
[a]Based on number of questions asked per section x 28 articles selected for neurocompression subgroup

with or without nerve root involvement (LDH being most frequent). Using MR or CT imaging, three studies assessed patients with facet arthrosis [49–51], four studies assessed patients with canal stenosis [20, 52–54], and two studies assessed both facet arthrosis and canal stenosis [31, 32]. These latter two studies (although eventually combined for analysis) reported outcomes separately for arthrosis and stenosis, allowing data to be assessed for each condition.

Risk of bias within studies

During initial risk of bias analysis, overall inter-rater agreement was weak (Table 2). However, complete agreement was reached on all items during the first consensus meeting, without the need for third reviewer arbitration.

The risk of bias indices showed a wide variation in potential study bias (Table 3). Studies utilizing imaging methods to assess muscle changes tended to show lower risk of bias than those using biopsy [13.9/19 (imaging) versus 12.1/19 (biopsy)].

Risk of bias across studies

Figure 2 provides a graphic breakdown of potential bias across studies. The four areas of risk most consistently identified related to: a) uncertainty regarding recruited population representation, with most studies failing to provide sufficient descriptive data to make a determination; b) lack of reporting of actual probability values, with newer studies more likely to provide these values; c) distribution of principal confounders, with nearly half the studies providing only partial details; and d) blinding. An inherent blinding challenge existed for the imaging-based studies – even if the examiner measuring the muscles was blinded to the imaging pathology report, the pathology would most likely be evident on the images if it was not specifically blocked from view.

Study findings with syntheses of results

For each of the following sections, a compilation of the relevant outcome details for the included studies is provided in Additional file 5. Attempts were made via email to contact authors when issues with study data required clarification. In two cases details were not obtained, one reporting anatomically improbable measurement ranges for some data [37], and one with missing error values for some outcomes [33]. In both instance these data were removed from analysis.

Paraspinal muscle morphology in patients with lumbar disc herniation (LDH) – assessed with imaging

Study characteristics and ROB Twelve studies assessed patients with unilateral LDH with radiculopathy; 11 using MRI and one using diagnostic ultrasound. Of these, six had a low risk of bias, three a moderate risk, and three a high risk; total sample sizes varied from 33 to 165 participants. In four studies, patients served exclusively as their own controls (involved vs uninvolved sides) [15, 18, 35, 41], two studies used both patients and healthy volunteers as controls [37, 42], and one study used the patients and healthy volunteers as controls plus included an LDH group without radiculopathy as a comparison [38]. One study compared acute versus chronic radiculopathy patients as well as using patients in each group as their own controls [16], while another study used healthy participants as the only control [39]. Two studies used low back pain patients without LDH or nerve root compression as a comparison – one chronic [36] and one non-specific [43], and the final study used chronic low back pain patients with degenerative disc disease (DDD) without LDH as a comparison [40]. All but one study assessed the lumbar multifidus muscles (LMM) (with or without including the erector spinae muscles (ESM)) and four studies included the psoas major muscles (PMM). Multiple measures of muscle morphology were used in most studies, with the total cross-sectional area (TCSA) and/or functional cross-sectional area (FCSA) being most consistently assessed.

Meta-analysis Four studies met our criteria for pooled data analysis assessing for differences in mean LMM TCSA [15, 16, 38, 41] (refer to Additional file 5 for study details). For those measures taken at the level of LDH, 166 patients with unilateral LDH where included but demonstrated no significant difference in the pooled SMD between sides (Figure 3a). A total of 90 patients were included for measurements below the level of LDH, also showing no differences (Figure 3b). As there were diverse outcomes between studies, subgroup analyses were undertaken to determine if this was dependent on the duration of symptoms; however, the pooled SMD remained non-significant [at the level of LDH – only acute included [0.14 (95% CI = −0.16, 0.45] and acute excluded [−0.17 (95% CI = −0.47, 0.14)]; below the level of LDH – only acute included [0.04 (95% CI = −0.38, 0.46)] and acute excluded [−0.03 (95% CI = −0.50, 0.44)]].

Three of these studies also met the criteria for assessing differences in the mean FCSA and FCSA:TCSA ratios [15, 38, 41]. For FCSA measures taken at or below the level of LDH, 90 patients with unilateral LDH where included; the pooled SMD again demonstrated no difference between sides (Figures 4a and 4b). A total of 90 patients were also included for FCSA:TCSA ratio measures at and below the level of LDH. While all studies demonstrated smaller mean measures on the affected side at both levels, no significant difference in the pooled SMD between sides was found (Figures 5a and 5b). Table 4 (section 1.0) reports the

Table 3 Risk of bias index

Article	Reporting[a]							
	1. Study hypothesis/ aim/objective clearly described?	2. Main outcome measures clearly described?	3. Characteristics of included patients clearly described?	4. Principal assessment parameters clearly described?	5. Distributions of principal confounders per group clearly described?	6. Main study findings clearly described?	7. Provides estimates of random variability for main outcomes?	10. Actual probability values reported?
Kalichman [31][c]	Y (1)	Y (1)	Y (1)	Y (2)	P (1)	Y (1)	Y (1)	Y (1)
Kalichman [32][c]	Y (1)	Y (1)	Y (1)	Y (2)	P (1)	Y (1)	Y (1)	Y (1)
Kim [16]	Y (1)	Y (1)	Y (1)	Y (2)	Y (2)	Y (1)	Y (1)	Y (1)
Battie [15]	Y (1)	Y (1)	Y (1)	Y (2)	Y (2)	Y (1)	Y (1)	Y (1)
Farshad [18]	Y (1)	Y (1)	Y (1)	Y (2)	Y (2)	Y (1)	Y (1)	Y (1)
Fortin [41]	Y (1)	Y (1)	Y (1)	Y (2)	Y (2)	Y (1)	Y (1)	Y (1)
Altinkaya [35]	Y (1)	Y (1)	Y (1)	Y (2)	Y (2)	Y (1)	N (0)	Y (1)
Jiang [53]	Y (1)	Y (1)	Y (1)	Y (2)	Y (2)	Y (1)	Y (1)	Y (1)
Kalichman [49]	Y (1)	Y (1)	Y (1)	Y (2)	N (0)	Y (1)	Y (1)	Y (1)
Abbas [52]	Y (1)	Y (1)	Y (1)	Y (2)	Y (2)	Y (1)	Y (1)	Y (1)
Boyaci [36]	Y (1)	Y (1)	Y (1)	Y (2)	P (1)	Y (1)	Y (1)	Y (1)
Zhao [47]	Y (1)	Y (1)	Y (1)	Y (2)	Y (2)	Y (1)	Y (1)	N (0)
Bhadresha [40]	Y (1)	Y (1)	Y (1)	Y (2)	P (1)	Y (1)	Y (1)	Y (1)
Mattila [46]	N (0)	Y (1)	Y (1)	Y (2)	P (1)	Y (1)	Y (1)	N (0)
Ogon [54]	Y (1)	Y (1)	Y (1)	Y (2)	Y (2)	Y (1)	Y (1)	Y (1)
Sebro [50]	Y (1)	Y (1)	Y (1)	Y (2)	Y (2)	N (0)	N (0)	Y (1)
Yarjanian [20]	Y (1)	Y (1)	Y (1)	P (1)	P (1)	Y (1)	Y (1)	Y (1)
Yoshihara [22]	Y (1)	Y (1)	N (0)	Y (2)	Y (2)	Y (1)	Y (1)	N (0)
Yu [51]	Y (1)	Y (1)	Y (1)	P (1)	P (1)	Y (1)	Y (1)	Y (1)
Hyun [38]	Y (1)	Y (1)	Y (1)	Y (2)	P (1)	Y (1)	Y (1)	N (0)
Yoshihara [33]	Y (1)	Y (1)	Y (1)	Y (2)	Y (2)	N (0)	N (0)	N (0)
Ford [45]	N (0)	Y (1)	N (0)	Y (2)	P (1)	Y (1)	Y (1)	N (0)
Frost [42]	Y (1)	Y (1)	Y (1)	Y (2)	Y (2)	N (0)	Y (1)	N (0)
Dangaria [37]	Y (1)	Y (1)	Y (1)	P (1)	P (1)	Y (1)	N (0)	N (0)
Kong [39]	Y (1)	Y (1)	Y (1)	P (1)	Y (2)	Y (1)	Y (1)	N (0)

Table 3 Risk of bias index *(Continued)*

Article	Reporting[a]							
	1. Study hypothesis/ aim/objective clearly described?	2. Main outcome measures clearly described?	3. Characteristics of included patients clearly described?	4. Principal assessment parameters clearly described?	5. Distributions of principal confounders per group clearly described?	6. Main study findings clearly described?	7. Provides estimates of random variability for main outcomes?	10. Actual probability values reported?
Bajek [44]	Y (1)	Y (1)	N (0)	Y (2)	P (1)	Y (1)	Y (1)	N (0)
Sun [43]	Y (1)	N (0)	Y (1)	P (1)	P (1)	Y (1)	N (0)	N (0)
Jowett [48]	Y (1)	Y (1)	N (0)	Y (2)	P (1)	N (0)	N (0)	N (0)
Total "Yes" (28)	26	27	24	23	14	24	22	16

[a]For items 4 & 5, articles that provided some but not all relevant criteria were rated as "partial". For item 10, articles were rated "yes" if actual values were provided for the majority of reported outcomes

[b]For items 11-25, articles were rated as "unable to be determined" if insufficient details were provided to make a determination. For item 15, articles were rated as "unable to be determined" if it was unclear regarding blinding when the same investigators were involved in obtaining the pathology details and performing the muscle evaluations; this was also the case when it was unclear if the clinical pathology and muscle assessments were performed by the same investigators

[c]These studies appeared to use different methodologies to analyse the same dataset so were combined for final analysis

Table 3 Risk of bias index *(Continued)*

Article	External Validity[b]						Internal Validity[b]			Total score (19)
	11. Subjects asked to participate represent entire recruited population?	12. Subjects prepared to participate represent entire recruited population?	15. Attempt made to blind those measuring main outcomes?	16. Any results based on data dredging made clear?	18. Statistical tests were appropriate?	20. Main outcome measures accurate?	21. Cases / controls recruited from same population?	22. Cases / controls recruited over same time period?	25. Adequate adjustment for confounding?	
Kalichman [31][c]	Y (1)	Y (1)	Y (1)	Y (1)	Y (1)	Y (1)	Y (1)	Y (1)	Y (1)	18
Kalichman [32][c]	Y (1)	Y (1)	Y (1)	Y (1)	Y (1)	Y (1)	Y (1)	Y (1)	Y (1)	18
Kim [16]	Y (1)	U (0)	Y (1)	Y (1)	Y (1)	Y (1)	Y (1)	Y (1)	Y (1)	18
Battie [15]	U (0)	U (0)	Y (1)	Y (1)	Y (1)	Y (1)	Y (1)	Y (1)	Y (1)	17
Farshad [18]	U (0)	U (0)	Y (1)	Y (1)	Y (1)	Y (1)	Y (1)	Y (1)	Y (1)	17
Fortin [41]	U (0)	U (0)	Y (1)	Y (1)	Y (1)	Y (1)	Y (1)	Y (1)	Y (1)	17
Altinkaya [35]	U (0)	U (0)	Y (1)	Y (1)	Y (1)	Y (1)	Y (1)	Y (1)	Y (1)	16
Jiang [53]	U (0)	U (0)	U (0)	Y (1)	Y (1)	Y (1)	Y (1)	Y (1)	Y (1)	16
Kalichman [49]	Y (1)	U (0)	Y (1)	Y (1)	Y (1)	Y (1)	Y (1)	Y (1)	Y (1)	16
Abbas [52]	U (0)	U (0)	U (0)	Y (1)	Y (1)	Y (1)	Y (1)	N (0)	Y (1)	15
Boyaci [36]	U (0)	U (0)	N (0)	Y (1)	Y (1)	Y (1)	Y (1)	Y (1)	Y (1)	15
Zhao [47]	U (0)	U (0)	U (0)	Y (1)	Y (1)	Y (1)	Y (1)	Y (1)	Y (1)	15
Bhadresha [40]	U (0)	U (0)	U (0)	Y (1)	Y (1)	Y (1)	Y (1)	Y (1)	N (0)	14
Mattila [46]	Y (1)	Y (1)	U (0)	Y (1)	Y (1)	Y (1)	Y (1)	U (0)	Y (1)	14
Ogon [54]	U (0)	U (0)	U (0)	Y (1)	Y (1)	Y (1)	U (0)	U (0)	Y (1)	14
Sebro [50]	U (0)	U (0)	U (0)	Y (1)	Y (1)	Y (1)	Y (1)	Y (1)	Y (1)	14
Yarjanian [20]	U (0)	U (0)	Y (1)	Y (1)	Y (1)	U (0)	Y (1)	Y (1)	Y (1)	14
Yoshihara [22]	U (0)	U (0)	U (0)	Y (1)	Y (1)	Y (1)	Y (1)	Y (1)	Y (1)	14
Yu [51]	U (0)	U (0)	Y (1)	Y (1)	U (0)	Y (1)	Y (1)	Y (1)	Y (1)	14
Hyun [38]	U (0)	U (0)	Y (1)	Y (1)	Y (1)	Y (1)	Y (1)	U (0)	N (0)	13
Yoshihara [33]	U (0)	U (0)	U (0)	Y (1)	Y (1)	Y (1)	Y (1)	Y (1)	Y (1)	13
Ford [45]	U (0)	U (0)	U (0)	Y (1)	Y (1)	Y (1)	Y (1)	Y (1)	Y (1)	12
Frost [42]	U (0)	U (0)	U (0)	Y (1)	Y (1)	Y (1)	U (0)	U (0)	Y (1)	12
Dangaria [37]	U (0)	U (0)	U (0)	Y (1)	Y (1)	Y (1)	Y (1)	U (0)	Y (1)	11

Table 3 Risk of bias index *(Continued)*

Article	External Validity[b]						Internal Validity[b]			
	11. Subjects asked to participate represent entire recruited population?	12. Subjects prepared to participate represent entire recruited population?	15. Attempt made to blind those measuring main outcomes?	16. Any results based on data dredging made clear?	18. Statistical tests were appropriate?	20. Main outcome measures accurate?	21. Cases / controls recruited from same population?	22. Cases / controls recruited over same time period?	25. Adequate adjustment for confounding?	Total score (19)
Kong [39]	U (0)	U (0)	U (0)	Y (1)	Y (1)	U (0)	U (0)	U (0)	Y (1)	11
Bajek [44]	U (0)	U (0)	U (0)	Y (1)	Y (1)	Y (1)	U (0)	U (0)	N (0)	10
Sun [43]	U (0)	U (0)	U (0)	Y (1)	Y (1)	Y (1)	Y (1)	Y (1)	U (0)	10
Jowett [48]	U (0)	U (0)	U (0)	Y (1)	U (0)	Y (1)	U (0)	U (0)	N (0)	7
Total "Yes" (28)	5	3	11	28	26	26	23	19	23	

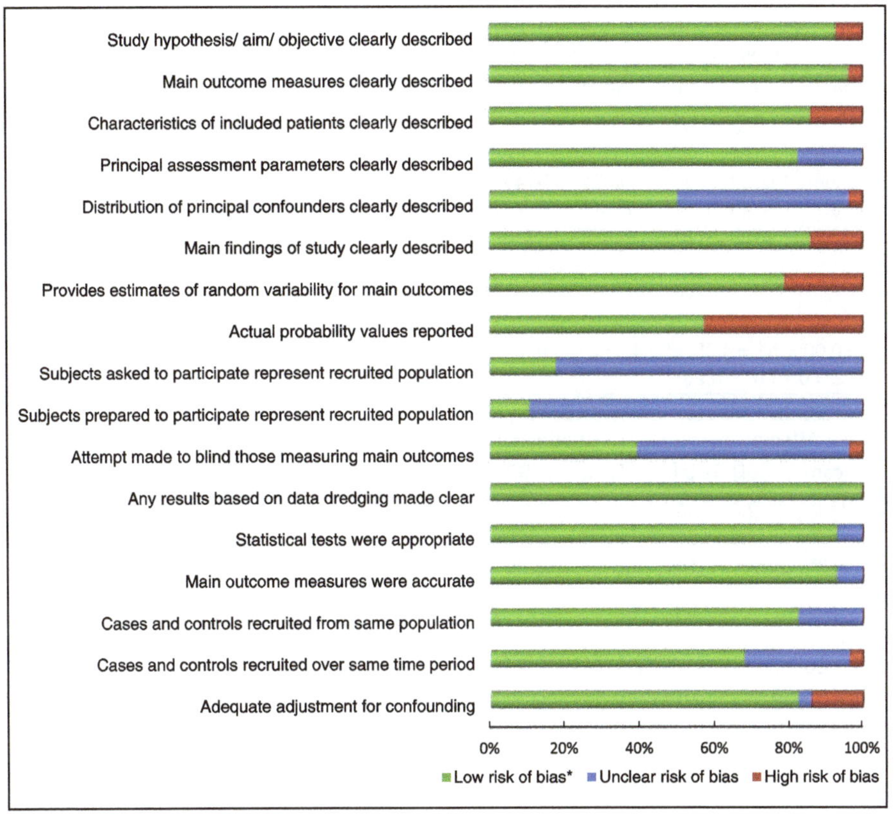

Fig. 2 Risk of bias across studies. *Low risk of bias: ROB tool criteria = Yes; Unclear risk of bias: ROB tool criteria = Partial or Unable to be determined; High risk of bias: ROB tool criteria = No

qualitative synthesis results from relevant studies not included in the meta-analyses.

Paraspinal muscle morphology in patients with lumbar disc herniation – assessed with biopsy

Study characteristics and ROB Six studies assessed patients with unilateral LDH with radiculopathy using muscle biopsy. Of these, one was of high quality, four of moderate quality, and one of low quality; study sample sizes ranged from 17 – 117. In four studies, patients served exclusively as their own controls (involved vs. uninvolved sides) [22, 33, 45, 47], and in two studies recently deceased persons who were previously healthy served as the control group [44, 46]. All studies assessed the LMM, with one study [45] also assessing the ESM. Although various measurement parameters were used across studies, they all included the mean fiber type distribution and diameter.

Meta-analysis All four studies with patients serving as their own control met the criteria for pooled data analysis when assessing mean fiber type diameter of the LMM. These studies measured type I and II fiber diameter (μm) at a total of 112 spinal levels in 83 unilateral LDH patients undergoing surgical intervention, with each study including both acute and chronic patients (refer to Additional file 5 for additional study details). The pooled analysis demonstrated a reduction of type I fiber diameter on the side of LDH (Figure 6a), which equated to the average mean diameter being 5.5% smaller on the side of LDH; similar results were seen for type II fiber diameter (Figure 6b), with the average mean diameter being 6.8% smaller on the side of LDH. The study by Ford et al. [45], contradicted the findings of the other three studies for both fiber types, but it was the lowest quality study and provided the least details regarding the relationship of the LDH to the muscle level biopsied.

Three of the above studies also met the criteria for pooling the assessment of differences in the mean fiber type distribution [22, 45, 47]. Although none of these studies reported a significant difference in fiber distribution individually, their pooled SMD demonstrated an increase in type I fiber distribution on the side of LDH (Figure 6c), which equated to a 7% greater average mean fiber distribution. The fourth study was not included in fiber distribution pooled data analysis due to the absence of a reported variance estimate which could not be obtained from the authors; however, consistent with the pooled data it did report a higher mean distribution of type I fibers on the side of LDH [33].

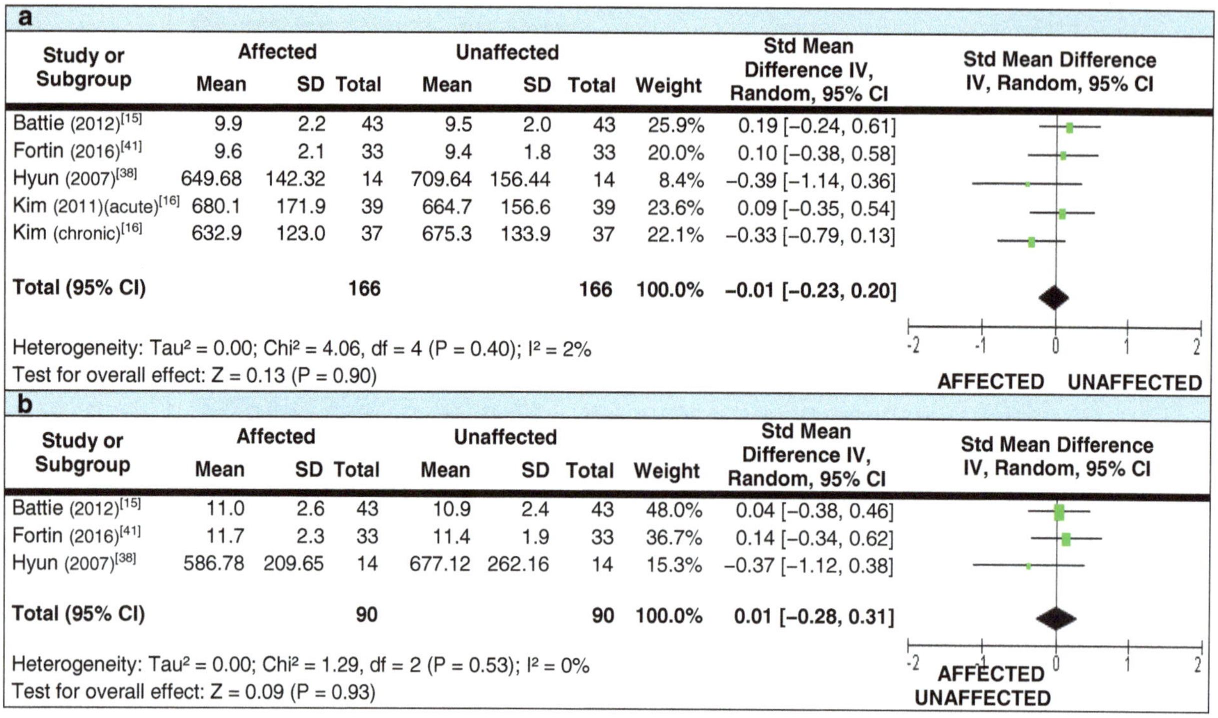

a

Study or Subgroup	Affected Mean	Affected SD	Affected Total	Unaffected Mean	Unaffected SD	Unaffected Total	Weight	Std Mean Difference IV, Random, 95% CI
Battie (2012)[15]	9.9	2.2	43	9.5	2.0	43	25.9%	0.19 [−0.24, 0.61]
Fortin (2016)[41]	9.6	2.1	33	9.4	1.8	33	20.0%	0.10 [−0.38, 0.58]
Hyun (2007)[38]	649.68	142.32	14	709.64	156.44	14	8.4%	−0.39 [−1.14, 0.36]
Kim (2011)(acute)[16]	680.1	171.9	39	664.7	156.6	39	23.6%	0.09 [−0.35, 0.54]
Kim (chronic)[16]	632.9	123.0	37	675.3	133.9	37	22.1%	−0.33 [−0.79, 0.13]
Total (95% CI)			**166**			**166**	**100.0%**	**−0.01 [−0.23, 0.20]**

Heterogeneity: Tau² = 0.00; Chi² = 4.06, df = 4 (P = 0.40); I² = 2%
Test for overall effect: Z = 0.13 (P = 0.90)

b

Study or Subgroup	Affected Mean	Affected SD	Affected Total	Unaffected Mean	Unaffected SD	Unaffected Total	Weight	Std Mean Difference IV, Random, 95% CI
Battie (2012)[15]	11.0	2.6	43	10.9	2.4	43	48.0%	0.04 [−0.38, 0.46]
Fortin (2016)[41]	11.7	2.3	33	11.4	1.9	33	36.7%	0.14 [−0.34, 0.62]
Hyun (2007)[38]	586.78	209.65	14	677.12	262.16	14	15.3%	−0.37 [−1.12, 0.38]
Total (95% CI)			**90**			**90**	**100.0%**	**0.01 [−0.28, 0.31]**

Heterogeneity: Tau² = 0.00; Chi² = 1.29, df = 2 (P = 0.53); I² = 0%
Test for overall effect: Z = 0.09 (P = 0.93)

Fig. 3 Pooled LMM imaging measurements – TCSA. Pooled total cross-sectional area (TCSA) measures for meta-analysis comparing the side affected by disc herniation to the unaffected side. 3**a**: at the level of herniation; 3**b**: below the level of herniation

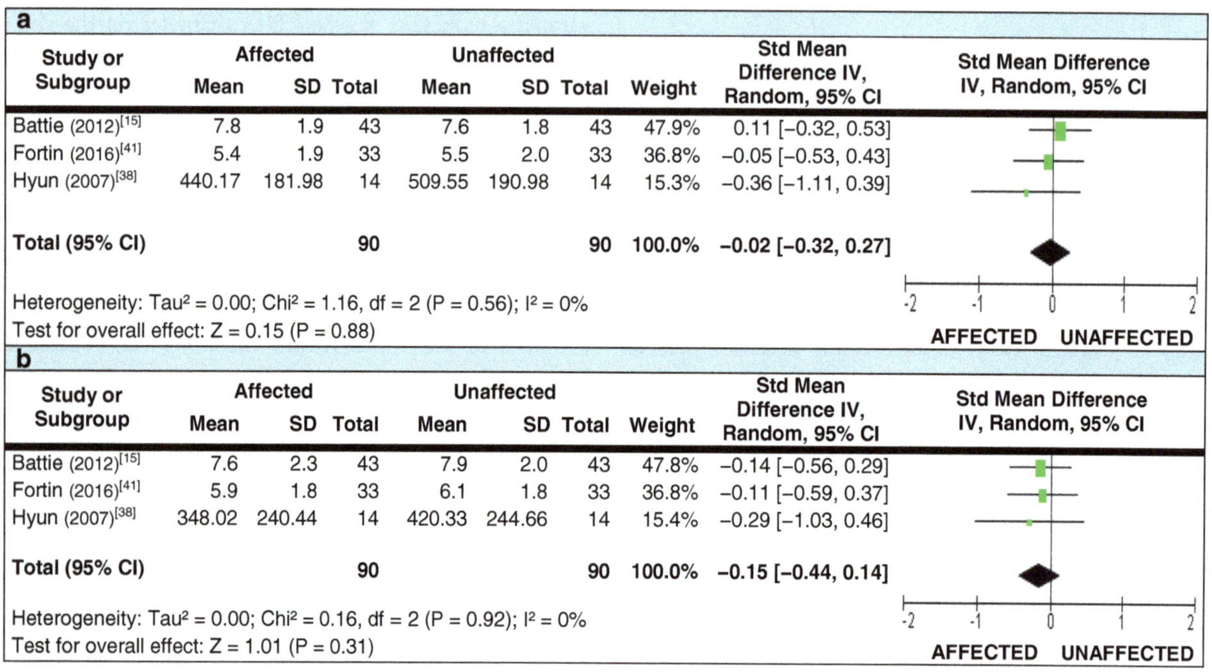

a

Study or Subgroup	Affected Mean	Affected SD	Affected Total	Unaffected Mean	Unaffected SD	Unaffected Total	Weight	Std Mean Difference IV, Random, 95% CI
Battie (2012)[15]	7.8	1.9	43	7.6	1.8	43	47.9%	0.11 [−0.32, 0.53]
Fortin (2016)[41]	5.4	1.9	33	5.5	2.0	33	36.8%	−0.05 [−0.53, 0.43]
Hyun (2007)[38]	440.17	181.98	14	509.55	190.98	14	15.3%	−0.36 [−1.11, 0.39]
Total (95% CI)			**90**			**90**	**100.0%**	**−0.02 [−0.32, 0.27]**

Heterogeneity: Tau² = 0.00; Chi² = 1.16, df = 2 (P = 0.56); I² = 0%
Test for overall effect: Z = 0.15 (P = 0.88)

b

Study or Subgroup	Affected Mean	Affected SD	Affected Total	Unaffected Mean	Unaffected SD	Unaffected Total	Weight	Std Mean Difference IV, Random, 95% CI
Battie (2012)[15]	7.6	2.3	43	7.9	2.0	43	47.8%	−0.14 [−0.56, 0.29]
Fortin (2016)[41]	5.9	1.8	33	6.1	1.8	33	36.8%	−0.11 [−0.59, 0.37]
Hyun (2007)[38]	348.02	240.44	14	420.33	244.66	14	15.4%	−0.29 [−1.03, 0.46]
Total (95% CI)			**90**			**90**	**100.0%**	**−0.15 [−0.44, 0.14]**

Heterogeneity: Tau² = 0.00; Chi² = 0.16, df = 2 (P = 0.92); I² = 0%
Test for overall effect: Z = 1.01 (P = 0.31)

Fig. 4 Pooled LMM imaging measurements – FCSA. Pooled functional cross-sectional area (FCSA) measures for meta-analysis comparing the side affected by disc herniation to the unaffected side. 4**a**: at the level of herniation; 4**b**: below the level of herniation

a

Study or Subgroup	Affected Mean	SD	Total	Unaffected Mean	SD	Total	Weight	Std Mean Difference IV, Random, 95% CI
Battie (2012)[15]	0.78	0.09	43	0.8	0.07	43	47.7%	−0.25 [−0.67, 0.18]
Fortin (2016)[41]	0.55	0.16	33	0.57	0.14	33	36.8%	−0.13 [−0.61, 0.35]
Hyun (2007)[38]	0.68	0.23	14	0.73	0.24	14	15.5%	−0.21 [−0.95, 0.54]
Total (95% CI)			**90**			**90**	**100.0%**	**−0.20 [−0.49, 0.10]**

Heterogeneity: $Tau^2 = 0.00$; $Chi^2 = 0.12$, df = 2 (P = 0.94); $I^2 = 0\%$
Test for overall effect: Z = 1.32 (P = 0.19)

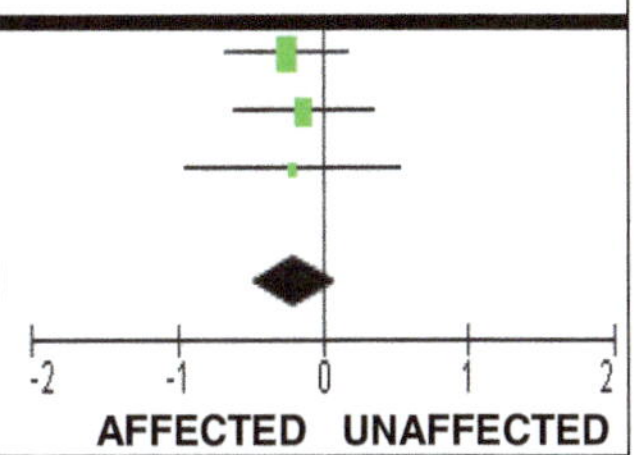

b

Study or Subgroup	Affected Mean	SD	Total	Unaffected Mean	SD	Total	Weight	Std Mean Difference IV, Random, 95% CI
Battie (2012)[15]	0.69	0.12	43	0.72	0.09	43	47.6%	−0.28 [−0.71, 0.14]
Fortin (2016)[41]	0.51	0.11	33	0.53	0.11	33	36.8%	−0.18 [−0.66, 0.30]
Hyun (2007)[38]	0.55	0.24	14	0.59	0.16	14	15.6%	−0.19 [−0.93, 0.55]
Total (95% CI)			**90**			**90**	**100.0%**	**−0.23 [−0.52, 0.06]**

Heterogeneity: $Tau^2 = 0.00$; $Chi^2 = 0.11$, df = 2 (P = 0.95); $I^2 = 0\%$
Test for overall effect: Z = 1.53 (P = 0.13)

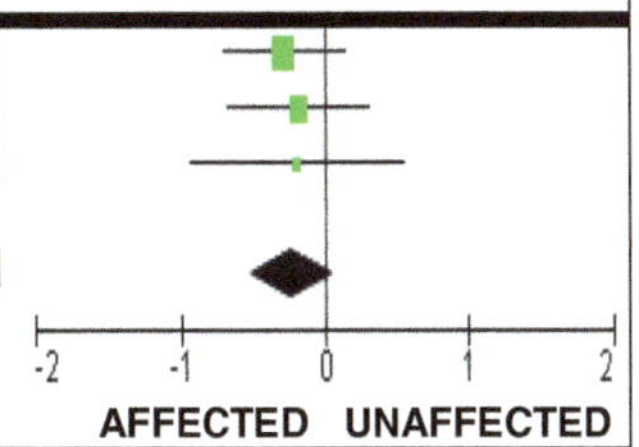

Fig. 5 Pooled LMM imaging measurements – FCSA:TCSA ratio. Pooled FCSA:TCSA ratio measures for meta-analysis comparing the side affected by disc herniation to the unaffected side. 5**a**: at the level of herniation; 5**b**: below the level of herniation

For the above analyses, only the measurements at the level below herniation were used from the Yoshihara et al. (2001) study [22]; results taken at the level of LDH were also available, but rather than combining the two sets of values, the latter dataset was included in a subsequent subgroup analysis based on the level of biopsy in relation to LDH. As the study by Ford et al., did not specify this relationship, it was excluded from further analysis. For biopsies acquired at [22, 47] or below [22, 33] the level of LDH, type I and II fiber diameter measures were only smaller on the affected side for muscles below the level of LDH: type I fiber diameter at the level of LDH (SMD [95% CI] = −0.27 [−0.68, 0.13]) and below the LDH (SMD [95% CI] = −0.53 [−0.95, −0.11]); type II fiber diameter at the level of LDH (SMD [95% CI] = −0.30 [−0.71, 0.10]) and below the LDH (SMD [95% CI] = −0.57 [−0.99, −0.16]). There was insufficient data to perform subgroup analysis on fiber type distribution. Table 4 (section 1.1) shows results from the qualitative synthesis for this section.

Paraspinal muscle morphology in patients with any spinal pathology and associated nerve root signs – assessed with biopsy

One study assessed the distribution of LMM fiber types in patients with spinal pathology with and without signs of NR involvement, along with a cadaveric control group [48]. The limited distinction of pathology types precluded pathology-based analysis. Although a significant difference was demonstrated in the percentage of type II fibers, both measures fell within the average type II fiber distribution of ~36% (±11%) noted by Mannion et al. [55], in a young, healthy population. This was the oldest and highest risk of bias study in this systematic review (7/19).

Paraspinal muscle morphology in patients with facet arthrosis – assessed with imaging

Study characteristics and ROB Four studies looked at three different data sets utilizing CT imaging to assess fatty infiltration of paraspinal muscles in individuals with facet arthrosis: two from the same general population [31, 32] and two from patient populations [49, 50]. Three studies were of high quality and one of moderate quality; total sample sizes varied from 100-187. Three studies assessed facet arthrosis and muscle changes at multiple spinal levels; one study evaluated the L4/5 level only [49]. Three studies evaluated the LMM and ESM and compared participants with arthrosis to those without; the remaining study assessed the LMM, PMM, and longissimus and assessed arthrosis on a summative grading scale [50]. A fifth, moderate quality study used MRI and CT to assess CSA and fatty infiltration of the LMM [51]. All studies applied different statistical analyses to the relationships between arthrosis and muscle changes, precluding data pooling. Table 4 (section 1.3) provides the results from the qualitative synthesis for this section.

Table 4 Detailed results analysis for non-pooled data

1.0 Paraspinal muscle morphology in patients with lumbar disc herniation – assessed with imaging:

1.0.1 Patients serving as own controls

- 3 studies assessed the TCSA of the PMM [15, 16, 37]:
  - [15]: acute patients: PMM was larger on side of LDH regardless of measurement relationship to LDH; not statistically significant.
  - [16]: acute and chronic patients at LDH level only: PMM CSA was insignificantly smaller on side of LDH for both groups.
  - [37]: chronic patients: PMM was smaller on side of LDH regardless of relationship to level of LDH; statistically significant at L4/5, L5/S1 ($P < 0.05$). Median % reduction of TCSA on side of LDH averaged 8.5% ($P < 0.05$) at L4/5, L5/S1.
- 2 high quality studies assessed the TCSA and FCSA of the ESM [15, 41]:
  - [15]: no significance to these differences at any level.
  - [41]: significantly smaller FCSA measures at L5/S1 (level below LDH) ($P = 0.04$), and significantly smaller ratios at L4/5, L5/S1 ($P = 0.04, 0.007$); TCSA on side of LDH was larger at the level above LDH ($P = 0.05$).
- 2 studies assessed MRI signal intensity of the LMM and ESM: one including acute [15], one chronic [41] patients. Both studies demonstrated:
  - significant increase in mean LMM signal (i.e., more fat) on side of LDH at the level below ($P = 0.014$ [15] and 0.04 [41]); no consistent or significant differences noted at or above the level of LDH.
  - higher mean ESM signal on side of LDH at the level of LDH in acute patients ($P = 0.017$) and the level below LDH (S1) in chronic ($P = 0.02$).
- 1 moderate quality study assessed the combined echo intensity of the LMM and ESM [42], and reported statstically non-significant results.
- 1 high quality study compared the affected to non-affected side to assess median TCSA and MLD of the LMM against duration of symptoms and severity of NR compression [35], reporting:
  - non-significant results for TSCA.
  - MLD larger on side of LDH across all *duration* groups ($P < 0.05$); MLD progressively enlarged as duration increased ($P = 0.021$).
  - non-significant results for MLD across all *severity* groups.
- 1 high quality study assessed FCSA and MLD ratios of the LMM, and their relationship to various clinical measures [18]:
  - no significant relationship found between FCSA or MLD ratios and severity of NR compression, symptom duration, or motor deficit.
  - 1 moderate quality study assessed TCSA, FCSA, and FCSA:TCSA ratios in LDH patients without radiculopathy [38], reporting no significant differences.

1.0.2 Compared to healthy controls without LDH or radiculopathy

- 4 LDH studies included a healthy control group [37–39, 42]:
  - [37]: measured side-to-side difference in TCSA of the PMM in a control group: no difference found between sides. Control group median TCSA was smaller than both LDH groups from L3/4 – L5/S1, but no statistical comparison was made between groups.
  - [38]: compared TCSA, FCSA, FCSA:TCSA ratio, and involved:uninvolved side FCSA ratios (IS:US) of control group LMM to patients with LDH – with and without radiculopathy.
    - TCSA smaller at L5/S1 on side of LDH in both patient groups ($P < 0.05$); FCSA significantly smaller in both patient groups at L4/5, L5/S1 ($P < 0.05$).
    - FCSA:TCSA ratio smaller in both patient groups at L3/4, L4/5 ($P < 0.05$).
    - IS:US ratio for radiculopathy group significantly smaller than controls at L4/5, L5/S1 ($P < 0.01$), and when all levels were combined ($P < 0.05$).
    - IS:US ratio abnormal in 79% of radiculopathy cases and 10% of controls ($P < 0.01$), but not between control group and uninvolved side of LDH.
  - [39]: assessed amount of combined fat infiltration of LMM and ESM (presumably bilaterally, but not defined). Fat infiltration was greater in the LDH group at all levels ($P < 0.05$ at L2/3; $P < 0.001$ from L3/4 – L5/S1).
  - [42]: assessed echo intensity of LMM and ESM combined, with no difference noted between any groups.

1.0.3 Compared to low back pain patients without LDH or radiculopathy

- 3 LDH studies included LBP comparison groups; 1 high quality [36], 1 moderate quality [40], and 1 low quality [43]:
  - [36]: compared TCSA and quantitative gradings of LMM, PVM, PMM, QLM for LDH with unilateral or bilateral radiculopathy to chronic LBP only patients.
    - smaller TCSA of right QLM only noted in the LDH group ($P = 0.01$).
    - higher grades of fat infiltration more prevalent in LDH group at all locations except PMM (P range: 0.02 – 0.04).
    - NB: 8 patients in the comparison group also had facet arthrosis, but no leg pain.
  - [40]: used point-of-contact calculations (Cavalieri approximation principle) to compare muscle:fat ratios of LMM, ESM, & PMM in single or multi-level LDH patients to same ratios in LBP patients (unknown symptom duration) with single or multi-level degenerative disc disease; individual muscles were combined bilaterally. No difference in ratios found between patient groups for any muscle at any level.
  - [43]: used quantitative muscle grading to assess the LMM bilaterally from L3/4 – L5/S1; greater atrophy, and more severe atrophy, reported in LDH group at all levels ($P < 0.01$). NB: no analyses made regarding side of LDH; unknown if differences in symptom chronicity present requiring adjustment.

1.0.4 Compared to LDH patients without radiculopathy

- 1 study compared the TCSA, FCSA, FCSA:TCSA ratio, and IS:US ratio (FCSA) of the LMM between LDH patients with and without radiculopathy [38]:
  - IS:US ratio for radiculopathy group smaller than LDH-only group at L4/5, L5/S1 ($P < 0.01$), and with all levels combined ($P < 0.05$).
  - IS:US ratio abnormal in 24% of LDH-only cases vs. 79% of radiculopathy cases ($P < 0.01$).
  - no differences in the remaining CSA measures were noted.

1.1 Paraspinal muscle morphology in patients with lumbar disc herniation – assessed with biopsy:

- 3 studies assessed mean fiber type diameter and distribution for the ESM [45] and the LMM [44, 46]:

Table 4 Detailed results analysis for non-pooled data *(Continued)*

- o [45]: compared the affected to non-affected side and found no difference for any measures.
- o [44]: compared to deceased controls: Type I fiber distribution in LMM higher for males with LDH ($P<0.05$); type I fiber diameter larger in males ($P<0.05$) and females ($P < 0.01$) with LDH; type IIA and IIB fiber diameter larger in male LDH patients ($P < 0.05$). NB: not adjusted for differences in age or sex.
- o [46]: compared to deceased controls: Type I fiber diameter was significantly larger in male LDH patients ($P < 0.01$).
- • 2 studies assessed mean muscle strength factor (MSF), one for the LMM and ESM [45], and one for the LMM only [47]:
- o [45]: non-significant results for both muscle groups.
- o [47]: type II fiber MSF was lower on the LDH side ($P < 0.05$).
- • 2 studies compared % frequencies of fiber type grouping and small angular fibers in the LMM [22, 33]:
- o [22]: higher grouping frequency on side of LDH at the level below LDH (L5): 27.6% vs.10.3%; higher angular fiber frequency noted on side of LDH at L5: 20.7% vs. 3.4% (no P values).
- o [33]: higher grouping frequency on side of LDH at L5 (level below LDH): 35% vs. 6%; higher angular fiber frequency noted on side of LDH at L5: 41% vs. 24% (no *P* values).
- • 1 study, using patients as their own control, measured mean fiber type CSA of the LMM, and fiber CSA with or without a +SLR [47], noting:
- o significantly and consistently smaller CSA for both fiber types on affected side of LDH ($P < 0.05$); this became more pronounced when considering +SLR patients only ($P < 0.01$), but non-significant with −SLR patients only.
- • 1 moderate quality study assessed mean atrophy/hypertrophy factors for type I & II fibers, and mean % core targetoid and moth-eaten change in the LMM against cadaveric controls [46]:
- o an increase in core-targetoid presence was found in male ($P < 0.01$) and female patients ($P < 0.001$), with higher type I fiber hypertrophy factor in male patients ($P < 0.01$) and an increase in moth-eaten change in female patients ($P < 0.001$).

1.3 Paraspinal muscle morphology in patients with facet arthrosis – assessed with imaging:

- • 4 studies assessed the association of facet arthrosis with paraspinal muscle density (2 using the same general population data set) [(31,32),49,50]:
- o [31]: reported severe arthrosis (grade 3) at L4/5 consistently associated with greater fat infiltration of the LMM and ESM (*P* range: 0.0002 – 0.056).
- o [32]: identified associations between reduced paraspinal muscle density and arthrosis [AOR: 3.68 [1.36 – 9.97] (LMM); 2.80 [1.10 – 7.16] (ESM)].
- o [49]: assessed L4/5, with AORs showing associations between arthrosis and muscle density ratios (*P* range: 0.001 – 0.009 (LMM); 0.002 – 0.01 (ESM)), as well as arthrosis and higher fat infiltration grades ($P <0.0001$ (LMM & ESM)). No associations found between arthrosis and mean muscle density only.
- o [50]: demonstrated negative correlations between LMM, PMM, and Longissimus muscle density and facet arthrosis with univariate analysis ($P <0.0001$ for all muscles), but non-significant correlations following multivariate analysis.
  - ▪ NB: this study grouped all measures rather than assessing muscle density or arthrosis by spinal level.
- • 1 study assessed arthrosis in relation to CSA and the muscle-fat index (MFI) [51], identifying:
- o smaller CSA and higher MFI (i.e., higher fat content) at all levels with arthrosis present ($P < 0.001$); increased MFI was independently associated with arthrosis at all levels (*P* range: <0.001 – 0.005).
- o differences in CSA asymmetry were greater for CSA with arthrosis present at L5/S1 only (*P* range: <0.001 – 0.005).

1.4 Paraspinal muscle morphology in patients with canal stenosis – assessed with imaging:

- • 4 studies assessed the association of canal stenosis with paraspinal muscle fat inflitration (2 using the same general population data set) [(31,32),52,53]:
- o [31, 32]: after adjusting for age, sex, and/or BMI, spinal stenosis was not associated with altered CT muscle density for the LMM or ESM (N = 15).
- o [52]: showed associations of stenosis with increased CT muscle density in LMM, ESM, and PMM in 165 patients with confirmed clinical symptoms of stenosis (*P* range = 0.036 to < 0.001).
  - ▪ NB: the lower fat content in the stenosis group may be the result of the muscles being measured above the level of reported stenosis.
- o [53]: assessed fat infiltration with MRI at the level of stenosis, with a greater fat infiltration ratio in the stenosis group (N = 40; $P = 0.004$).
- • 3 studies assessed the relationship of stenosis to muscle atrophy [20, 52, 53]:
- o [20]: reported a reduction in FCSA of LMM between stenosis and healthy control groups ($P = 0.04$), but not stenosis and LBP groups.
- o [52]: demonstrated greater FCSA of the ESM in male ($P = 0.011$) and female ($P = 0.014$) stenosis patients, and PMM in male stenosis patients ($P = 0.042$), but no significant difference for the LMM. NB: acquired measurements at L3, which could account for conflicting results with other studies.
- o [53]: evaluated muscle asymmetry and TCSA measures of the LMM at L4/5;with greater asymmetry ($P = 0.006$) and lower TCSA:body ratios ($P = 0.006$) reported in the stenosis group.
- • 1 study used MR spectroscopy to assess extramyocellular lipids (EMCL) and intramyocelluar lipds (IMCL) [54]:
- o when assessing EMCL content (i.e, the fat tissue deposits visible on standard MR imaging), no difference was found between the stenosis and CLBP groups; this is in agreement with the study by Yarjanian above [20].
- o IMCL content was higher in the CLBP vs. stenosis group ($P =< 0.01$).
  - ▪ NB: IMCL deposits not are seen on standard imaging, being more likely to increase due to metabolic changes associated with inactivity; significantly higher VAS scores in the CLBP group would be a more important contributor than potential NR compression.
  - ▪ NB: this study also analysed postural changes between each group but found no differences; alignment was not a confounding factor in this analysis.

LMM **Lumbar multifidus muscle,** ***PMM*** **Psoas major muscle,** ***PVM*** **Paravertebral (paraspinal) muscle,** ***ESM*** **Erector spinae muscle,** ***QLM*** **Quadratus lumborum muscle,** ***LBP*** **Low back pain,** ***SLR*** **Straight leg raise,** ***NR*** **Nerve root,** ***LDH*** **lumbar disc herniation,** ***CSA*** **Cross-sectional area,** ***TCSA*** **Total CSA,** ***FCSA*** **Functional CSA,** ***MLD*** **Muscle laminar distance,** ***IS US ratio*** **Involved side to uninvolved side ratio,** ***VAS*** **Visual analogue scale,** ***AOR*** **Adjusted odds ratio,** ***BMI*** **body mass index,** ***CT*** **Computed tomography,** ***MRI*** **Magnetic resonance imaging**

a

Study or Subgroup	Affected Mean	Affected SD	Affected Total	Unaffected Mean	Unaffected SD	Unaffected Total	Weight	Std Mean Difference IV, Random, 95% CI
Ford (1983)[45]	58.9	16.7	18	58.8	8.3	18	22.3%	0.01 [−0.65, 0.66]
Yoshihara (2001)[22]	59.1	7.2	29	63.1	10.0	29	35.0%	−0.45 [−0.97, 0.07]
Yoshihara (2003)[33]	58.1	7.5	17	63.6	8.5	17	19.8%	−0.67 [−1.36, 0.02]
Zhao (2000)[47]	45.3	7.1	19	48.6	6.8	19	22.9%	−0.46 [−1.11, 0.18]
Total (95% CI)			**83**			**83**	**100.0%**	**−0.40 [−0.70, −0.09]**

Heterogeneity: $Tau^2 = 0.00$; $Chi^2 = 2.15$, df = 3 (P = 0.54); $I^2 = 0\%$
Test for overall effect: Z = 2.51 (P = 0.01)

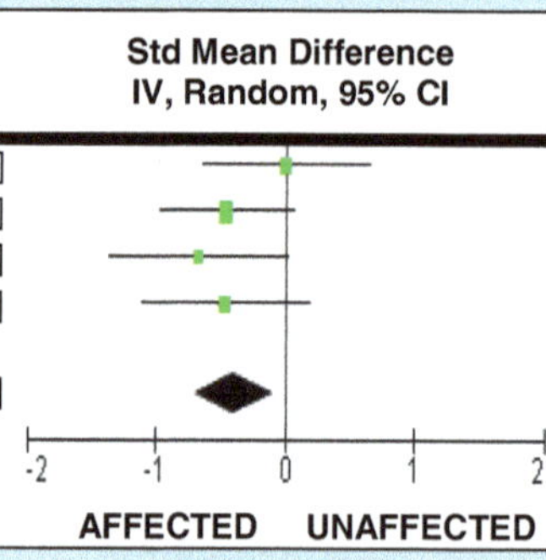

b

Study or Subgroup	Affected Mean	Affected SD	Affected Total	Unaffected Mean	Unaffected SD	Unaffected Total	Weight	Std Mean Difference IV, Random, 95% CI
Ford (1983)[45]	42.5	14.2	18	40.8	12.8	18	22.4%	0.12 [−0.53, 0.78]
Yoshihara (2001)[22]	40.5	8.1	29	44.9	7.3	29	34.2%	−0.56 [−1.09, −0.04]
Yoshihara (2003)[33]	39.3	8.7	17	44.5	8.5	17	20.3%	−0.59 [−1.28, 0.10]
Zhao (2000)[47]	33.3	7.0	19	36.5	8.6	19	23.2%	−0.40 [−1.04, 0.24]
Total (95% CI)			**83**			**83**	**100.0%**	**−0.38 [−0.69, −0.06]**

Heterogeneity: $Tau^2 = 0.00$; $Chi^2 = 3.10$, df = 3 (P = 0.38); $I^2 = 3\%$
Test for overall effect: Z = 2.35 (P = 0.02)

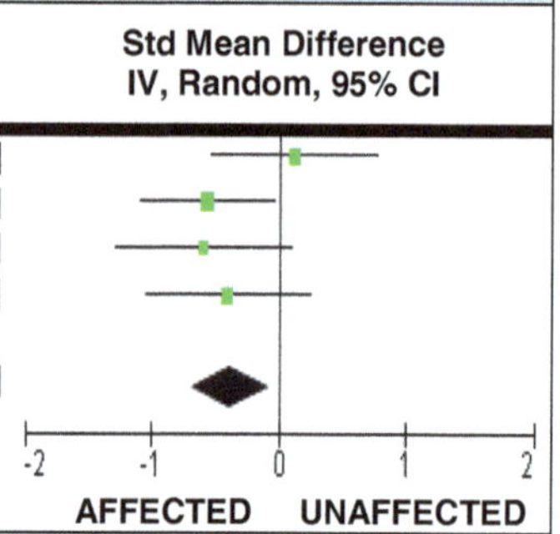

c

Study or Subgroup	Affected Mean	Affected SD	Affected Total	Unaffected Mean	Unaffected SD	Unaffected Total	Weight	Std Mean Difference IV, Random, 95% CI
Ford (1983)[45]	53.0	15.0	18	49.0	19.5	18	29.3%	0.22 [−0.43, 0.88]
Yoshihara (2001)[22]	66.0	6.7	29	60.6	7.1	29	40.0%	0.77 [0.24, 1.31]
Yoshihara (2003)[33]	60.2	12.9	19	58.1	11.6	19	30.7%	0.17 [−0.47, 0.80]
Total (95% CI)			**66**			**66**	**100.0%**	**0.43 [0.03, 0.82]**

Heterogeneity: $Tau^2 = 0.03$; $Chi^2 = 2.59$, df = 2 (P = 0.27); $I^2 = 23\%$
Test for overall effect: Z = 2.10 (P = 0.04)

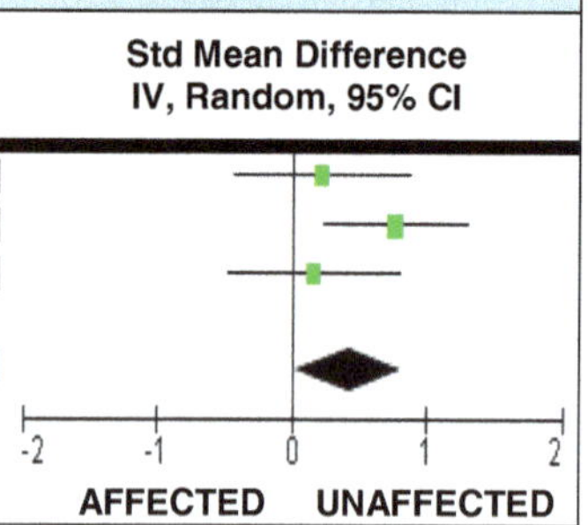

Fig. 6 Pooled LMM biopsy measurements. Pooled biopsy measures for meta-analysis comparing the side affected by disc herniation to the unaffected side. 6**a**: type I fiber size; 6**b**: type II fiber size; 6**c**: type I fiber distribution

Paraspinal muscle morphology in patients with canal stenosis – assessed with imaging

Study characteristics and ROB Six studies looked at five different data sets to assess relationships between central stenosis and muscle morphology, with four being of high quality and two of moderate quality; total sample sizes ranged from 35 – 345. Two studies used the same CT data set to assess fatty infiltration of the LMM and ESM in a general volunteer population [31, 32]. The remaining studies evaluated patients with clinical and/or imaging findings consistent with stenosis; one used CT [52], two used MRI [20, 53], and one used MR spectroscopy [54]. Of these latter four studies, one compared spinal stenosis patients to LBP patients without spinal stenosis as well as asymptomatic volunteers [20], one compared stenosis to chronic LBP patients only [54], while to remaining two studies compared patients with and without stenosis only. Muscle analysis utilized a variety of approaches and statistical analyses were also quite variable, precluding the pooling of data. Table 4 (section 1.4) reports the results from the qualitative synthesis data for this section.

Discussion

This systematic review is the first to synthesize studies examining the relationships between paraspinal muscle morphology and spinal pathologies associated with neurocompression in patients with specific LBP. We found LDH to be associated with muscle morphological changes comprising fiber size, fiber type, and fiber distribution. Specifically, the findings of our meta-analyses demonstrated that when patients served as their own controls, LDH was associated with decreased type I and II fiber size, and an increased proportion of type I fibers, in the LMM at the level below the herniation; this could be related to compressive nerve root damage leading to muscle fiber denervation [46]. From the qualitative synthesis of individual studies (Table 4), we found a higher frequency of small angular fibers (indicating denervation of single motor neuron muscle fibers [46]) and fiber type grouping (indicating collateral re-innervation of these fibers [46]) on the side of and below LDH, which correlated with the more significant amount of fiber atrophy found at the level below herniation in the pooled data. A higher percentage of core targetoid change was also identified at the level below LDH in one study, which is a non-specific indicator of underlying muscle disease, including denervation [46]. The findings from the pooled and non-pooled data suggest that persistent compression of the nerve roots may be contributing to atrophy of muscle fibers supplied by that nerve. Whether these changes are permanent or reversible is unclear.

Pooling of data from studies that used imaging modalities to measure the cross-sectional area of paraspinal muscles did not identify associations with spinal pathology. However, several individual studies did report associations between spinal pathology and imaging derived measures of paraspinal muscle morphology, particularly regarding LDH with chronic radiculopathy, and facet arthrosis [31, 32, 35, 36, 38, 39, 43, 49, 51]. Increased fatty infiltration of the PVM occurred with higher grades of facet degeneration, particularly at L4/5 (where facet joint arthrosis is most commonly found [56]). For central canal stenosis, the limited number of studies, conflicting outcomes, and key variations in study methodology precluded a definitive conclusion.

The absence of findings of a consistent reduction of muscle CSA in the presence of these specific pathological conditions may indicate that no significant relationships exist; however, it may also be possible that the variability in study designs is partially concealing the impact of the changes. For example, mixing measures across spinal levels rather than specifically measuring "at" and "below" the herniation, measuring above the level of pathology, grouping all spinal levels instead of individual analysis, or mixing acute and chronic back pain patients in the same analysis. Conversely, any number of study design or measurement variations could also have resulted in the apparent mismatch between the biopsy and imaging findings; however, actual morphological reasons for this difference may relate to fiber type distribution being less apparent anatomically and thus only notable with biopsy, or the internal complexity of the gross anatomy of the LMM masking microscopic changes to individual fiber size on imaging. Additionally, imaging modalities cannot provide the same level of precision as histological studies.

Potential confounders to be considered when interpreting the outcomes of this review include the neurological supply of the multifidus muscles, how muscle atrophy presents, and the types of controls used between studies. When considering uni-segmental versus multi-segmental nerve supply to the LMM, it is physiologically apparent that muscle activation (whether normal or pathological) can occur well above or below the level of primary nerve root involvement, even if the anatomical data suggests level-specific innervation [57]; however, Kottlors et al. [57], have suggested that this effect reduces the further away the level of muscle origin is from the nerve root affected. If that is the case, the primary alteration to the LMM from any nerve root lesion should be most profound at the level supplied by the medial branch of the dorsal ramus of the affected nerve root, with progressively less change occurring to the muscles farther away. This may help explain the occasional finding of reduced LMM FCSA (albeit insignificantly) of the muscle above an affected nerve root, but the greater likelihood of significant FCSA reduction of muscles supplied primarily by a compressed nerve root.

Within several studies, the side-to-side differences in the reported TCSA were less consistent than those noted for the FCSA. While muscle atrophy is most simply assessed by imaging as a reduction in the overall size of a muscle's TCSA, this does not take into account the possibility that individual muscle fascicles may atrophy and be replaced by fat infiltration [58] without reducing the muscle's total cross-section. This change may manifest most clearly in the multifidus muscle fascicles closest to the spinolaminar margins (as visualized on axial cross-sections from L4-S1), which are directly innervated by an affected L4 or L5 nerve root. This variability could be accounted for in the assessment of atrophy if a muscle-to-fat ratio component is included, and by including all tissue within the epimysial boundaries.

The issue of using patients as their own controls, versus healthy (with imaging studies) or cadaveric controls (for biopsy studies) was considered. The advantages of using patients as their own controls includes consistency of image parameters, quality, spinal level selection and patient parameters (e.g., matching size, age, sex variables), as well as being generally more convenient since fewer participants are required. Disadvantages include the potential for inherent confounders, such as normal asymmetry, any effect of the pathologic variable on the contralateral side, or the potential for neurological alterations contralateral to the side of pathology [57]. However, our review did not show outcomes to be greatly varied between studies based on the type of control group, except with biopsies using cadaveric controls.

Limitations

A key challenge for undertaking this review was the inherent difficulty in assessing paraspinal muscle morphology by any study looking at these muscle groups, due to a lack of agreement on multifidus muscle gross and neuroanatomy; at least ten published variations are described. The 2008 study by Lonnemann et al. [59], provides a clear overview of these descriptions, but also offers a new one. This is further complicated by a 2011 article by Cornwall et al. [60], describing anatomy more closely found in the seminal study by Macintosh et al. [61], but with their own distinct alternations to that description. Nevertheless, the Lonnemann [59] and Cornwall [60] studies both agree on the complex inter-digitation or blending of the different fascicles of the LMM, which makes distinction of individual fascicles on imaging exceedingly challenging. For our review, this underlying anatomical complexity was further compounded by a lack of focused measurement methodologies or agreed muscle degeneration criteria used in the included studies. This resulted in a wide variety of approaches to investigate for associations between spinal pathology and paraspinal muscles changes, with outcomes that were difficult to compare or amalgamate for a more robust statistical analysis. In this regard, our findings were consistent with a recent narrative review by Kalichman et al. [62], and a proposed paraspinal muscle analysis methodology by Crawford et al. [63], each identifying a strong need to establish uniform methods for evaluating paraspinal muscle degeneration.

The limited quality assessment tool options for cross-sectional studies created a challenge, and while no generally accepted and valid tool was identified for looking at the associations between pathology and muscle changes, two options presented with the best potential: that developed by Downs and Black [28], and the Newcastle-Ottawa scale [64]. Although the Newcastle-Ottawa scale was designed specifically for observational studies, it was lacking in several reporting items we felt were important, was initially focussed on cohort and case control studies, and was still in the validation process. As both potential tools required modification, we determined to use a modified version of the Downs and Black risk of bias tool following the protocols of other similar published reviews [29, 30]. We also incorporated one additional modification by replacing a "clearly described intervention" item with a "clearly described assessment parameters" item, as we determined this to be an important and equivalent quality issue for our topic. These modifications may have had a small impact on overall risk of bias analysis, but this should have equally affected all studies. Varying degrees of familiarity with the tool between examiners may also have contributed to some of the initial non-agreement in the ROB analysis.

An insufficient number of studies were available to statistically assess for publication bias (e.g., funnel plots). However, while there is a potential for positive publication bias, the risk would seem fairly low in this review since the studies were observational and non-interventional, with no particular outcome from which those authors would benefit. Additionally, the moderate level of initial agreement for full text screening, and weak to moderate level of initial agreement for ROB analysis may have contributed to potential selection and/or quality bias; however, in the majority of cases the disagreement was either due to one examiner overlooking or misinterpreting a small inclusion/exclusion detail in a study, or related to complexities regarding how information was reported in relation to the ROB analysis criteria. In every case, full consensus was reached at the first meeting, with a relatively even mix of altered input between each examiner such that no one assessor dominated the review outcome.

The small number of studies included in each meta-analysis can reduce the precision of the estimate of the between-studies variance; the summary effect size results should be not be considered in isolation from the qualitative analysis.

Finally, this review does not address the issue of causality between pathology or altered muscle morphology and clinical findings. Additionally, in those instances where an association between spinal pathology and altered morphology was identified, no conclusions can be reached regarding the potential future clinical impact of these relationships.

Recommendations

The high variability of approaches utilized to measure muscle morphology via imaging modalities created challenges for identifying any clear trends. In an attempt to promote some level of uniformity to muscle measurement techniques, in addition to and in conjunction with the protocols proposed by Crawford et al. [63], the following are recommended: 1) measurement ratios are preferable to standalone total or functional cross-sectional area measures, as they help to account for variations in individual patient anatomy and imaging parameters; 2) when calculating total cross-sectional area, measures should still include any central fat (i.e., measure to the vertebral arch boundaries for the multifidus), as this accounts for the total replacement of intra-epimysial muscle by fat; 3) when measuring functional muscle area, all obvious intramuscular fat should be excluded – this is potentially more time consuming, but provides a truer indication of functional muscle; 4) use of raw data from assessing muscle brightness (e.g., signal/density/echogenicity) is subject to variability between equipment and facilities – ratio differences in brightness may help overcome this limitation; 5) measurements should be analysed by individual spinal levels and specified in relation to the level of spinal pathology, as the data suggests this relationship to be of potential importance; 6) although measurements at any spinal level are acceptable, studies should at minimum include measures below the level of spinal pathology, particularly for disc herniations; 7) as an individual's age, sex, and to a lesser degree BMI, all appear to have the potential to influence the morphology and/or appearance of the various paraspinal muscle groups, these three parameters should be clearly identified and accounted for during any analysis.

Conclusions

Histologically, there was recurring evidence that fiber changes consistent with muscle denervation and re-innervation were associated with LDH when the uninvolved side muscles were used as the control. Insufficient biopsy evidence was available to analyse for relationships between arthrosis or stenosis and altered muscle fiber morphology. With imaging, the only relatively consistent finding was the apparent reduction in LMM functional muscle on the side of LDH and radiculopathy as symptoms became more chronic; however, several studies failed to separate acute from chronic patients in their analysis so the true differences relating to chronicity are unclear. Future studies should attempt to report and analyse chronic and acute patients separately to address this issue. No consistent imaging findings associated with LDH-related changes to the PMM were identified. Increased severity of facet arthrosis appeared to correlate with increased fatty infiltration of the PVM at the level of arthrosis. Any associations between spinal canal stenosis and altered muscle morphology were inconclusive.

Although a number of studies have looked at the potential impact of neurocompressive conditions on paraspinal muscle morphology, uncertainty remains – in large part due to the publication of a significant number of moderate to high risk of bias studies, and the variability of approaches used by these studies to assess for relationships. In patients with chronic radiculopathy, neurocompressive disorders seem to alter muscle morphology at or below the affected level. Future research should include more uniform methods and our proposed criteria may potentially improve the chance of determining if there are any clinically relevant associations between spinal pathology and muscle atrophy.

Additional files

Additional file 1: Appendix 1. Database search parameters.

Additional file 2: Appendix 2. Systematic review selection/extraction form

Additional file 3: Appendix 3. Checklist for measuring risk of bias

Additional file 4: Appendix 4. Articles excluded at full-text review

Additional file 5: Extracted data and outcomes broken down by pathology and assessment methodology†

Abbreviations

CLBP: Chronic low back pain; CSA: Cross-sectional area; DDD: Degenerative disc disease; EMCL: Extramyocellular lipids; ESM: Erector spinae muscle; FCSA: Functional cross-sectional area; IMCL: Intramyocellular lipids; IS:US: Involved side : uninvolved side; LBP: Low back pain; LDH: Lumbar disc herniation; LMM: Lumbar multifidus muscle; MFI: Muscle-fat index; MLD: Muscle-laminar distance; MSF: Muscle strength factor; NR: Nerve root; PMM: Psoas major muscle; PVM: Paravertebral / Paraspinal muscle; QLM: Quadratus lumborum muscle; ROB: Risk of bias; SLR: Straight leg raise; SMD: Standardised mean difference; TCSA: Total cross-sectional area

Acknowledgements

The authors are greatly indebted to Margaret Solosy, Health Sciences Librarian, Murdoch University, and Majbritt Ursula Johansen, Research Librarian, University Library of Southern Denmark, for their assistance in designing the various database search parameters for this review.

Funding

This project was partially funded through a PhD scholarship from the Chiropractic and Osteopathic College of Australasia (COCA Research Ltd.). The funding body made no other contributions to any aspects of this study.

Authors' contributions

JRC was responsible for primary study logistics, and contributed to the conception and protocol design, the acquisition, analysis and interpretation of data, the drafting and revising of content, and preparation for submission. BFW contributed to the study conception and protocol design, acquisition and interpretation of data, and content revision. EA contributed to the protocol design, acquiring data, and revising content. PK contributed to the protocol design, acquisition and interpretation of data, and revising content. TSJ contributed to the protocol design, interpretation of data, and revising content. JJH contributed to the study conception, protocol and statistical design, acquisition, analysis and interpretation of data, and revision of content. All authors have read and approved the final manuscript.

Consent for publication

Not applicable

Competing interests

PK is a member of the Editorial Board of BMC Musculoskeletal Disorders. The other authors declare that they have no competing interests.

Author details

[1]School of Health Professions, Murdoch University, 90 South Street, Murdoch, Western Australia 6150, Australia. [2]Department of Sports Science and Clinical Biomechanics, University of Southern Denmark, Campusvej 55, 5230, Odense M, DK, Denmark. [3]Spine Centre of Southern Denmark, Ostre Hougvej 55, 5500 Middelfart, DK, Denmark. [4]Nordic Institute of Chiropractic and Clinical Biomechanics, Campusvej 55, 5230 Odense M, DK, Denmark. [5]Department of Diagnostic Imaging, Regional Hospital Silkeborg, Falkevej 1-3, 8600 Silkeborg, DK, Denmark. [6]Faculty of Kinesiology, University of New Brunswick, 3 Bailey Drive, Fredericton, New Brunswick E3B 5A3, Canada. [7]School of Psychology and Exercise Science, Murdoch University, 90 South Street, Murdoch, Western Australia 6150, Australia.

References

1. Collaborators GDallaP. Global, regional, and national incidence, prevalence, and years lived with disability for 328 diseases and injuries for 195 countries, 1990-2016: A systematic analysis for the global burden of disease study 2016. Lancet. 2017;390(10100):1211-1259.

2. Walker BF. The prevalence of low back pain: A systematic review of the literature from 1966 to 1998. J Spinal Disord. 2000;13(3):205–17.
3. Hoy D, Bain C, Williams G, March L, Brooks P, Blyth F, et al. A systematic review of the global prevalence of low back pain. Arthritis Rheum. 2012; 64(6):2028–37.
4. Walker BF, Muller R, Grant WD. Low back pain in Australian adults: The economic burden. Asia Pac J Public Health. 2003;15(2):79–87.
5. Montgomery W, Sato M, Nagasaka Y, Vietri J. The economic and humanistic costs of chronic lower back pain in Japan. ClinicoEconomics and Outcomes Research: CEOR. 2017;9:361–71.
6. Koes BW, van Tulder MW, Thomas S. Diagnosis and treatment of low back pain. BMJ. 2006;332(7555):1430-1434.
7. Lee S, Chan C, Lam T, Lam C, Lau N, Lau RW, et al. Relationship between low back pain and lumbar multifidus size at different postures. Spine (Phila Pa 1976). 2006;31(19):2258–62.
8. Kjaer P, Bendix T, Sorensen JS, Korsholm L, Leboeuf-Yde C. Are MRI-defined fat infiltrations in the multifidus muscles associated with low back pain? BMC Med. 2007;5(2).
9. Kamaz M, Kiresi D, Oguz H, Emlik D, Levendoglu F. CT measurement of trunk muscle areas in patients with chronic low back pain. Diagn Interv Radiol. 2007;13(3):144–8.
10. Hides J, Gilmore C, Stanton W, Bohlscheid E. Multifidus size and symmetry among chronic LBP and healthy asymptomatic subjects. Man Ther. 2008; 13(1):43–9.
11. Wallwork TL, Stanton WR, Freke M, Hides JA. The effect of chronic low back pain on size and contraction of the lumbar multifidus muscle. Man Ther. 2009;14(5):496–500.
12. Fortin M, Macedo LG. Multifidus and paraspinal muscle group cross-sectional areas of patients with low back pain and control patients: A systematic review with a focus on blinding. Phys Ther. 2013;93(7):873–88.
13. Wong AYL, Parent EC, Funabashi M, Stanton TR, Kawchuk GN. Do various baseline characteristics of transversus abdominis and lumbar multifidus predict clinical outcomes in nonspecific low back pain? A systematic review. Pain. 2013;154(12):2589–602.
14. Wong AY, Parent EC, Funabashi M, Kawchuk GN. Do changes in transversus abdominis and lumbar multifidus during conservative treatment explain changes in clinical outcomes related to nonspecific low back pain? A systematic review. J Pain. 2014;15(4):377 e1-35.
15. Battie MC, Niemelainen R, Gibbons LE, Dhillon S. Is level- and side-specific multifidus asymmetry a marker for lumbar disc pathology? Spine Journal. 2012;12(10):932–9.
16. Kim WH, Lee SH, Lee DY. Changes in the cross-sectional area of multifidus and psoas in unilateral sciatica caused by lumbar disc herniation. Journal of Korean Neurosurgical Society. 2011;50(3):201–4.
17. Chen YY, Pao JL, Liaw CK, Hsu WL, Yang RS. Image changes of paraspinal muscles and clinical correlations in patients with unilateral lumbar spinal stenosis. Eur Spine J. 2014;23(5):999–1006.
18. Farshad M, Gerber C, Farshad-Amacker NA, Dietrich TJ, Laufer-Molnar V, Min K. Asymmetry of the multifidus muscle in lumbar radicular nerve compression. Skeletal Radiol. 2014;43(1):49–53.
19. Ploumis A, Michailidis N, Christodoulou P, Kalaitzoglou I, Gouvas G, Beris A. Ipsilateral atrophy of paraspinal and psoas muscle in unilateral back pain patients with monosegmental degenerative disc disease. Br J Radiol. 2011; 84(1004):709–13.
20. Yarjanian JA, Fetzer A, Yamakawa KS, Tong HC, Smuck M, Haig A. Correlation of paraspinal atrophy and denervation in back pain and spinal stenosis relative to asymptomatic controls. PM and R. 2013;5(1):39–44.
21. Kang CH, Shin MJ, Kim SM, Lee SH, Lee CS. MRI of paraspinal muscles in lumbar degenerative kyphosis patients and control patients with chronic low back pain. Clin Radiol. 2007;62(5):479–86.
22. Yoshihara K, Shirai Y, Nakayama Y, Uesaka S. Histochemical changes in the multifidus muscle in patients with lumbar intervertebral disc herniation. Spine (Phila Pa 1976). 2001;26(6):622–6.
23. Dulor JP, Cambon B, Vigneron P, Reyne Y, Nougues J, Casteilla L, et al. Expression of specific white adipose tissue genes in denervation-induced skeletal muscle fatty degeneration. FEBS Lett. 1998;439(1-2):89–92.
24. Carlson BM. The biology of long-term denervated skeletal muscle. European Journal of Translational Myology. 2014;24(1):3293.
25. Steffens D, Hancock MJ, Maher CG, Williams C, Jensen TS, Latimer J. Does magnetic resonance imaging predict future low back pain? A systematic review. Eur J Pain. 2014;18(6):755–65.
26. Moher D, Liberati A, Tetzlaff J, Altman DG. Preferred reporting items for systematic reviews and meta-analyses: The PRISMA statement. Ann Intern Med. 2009;151(4):264–9 w64.
27. Stroup DF, Berlin JA, Morton SC, et al. Meta-analysis of observational studies in epidemiology: A proposal for reporting. JAMA. 2000;283(15):2008–12.
28. Downs SH, Black N. The feasibility of creating a checklist for the assessment of the methodological quality both of randomised and non-randomised studies of health care interventions. J Epidemiol Community Health. 1998; 52(6):377–84.
29. Mills K, Hunt MA, Leigh R, Ferber R. A systematic review and meta-analysis of lower limb neuromuscular alterations associated with knee osteoarthritis during level walking. Clin Biomech (Bristol, Avon). 2013;28(7):713–24.
30. Munn J, Sullivan SJ, Schneiders AG. Evidence of sensorimotor deficits in functional ankle instability: A systematic review with meta-analysis. J Sci Med Sport. 2010;13(1):2–12.
31. Kalichman L, Hodges P, Li L, Guermazi A, Hunter DJ. Changes in paraspinal muscles and their association with low back pain and spinal degeneration: CT study. Eur Spine J. 2010;19(7):1136–44.
32. Kalichman L, Kim DH, Li L, Guermazi A, Hunter DJ. Computed tomography-evaluated features of spinal degeneration: Prevalence, intercorrelation, and association with self-reported low back pain. The Spine Journal : Official Journal of the North American Spine Society. 2010;10(3):200–8.
33. Yoshihara K, Nakayama Y, Fujii N, Aoki T, Ito H. Atrophy of the multifidus muscle in patients with lumbar disk herniation: Histochemical and electromyographic study. Orthopedics. 2003;26(5):493–5.
34. McHugh ML. Interrater reliability: The kappa statistic. Biochemia Medica. 2012;22(3):276–82.
35. Altinkaya N, Cekinmez M. Lumbar multifidus muscle changes in unilateral lumbar disc herniation using magnetic resonance imaging. Skeletal Radiol. 2015. https://doi.org/10.1007/s00256-015-2252-z.
36. Boyacı A, Tutoğlu A, Boyacı N, Dokumacı DŞ. MRI evaluation of fatty degeneration of paravertebral muscles in the patients with lumbar disc herniation with nerve root compression [Turkish]. Journal of Physical Medicine & Rehabilitation Sciences / Fiziksel Tup ve Rehabilitasyon Bilimleri Dergisi. 2015;18(1):7–12.
37. Dangaria TR, Naesh O. Changes in cross-sectional area of psoas major muscle in unilateral sciatica caused by disc herniation. Spine (Phila Pa 1976). 1998;23(8):928–31.
38. Hyun JK, Lee JY, Lee SJ, Jeon JY. Asymmetric atrophy of multifidus muscle in patients with unilateral lumbosacral radiculopathy. Spine (Phila Pa 1976). 2007;32(21):E598–602.
39. Kong BJ, Lim JS, Kim K. A study on dispersion and rate of fat infiltration in the lumbar spine of patients with herniated nucleus polpusus. Journal of Physical Therapy Science. 2014;26(1):37–40.
40. Bhadresha A, Lawrence OJ, McCarthy MJ. A comparison of magnetic resonance imaging muscle fat content in the lumbar paraspinal muscles with patient-reported outcome measures in patients with lumbar degenerative disk disease and focal disk prolapse. Global Spine Journal. 2016;6(4):401–10.
41. Fortin M, Lazary A, Varga PP, McCall I, Battie MC. Paraspinal muscle asymmetry and fat infiltration in patients with symptomatic disc herniation. Eur Spine J. 2016;25(5):1452–9.
42. Frost LR, Brown SH. Neuromuscular ultrasound imaging in low back pain patients with radiculopathy. Man Ther. 2016;21:83–8.
43. Sun D, Liu P, Cheng J, Ma Z, Liu J, Qin T. Correlation between intervertebral disc degeneration, paraspinal muscle atrophy, and lumbar facet joints degeneration in patients with lumbar disc herniation. Trials. 2017;18(1):167.
44. Bajek S, Bobinac D, Bajek G, Vranić TS, Lah B, Dragojević DM. Muscle fiber type distribution in multifidus muscle in cases of lumbar disc herniation. Acta Medica Okayama. 2000;54(6):235–41.
45. Ford D, Bagnall KM, McFadden KD. Analysis of vertebral muscle obtained during surgery for correction of a lumbar disc disorder. Acta Anat (Basel). 1983;116(2):152–7.
46. Mattila M, Hurme M, Alaranta H, Paljarvi L, Kalimo H, Falck B, et al. The multifidus muscle in patients with lumbar disc herniation. A histochemical and morphometric analysis of intraoperative biopsies. Spine (Phila Pa 1976). 1986;11(7):732–8.
47. Zhao WP, Kawaguchi Y, Matsui H, Kanamori M, Kimura T. Histochemistry and morphology of the multifidus muscle in lumbar disc herniation - comparative study between diseased and normal sides. Spine (Phila Pa 1976). 2000;25(17):2191–9.

48. Jowett RL, Fidler MW, Troup JD. Histochemical changes in the multifidus in mechanical derangements of the spine. The Orthopedic Clinics of North America. 1975;6(1):145–61.
49. Kalichman L, Klindukhov A, Li L, Linov L. Indices of paraspinal muscles degeneration: Reliability and association with facet joint osteoarthritis: Feasibility study. J Spinal Disord Tech. 2013. https://doi.org/10.1097/BSD.0b013e31828be943.
50. Sebro R, O'Brien L, Torriani M, Bredella MA. Assessment of trunk muscle density using CT and its association with degenerative disc and facet joint disease of the lumbar spine. Skeletal Radiol. 2016;45(9):1221–6.
51. Yu B, Jiang K, Li X, Zhang J, Liu Z. Correlation of the features of the lumbar multifidus muscle with facet joint osteoarthritis. Orthopedics. 2017;40(5): e793–800.
52. Abbas J, Slon V, May H, Peled N, Hershkovitz I, Hamoud K. Paraspinal muscles density: A marker for degenerative lumbar spinal stenosis? BMC Musculoskelet Disord. 2016;17(1):422.
53. Jiang J, Wang H, Wang L, Zhang B, Guo Q, Yuan W, et al. Multifidus degeneration, a new risk factor for lumbar spinal stenosis: A case-control study. World Neurosurg. 2017;99:226–31.
54. Ogon I, Takebayashi T, Takashima H, Morita T, Yoshimoto M, Terashima Y, et al. Magnetic resonance spectroscopic analysis of multifidus muscles lipid content and association with spinopelvic malalignment in chronic low back pain. Br J Radiol. 2017;90(1073):20160753.
55. Mannion AF, Dumas GA, Cooper RG, Espinosa FJ, Faris MW, Stevenson JM. Muscle fibre size and type distribution in thoracic and lumbar regions of erector spinae in healthy subjects without low back pain: Normal values and sex differences. J Anat. 1997;190(4):505–13.
56. Kalichman L, Li L, Kim DH, Guermazi A, Berkin V, O'Donnell CJ, et al. Facet joint osteoarthritis and low back pain in the community-based population. Spine (Phila Pa 1976). 2008;33(23):2560–5.
57. Kottlors M, Glocker FX. Polysegmental innervation of the medial paraspinal lumbar muscles. Eur Spine J. 2008;17(2):300–6.
58. Hodges PW, James G, Blomster L, Hall L, Schmid A, Shu C, et al. Multifidus muscle changes after back injury are characterized by structural remodeling of muscle, adipose and connective tissue, but not muscle atrophy: Molecular and morphological evidence. Spine (Phila Pa 1976). 2015;40(14): 1057–71.
59. Lonnemann ME, Paris SV, Gorniak GC. A morphological comparison of the human lumbar multifidus by chemical dissection. J Man Manip Ther. 2008; 16(4):E84–92.
60. Cornwall J, Stringer MD, Duxson M. Functional morphology of the thoracolumbar transversospinal muscles. Spine (Phila Pa 1976). 2011;36(16): E1053–61.
61. Macintosh JE, Valencia F, Bogduk N, Munro RR. The morphology of the human lumbar multifidus. Clin Biomech (Bristol, Avon). 1986;1(4):196–204.
62. Kalichman L, Carmeli E, Been E. The association between imaging parameters of the paraspinal muscles, spinal degeneration, and low back pain. BioMed research international. 2017. https://doi.org/10.1155/2017/2562957.
63. Crawford RJ, Cornwall J, Abbott R, Elliott JM. Manually defining regions of interest when quantifying paravertebral muscles fatty infiltration from axial magnetic resonance imaging: A proposed method for the lumbar spine with anatomical cross-reference. BMC Musculoskelet Disord. 2017;18(1):25.
64. Wells G, Shea B, O'Connell D, Peterson J. Welch V et al. In: The Newcastle-Ottawa Scale (NOS) for assessing the quality of nonrandomised studies in meta-analyses Ottawa Hospital Research Institute; 2014. http://www.ohri.ca/programs/clinical_epidemiology/oxford.asp.

16

Kinesio taping reduces elbow pain during resisted wrist extension in patients with chronic lateral epicondylitis

Yen-Ting Cho[1], Wen-Yen Hsu[1], Li-Fong Lin[2] and Yen-Nung Lin[1,3*]

Abstract

Background: Lateral epicondylitis is frequently seen in racquet sport players and the treatments are usually symptomatic rather than curative. Taping therapy is cheap and easy to apply in the sport field. In this study we valued the effectiveness of Kinesio taping (KT) on immediate pain control for patients with chronic lateral epicondylitis.

Methods: We conducted a randomized, double-blinded, cross-over study with 15 patients with chronic lateral epicondylitis. All participants received two taping sessions in a random order with a 3-day interval in between: one with KT and the other with sham taping (ST). Pain perceived during resisted wrist extension and at rest using numeric rating scale (NRS), the pain-free grip strength, and the pressure pain threshold, were measured before and 15 min after the tape was applied.

Results: A significant reduction of 2.1 ± 1.6 ($Z = -3.081$, $P = 0.002$) and 0.7 ± 0.8 ($Z = -2.428$, $P = 0.015$) was found on a NRS with KT and ST, respectively, indicating that both taping sessions produced immediate pain relief for resisted wrist extension. Both taping sessions significantly improved the pain-free grip strength with increases of 3.31 ± 5.05 ($Z = -2.615$, $P = 0.009$) and 2.43 ± 3.31 ($Z = -2.783$, $P = 0.005$) kg found with KT and ST, respectively. Compared with ST, KT exhibited superiority in controlling pain experienced during resisted wrist extension ($Z = -2.168$, $P = 0.030$).

Conclusions: Taping produced unneglectable placebo effects on pain relief and painf-free grip strength for patients with lateral epicondylitis, and KT seemed to have additional effects on controlling pain that was elicited by resisted wrist extension.

Keywords: Tennis elbow, Physiotherapy, Tape, Epicondylopathy, Tendinopathy

Background

Lateral epicondylitis (tennis elbow) is the most common cause of elbow pain [1], and is commonly seen in racquet sports players with a reported incidence of 9~ 35% and a prevalence of 14~ 41% among tennis players [2]. The dominant upper limb is much more often involved [3]. It typically presents with pain around the lateral epicondyle elicited by forceful wrist extension. This is the result of the degenerative angiofibroblastic hyperplasia of wrist extensor tendons due to repeated microtraumas [4]. Although treatments are usually non-surgical (e.g., oral medications, steroid injections, and physiotherapy), many of them lack sufficient evidence of beneficial effects [5–7]. In some cases, the recovery phase can be as long as several months [8], potentially impacting the quality of life and sports performance of affected individuals [9].

* Correspondence: semitune@gmail.com
[1]Department of Physical Medicine and Rehabilitation, Wan Fang Hospital, Taipei Medical University, No.111, Hsing-Long Road, Section 3, Taipei 116, Taiwan
[3]Graduate Institute of Injury Prevention and Control, Taipei Medical University, Taipei, Taiwan

Kinesio taping (KT) is widely used to manage various musculoskeletal problems. Invented by the Japanese chiropractor Kenzo Kase in the 1970s, the tape is an elastic woven-cotton strip with heat-sensitive acrylic adhesive and the maximum available tension of about 40–60% its overall length [10]. Numerous effects of KT are hypothesized, including pain reduction, normalizing muscle function, improving proprioceptive feedback, and correcting articular malalignment [11, 12]. Various clinical effects of KT have been reviewed in a diversity of conditions and populations [13–18]. Various quality and methodology of the trials has influenced the consistency of results in these reviews. The results has been interpreted as either trivial [13] or no effects [14] on muscle strength in healthy adults. KT may [17, 18] or may not [16] reduce pain in the short-term use when compared with minimal treatment, and not be superior when compared with other interventions [17, 18] in patients with musculoskeletal disorders. Despite the inconsistencies, some randomized controlled trials have reported that the KT is beneficial in controlling pain in certain conditions such as acute [19] and chronic low-back pain [20], cervical whiplash [21], and knee pain after joint replacement [22]. Certainly, well-designed research is warranted so that the practitioners can be confident that KT is beneficial for their patients.

The effectiveness of KT in managing lateral epicondylitis has not been adequately explored. In a non-control study with before-after design, Dilek et al. reported that patients' pain and grip strength significantly improved after applying KT [23]. However, without a control group, those positive findings can be due to the placebo effect. We therefore designed this study with a placebo control to investigate the effectiveness of KT on pain relief. We also focused on the immediate effects on pain reduction during dynamic motions in hope of applying the results to the sport fields. Considering that pain measures are usually subjective and might have great inter-individual variability, we used a randomized cross-over design with self-comparator to maximize statistical power from our sample size. We hypothesized that KT could provide immediate effects on pain reduction in patients with lateral epicondylitis.

Methods

Participants

We screened for eligible patients from the rehabilitation outpatient department of Wan-Fang Hospital with a diagnosis of chronic lateral epicondylitis. The criteria for the diagnosis of chronic lateral epicondylitis was based on the clinical presentation and included: (1) typical pain over the lateral epicondyle elicited by resisted wrist extension; (2) tenderness at the lateral epicondyle; and (3) symptoms lasting for at least 2 months. Patients were excluded if they previously had had experience with KT treatment, had had a steroid injection for lateral epicondylitis within the past 3 months, were suspected of having elbow arthritis, or had a wound where the taping was to be applied. If pain was reported in both elbows, the one with more-severe pain was used in our experiment.

Design

Participants who met the enrollment criteria and completed the consent form were assigned to receive two taping sessions with different tapes: one with KT and the other one with sham taping (ST). A 2 (treatment) × 2 (period) crossover design was used (Fig. 1). Participants received the two taping sessions in a random order with a 3-day washout interval in between. The physiatrist performing the taping conducted the randomization by coin toss. Oral medications (e.g., nonsteroid anti-inflammatory agents and acetaminophen) and physiotherapy were not allowed since 2 days before the pretest. The Institutional Review Board of Taipei Medical University reviewed and approved the research protocol in the spirit of the *Helsinki Declaration*.

Taping procedure

The Kinesio Tex Tape was used for KT and the Elastic Adhesive Tape (3 M™) for ST. The color and width of the two tapes were very similar, appearance-wise making it hard to differentiate between them (Fig. 2). The taping was performed by an experienced physical therapist. We used two Y-shaped Kinesio strips for the KT procedure for lateral epicondylitis as proposed by Kaze et al. [10], with the main strip applied along the extensor muscles and the second strip vertical to the first one on the proximal forearm (Fig. 2). The main strip was used to inhibit the targeted muscles while the second strip correct the fascia. The patient was positioned with the elbow extended and the wrist ulnar deviated and flexed. After cutting the tape into a Y-shape, we applied the tape head (anchor) of the first strip to the wrist, stretched the tape slightly with approximately 30% of available tension to the tails, laid down the tape ends with no tension, and applied pressure to the tape surface to initiate adhesion. We then applied the anchor of the second strip 1 in. distal and anterio-medial to the lateral epicondyle with no tension, applied approximately 30% tension to each tail across the wrist extensors, laid down the ends at the border of ulnar with no tension, and applied pressure to the tape surface to initiate adhesion. The applied tension was estimated according to the length stretched. For example, if a segment of tape is 4 cm in length under no tension and can be stretched up to 6 cm, the tension when stretched to 5 cm would be $(5–4) / (6–4) = 50\%$. The ST procedure was very similar to that of KT except that the wrist was placed in a neutral rather than a

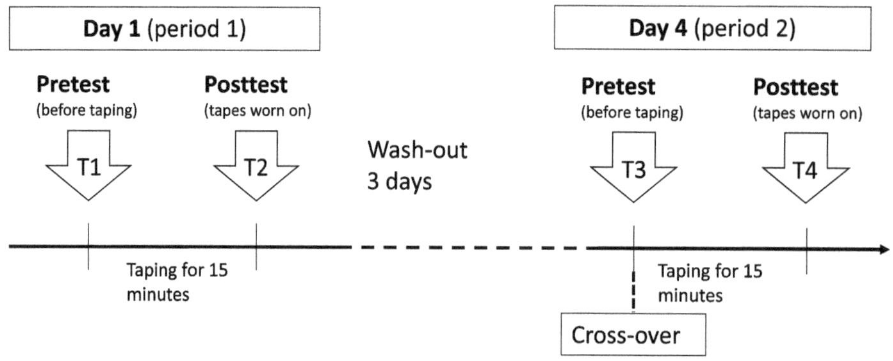

Fig. 1 Study process

flexed position when applying the tape. ST was also carefully applied tension-free during the entire procedure.

Basic information

Basic participant characteristics, such as gender, age, duration of disease and affected side were obtained through a short interview with a structured questionnaire including the Patient-Rated Tennis Elbow Evaluation (PRTEE). PRTEE (0~ 100) assessed the pain and disabilities caused by lateral epicondylitis with a higher score indicating more significant impacts [24].

Outcome measurements

The primary outcome was the pain experienced during resisted wrist extension, as it had been in other lateral epicondylitis trials [25]. We standardized the pain measuring procedure by having the participant hold an 1-kg weight in a standing posture with the arm relaxed (pain-1 kg). The participant was then asked to slowly lift the weight while flexing the elbow from 0 to 120 degrees and then slowly returning to the starting position (Fig. 3). The wrist was kept pronated during the process to ensure that the wrist extensor muscles were isometrically contracted to counter gravity. The participant repeated the process three times and then reported the degree of perceived pain during the process using an 11-point numerical rating scale (NRS) [26] with 0 = "no pain" and 10 = "worst possible pain". In a pre-study test with 5 participants, we found the test-retest reliability was good with an intra-class correlation coefficient of 0.91. A reduction of 2 points is thought to be the minimal clinically important difference (MCID) [26].

Other outcomes of interest included pain at rest using the NRS (pain-rest), the pain-free grip strength, (PFG)

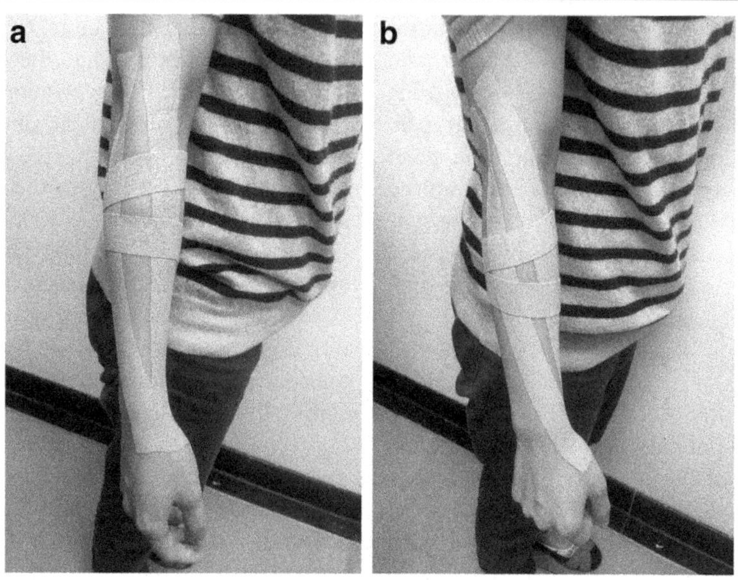

Fig. 2 Application of Kinesio taping (KT) and sham taping (ST) for lateral epicondylitis in this study. **a** Kinesio taping. **b** Sham taping with Elastic Adhesive Tapes (3 M™). Note that the soft tissue is bulging between the tape tails from being squeezed by the tension (**a**), and the skin is completely smooth between the tails (**b**). It was difficult to differentiate between the two tape types by their appearance

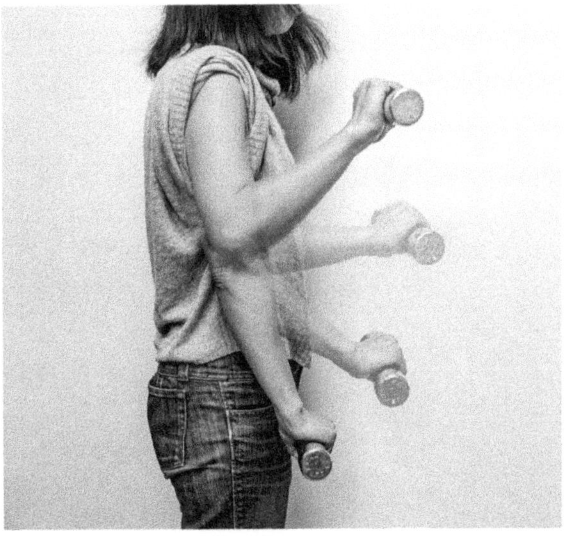

Fig. 3 The pain-1 kg test. During the test, participants lifted the weight while flexing the elbow from 0 to 120 degrees and returned the weight to starting position. The wrist was kept pronated during this process so that the wrist extensor muscles were isometrically contracted to counter gravity throughout the process

and the pressure pain threshold (PPT). When measuring the PFG, the subject stood with the elbow in complete extension and the shoulder and radioulnar joints in neutral rotation. The subject then began to squeeze a dynamometer (JAMAR Plus, Patterson Medical, Canada) with increasing force until he/she felt elbow pain [27]. The PPT (i.e., minimum amount of pressure that triggered pain) was quantified by applying the 1-cm^2 rubber probe tip of a digital algometer (Force Ten FDX Force Gage, Wagner Instruments, USA) to the most palpably tender site over the lateral epicondyle [28]. The PFG and PPT were measured three times and average values used for analysis. An assessor blinded to the treatment assignment performed all measurements before taping (pretest) and 15 min after taping with the tape in situ (posttest). We removed tapes after the posttest. Despite the similar appearances of the KT and ST, participants were asked to wear a long-sleeved shirt to cover the taping so that the assessor was sufficiently blinded to the taping type at the posttest.

Data analysis

We used non-parametric tests for this small-sample study. Carryover effects were investigated by comparing the outcomes at T1 and T3 with Wilcoxon signed-rank test. The changes caused by taping were assessed using Wilcoxon signed-rank test. To compare the effects between the two taping, we divided the participants by sequence as KT-ST and ST-KT groups. We defined the differences between the two periods for KT-ST group as μ(KT-ST) = μ(KT)- μ(ST); and for ST-KT group as μ(ST-KT) = μ(ST)- μ(KT). Then we compared the μ(KT-ST) and μ(ST-KT) using Mann-Whitney U test, with the H_0: μ(KT-ST)- μ(ST-KT) = 0, which is equal to test the H_0: μKT - μST = 0. We also tested the sequence effects by comparing "μ(KT) + μ(ST)" between the two groups. A two-tailed $P < 0.05$ represented the level of significance. Based on a previous KT study [21] that showed an effect size of 0.9 on visual analog scale for pain, a total sample size of 15 participants in this study would provide a power of 0.9 to detect the between-group difference with an level of 0.05. All analyses were performed using the SPSS statistical package version 17.0.

Results

Table 1 showed the characteristics of the participants. Fifteen participants who completed the study had a mean age of 52.3 years (SD 8.8) and a disease duration of 4.9 months (SD 2.7). Twelve right hands and three left hands were tested. The PRTEE questionnaire ranged from 24~ 78 with a mean of 46.3 (SD 17.5), indicating a wide range of severity of pain symptoms and disabilities that were caused by lateral epicondylitis.

No significant differences existed between T1 and T3 regarding all the outcomes, with a Z value of – 1.540, – 1.469, – 1.051, – 0.511 for pain-1 kg, pain-rest, PFG, and PPT respectively (all $P > 0.05$, not shown in Tables), indicating no significant carryover/period effects. The pretest, posttest, and changes in outcome parameters regarding the taping types were shown in Table 2. After taping, both taping sessions significantly produced immediate pain relief during resisted wrist extension ($P = 0.002$ and 0.015 for KT and ST respectively) and increases in pain-free grip strength ($P = 0.009$ and 0.005 for KT and ST respectively). In addition, the ST significantly decreased the pain at rest ($P = 0.014$) and the KT increased the PPT ($P = 0.016$).

The results of comparison for taping and sequence effects were shown in Table 3. Significant between-taping difference was noted in pain-1 kg ($P = 0.030$), indicating the KT was superior to ST in controlling the pain experienced during resisted wrist extension. No significant differences were found regarding the other parameters, and no significant sequence effect was found in the pain parameters (all $P > 0.05$).

Discussion

In this study, we explored the effects of KT on pain relief by measuring several pain parameters in patients with lateral epicondylitis. Our results showed that both taping sessions (KT and ST) produced significant improvement in pain experienced during resisted wrist extension and pain-free grip strength. However, KT was superior to ST in reducing pain elicited by resisted wrist extension, while producing an average reduction of 2.1 points on the NRS, reaching the MCID. Our results

Table 1 Basic characteristics of participants

No.	Gender (M/F)	Age (y)	Duration of disase (months)	Affected elbow (R/L)	PRTEE -pain	PRTEE -ADL	PRTEE -total	Treatment order
1	F	5X	6	R	36	37.5	73.5	ST-KT
2	M	5X	5	R	15	9.5	24.5	KT-ST
3	F	7X	9	R	36	21	57	ST-KT
4	F	4X	3	R	22	13	35	KT-ST
5	F	5X	4	R	25	17	42	KT-ST
6	F	5X	2	L	25	25.5	50.5	ST-KT
7	F	4X	6	L	38	40	78	KT-ST
8	M	6X	4	R	23	23.5	46.5	KT-ST
9	F	5X	5	R	28	12.5	40.5	KT-ST
10	M	4X	3	L	15	15.5	30.5	ST-KT
11	M	4X	2	R	42	33.5	75.5	KT-ST
12	F	6X	3	R	22	20	42	ST-KT
13	M	6X	3	R	19	20	39	KT-ST
14	F	4X	6	R	15	9	24	ST-KT
15	F	4X	12	R	29	7.5	36.5	KT-ST

M male, *F* female, *BMI* body mass index, *R* right, *L* left, *PRTEE* patient-rated tennis elbow evaluation, *ADL* activity of daily living, *KT* Kinesio taping, *ST* sham taping

supported the use of KT as a temporary pain management for lateral epicondylitis.

Lateral epicondylitis is commonly seen in racquet sports. Substantial eccentric contractions of the extensor carpi during the backhand stroke are likely the cause of repetitive microtrauma leading to the lateral epicondylitis [29]. Lateral epicondylitis also has a high prevalence among the general population, affecting about 1~3% of people of working age [30]. Traditionally, the management usually relies on conservative treatments, such as oral non-steroidal anti-inflammatory drugs, physical agents (eg, ultrasound, electrical stimulation), therapeutic exercise, or steroid injection. Even with these treatments, patients usually have to endure symptoms for several months. Therefore, an effective temporary management, such as taping, can potentially improve the quality of life and sport performance.

As shown in Table 2, KT significantly improved the pain-1 kg, PFG, and PPT, yet the mechanism is unclear. The initial concept of applying KT when introduced is to reduce the build-up of fluid between and within the layers of the soft tissue [10]. However, the correlation between this concept and the effects on pain relief is not well explained. Therefore, some other mechanisms for pain relief have been hypothesized. For one, it was

Table 2 Means (SD) for pretest, posttest, and changes in outcomes by tapings

	Pretest	Posttest	Difference (Posttest - pretest)	[a]Significance for the changes Z-value	*P*-value
Pain-1 kg (0~ 10)					
Kinesio taping	4.4 (2.4)	2.3 (2.0)	−2.1 (1.6)	−3.081	0.002
Sham taping	3.3 (2.3)	2.7 (2.1)	−0.7 (0.8)	− 2.428	0.015
Pain-at rest (0~ 10)					
Kinesio taping	1.7 (2.1)	1.0 (1.3)	−0.7 (1.5)	−1.633	0.102
Sham taping	2.1 (2.1)	1.5 (1.6)	−0.6 (0.7)	−2.460	0.014
PFG (kg)					
Kinesio taping	10.70 (8.03)	14.02 (10.56)	3.31 (5.05)	−2.615	0.009
Sham taping	12.59 (8.44)	15.01 (10.47)	2.43 (3.31)	−2.783	0.005
PPT(lbf)					
Kinesio taping	3.1 (2.6)	3.9 (4.1)	0.8 (1.6)	−2.414	0.016
Sham taping	2.5 (1.7)	3.5 (4.1)	1.0 (3.2)	−1.162	0.245

Pain-1 kg pain when holding a 1-kg weight, *PFG* pain-free grip strength, *PPT* pressure pain threshold
[a]Significance was assessed with Wilcoxon signed-rank test

Table 3 Between-group differences regarding the outcome measurements

	[a]Effect at	[b]Effect at	Comparison for taping effects			Comparison for sequence effects		
	Period 1	Period 2	Period 1-Period 2	Z-value	[c]*P*-value	Period 1+ Period 2	Z-value	[c]*P*-value
Pain-1 kg (0~ 10)								
KT-ST (*n* = 9)	−1.9 (1.4)	−0.8 (1.0)	− 1.1 (1.8)	−2.168	0.030	−2.7 (1.5)	−0.240	0.811
ST-KT (*n* = 6)	−0.5 (0.5)	−2.3 (2.1)	1.8 (2.2)			−2.8 (2.0)		
Pain-at rest (0~ 10)								
KT-ST (*n* = 9)	−1.0 (1.7)	−0.9 (0.8)	−0.1 (1.8)	0	1.000	−1.9 (2.0)	−1.538	0.124
ST-KT (*n* = 6)	−0.2 (0.4)	−0.5 (0.8)	0.3 (0.5)			−0.7 (1.2)		
PFG (kg)								
KT-ST (*n* = 9)	3.3 (6.3)	2.9 (3.4)	0.4 (5.3)	−0.589	0.556	6.2 (8.7)	−0.059	0.953
ST-KT (*n* = 6)	1.7 (3.3)	3.3 (2.8)	−1.6 (2.2)			5.0 (5.7)		
PPT(lbf)								
KT-ST (*n* = 9)	0.6 (0.5)	0.1 (0.6)	0.5 (0.4)	−0.354	0.723	0.6 (1.0)	−0.707	0.480
ST-KT (*n* = 6)	2.3 (4.9)	1.2 (2.6)	1.1 (2.5)			3.5 (7.5)		

Pain-1 kg pain when holding a 1-kg weight, *PFG* pain-free grip strength, *PPT* pressure pain threshold
[a]Effect at Period 1 = Posttest (T2)- Pretest (T1)
[b]Effect at Period 2 = Posttest (T4)- Pretest (T3)
[c]Significance was assessed with Mann-Whitney U test

suggested that non-neuronal cells may act as a key signaling pathway for sensory modalities by triggering adjacent nerve terminals [31]. As we understand, somatic pain is perceived when noxious stimuli activate specific receptors (nociceptors) of thinly myelinated Aδ- and unmyelinated C-fibers. Some studies suggested that keratinocytes may represent non-neuronal primary transducers of mechanical stimuli, probably via a signal transduction cascade mechanism, to evoke a response in adjacent C-fibers [31, 32]. If so, cutaneous stretching produced by KT may possibly affect pain processing via keratinocytes. Furthermore, stimulation by cutaneous stretching may also interfere with the transmission of pain by facilitating a pain inhibitory mechanism. By gate control theory, the constant somatosensory input by cutaneous stretching could potentially close the "gates" to painful input, which prevents pain sensation from traveling to the central nervous system [33].

Another possible explanation is related to muscle activities modulation. Several studies suggested that KT can potentially modulate muscle activities [34–36]. A study conducted by Hsu et al. revealed that the muscle activity was decreased in lower trapezius but increased in serratus anterior and upper trapezius after taping on the lower trapezius [34]. Wong et al. and Yeung et al. also found that taping on the vastus medialis shortened the time to generate peak torque of knee extension [35, 36]. These preliminary reports may lead to the hypothesis that KT reduces pain through modulating muscle activities, possibly accounting for why KT was superior to the ST in reducing pain during resisted wrist extension but not at rest. Therefore, we speculate that the benefits of KT may partly come from the decreased load on the lateral epicondyle during the contraction of wrist extensors. For example, the main strip applied parallel to the forearm may inhibit the muscle activity with its elasticity and reduce the irritation of the enthesis. Meanwhile, it is our hypothesis that the second strip applied vertical to the forearm may act in a similar way to the commonly used elbow brace which produces a wider muscle origin thereby decreasing the stress at the lateral epicondyle [27]. However, further studies are needed to explore the possible mechanisms.

It is interesting to note that ST also exhibited significant improvements in pain-1 kg and the PFG (Table 2). In our study, we used elastic tape for ST, which might have had some effects when the tape was stretched and a traction force was created. However, the treatment effect should have been minimal, as we carefully avoided any tension when applying ST over the forearm. Therefore, those improvements may be attributed to the placebo effect.

Our findings were similar to a recently published study conducted by Shakeri et al. [37] The authors designed a 4-day intervention to compare the KT with the placebo (KT without tension) and evaluate the effectiveness for patients with lateral epicondylitis. Both tapings resulted in reduced pain during activities and the degree of arm disabilities after 4 days of intervention but KT exhibited significantly greater improvement. The authors also found no difference between the KT and placebo groups regarding the grip strength and pain threshold. Different from Shakeri's work, our study was intended to understand the potential benefits of applying the KT in the sport field. This is the reason we measured the immediate effects on dynamic motion by lifting a 1-kg weight to simulate the backhand stroke of racquet sports.

In contrast, a Chinese study group published a series of researches recently and provided negative evidence. They conducted two crossover studies to assess the effects of KT applied to wrist extensors at different taping conditions (eg, facilitatory KT, inhibitory KT, no KT) among healthy adults [38] and patients with lateral epicondylitis [39]. The authors found no difference between these different conditions regarding maximal grip strength and electromyographic activities in both populations [38, 39]. They also found no significant effects on pain intensity and PFG, in patients with lateral epicondylitis [39]. While the authors reported null effects, they did not consider the carryover and sequence effects which are essential methodological issues for a crossover study, so that the interference between the conditions could possibly lead to the negative results. Considering that KT is a cheap and convenient option that can potentially manage pain instantly, further exploration of its treatment mechanism and effects with well-designed researches is certainly worthwhile.

Several study limitations should be addressed. First, the sample size was small. Second, only the immediate effects of KT were evaluated. Whether these effects lasted beyond 15 min is unknown. Third, we only explored the effects on pain elicited by isometric wrist extension with 1-kg resistance, so whether KT is effective at higher resistance is also unknown. These issues are important to consider before applying taping in the sport field. Fourth, placebo effect of any kind of taping that the subjects might expect benefit on that cannot be ruled out. And finally, although we would like to project our results onto people who sustain lateral epicondylitis from sport injuries, we did not specifically limit our patient selection to athletes.

Conclusions

Taping produced unneglectable placebo effects on pain relief and PFG for patients with lateral epicondylitis, and KT seemed to have additional effects on controlling pain that was elicited by resisted wrist extension.

Abbreviations

KT: Kinesio taping; MCID: Minimal clinically important difference; NRS: Numerical rating scale; PFG: Pain-free grip strength; PPT: Pressure pain threshold; PRTEE: Patient-rated tennis elbow evaluation; ST: Sham taping

Acknowledgements

We thanked Dr. Chih-Yang Hsu for English editing.

Funding

This study was supported by a grant (no. 105-wf-eva-24) from Wan Fang Medical Center, Taipei Medical University.

Authors' contributions

YTC, WYH, LFL, and YNL all contributed to the method designing, YNL and YTC conducted data analyses and wrote the first draft of the report with input from the other authors. All authors have read and approved the manuscript.

Competing interests

The authors declare that they have no competing interests.

Author details

[1]Department of Physical Medicine and Rehabilitation, Wan Fang Hospital, Taipei Medical University, No.111, Hsing-Long Road, Section 3, Taipei 116, Taiwan. [2]Department of Physical Medicine and Rehabilitation, Shuang-Ho Hospital, Taipei Medical University, New Taipei City, Taiwan. [3]Graduate Institute of Injury Prevention and Control, Taipei Medical University, Taipei, Taiwan.

References

1. Walker-Bone K, Palmer KT, Reading I, Coggon D, Cooper C. Prevalence and impact of musculoskeletal disorders of the upper limb in the general population. Arthritis Rheum. 2004;51:642–51.
2. Pluim BM, Staal JB, Windler GE, Jayanthi N. Tennis injuries: occurrence, aetiology, and prevention. Br J Sports Med. 2006;40:415–23.
3. Smidt N, Lewis M, Van Der Windt DA, Hay EM, Bouter LM, Croft P. Lateral epicondylitis in general practice: course and prognostic indicators of outcome. J Rheumatol. 2006;33:2053–9.
4. Faro F, Wolf JM. Lateral epicondylitis: review and current concepts. J Hand Surg Am. 2007;32:1271–9.
5. Smidt N, Assendelft WJ, Arola H, Malmivaara A, Greens S, Buchbinder R, van der Windt DA, Bouter LM. Effectiveness of physiotherapy for lateral epicondylitis: a systematic review. Ann Med. 2003;35:51–62.
6. Labelle H, Guibert R, Joncas J, Newman N, Fallaha M, Rivard CH. Lack of scientific evidence for the treatment of lateral epicondylitis of the elbow. An attempted meta-analysis. J Bone Joint Surg Br. 1992;74:646–51.
7. Smidt N, Assendelft WJ, van der Windt DA, Hay EM, Buchbinder R, Bouter LM. Corticosteroid injections for lateral epicondylitis: a systematic review. Pain. 2002;96:23–40.
8. Smidt N, Van Der Windt DA, Assendelft WJ, Devillé WL, Korthals-de Bos IB, Bouter LM. Corticosteroid injections, physiotherapy, or a wait-and-see policy for lateral epicondylitis: a randomised controlled trial. Lancet. 2002;359:657–62.
9. Alizadehkhaiyat O, Fisher AC, Kemp GJ, Frostick SP. Pain, functional disability, and psychologic status in tennis elbow. Clin J Pain. 2007;23:482–9.
10. Kase K, Wallis J, Kase T. Clinical therapeutic applications of the Kinesio taping. 3rd ed. USA: Kinesio; 2013.
11. Kase K, Tatsuyuki H, Tomoko O. Development of kinesio tape. Kinesio taping perfect manual. Kinesio Taping Association. 1996;6–10:117–8.
12. Ouyang JH, Chang KH, Hsu WY, Cho YT, Liou TH, Lin YN. Non-elastic taping, but not elastic taping, provides benefits for patients with knee osteoarthritis: systemic review and meta-analysis. Clin Rehabil. 2018;32:3–17.
13. Williams S, Whatman C, Hume PA, Sheerin K. Kinesio taping in treatment and prevention of sports injuries: a meta-analysis of the evidence for its effectiveness. Sports Med. 2012;42:153–64.
14. Csapo R, Alegre LM. Effects of Kinesio(®) taping on skeletal muscle strength-a meta-analysis of current evidence. J Sci Med Sport. 2015;18:450–6.
15. Kalron A, Bar-Sela S. A systematic review of the effectiveness of Kinesio taping–fact or fashion? Eur J Phys Rehabil Med. 2013;49:699–709.
16. Parreira PCS, Costa LCM, Hespanhol Junior LC, Lopes AD, Costa LO. Current evidence does not support the use of Kinesio taping in clinical practice: a systematic review. J Physiother. 2014;60:31–9.
17. Lim EC, Tay MG. Kinesio taping in musculoskeletal pain and disability that lasts for more than 4 weeks: is it time to peel off the tape and throw it out with the sweat? A systematic review with meta-analysis focused on pain and also methods of tape application. Br J Sports Med. 2015;49:1558–66.
18. Montalvo AM, Cara EL, Myer GD. Effect of kinesiology taping on pain in individuals with musculoskeletal injuries: systematic review and meta-analysis. Phys Sportsmed. 2014;42:48–57.

19. Kelle B, Guzel R, Sakalli H. The effect of Kinesio taping application for acute non-specific low back pain: a randomized controlled clinical trial. Clin Rehabil. 2016;30:997–1003.
20. Castro-Sánchez AM, Lara-Palomo IC, Matarán-Peñarrocha GA, Fernández-Sánchez M, Sánchez-Labraca N, Arroyo-Morales M. Kinesio taping reduces disability and pain slightly in chronic non-specific low back pain: a randomised trial. J Physiother. 2012;58:89–95.
21. González-Iglesias J, Fernández-de-Las-Peñas C, Cleland JA, Huijbregts P, Del Rosario Gutiérrez-Vega M. Short-term effects of cervical kinesio taping on pain and cervical range of motion in patients with acute whiplash injury: a randomized clinical trial. J Orthop Sports Phys Ther. 2009;39:515–21.
22. Donec V, Krisciunas A. The effectiveness of Kinesio taping(R) after total knee replacement in early postoperative rehabilitation period. A randomized controlled trial. Eur J Phys Rehabil Med. 2014;50:363–71.
23. Dilek B, Batmaz I, Sarıyıldız MA, Sahin E, Ilter L, Gulbahar S, Cevik R, Nas K. Kinesio taping in patients with lateral epicondylitis. J Back Musculoskelet Rehabil. 2016;29:853–8.
24. Rompe JD, Overend TJ, MacDermid JC. Validation of the patient-rated tennis elbow evaluation questionnaire. J Hand Ther. 2007;20:3–10.
25. Mishra AK, Skrepnik NV, Edwards SG, Jones GL, Sampson S, Vermillion DA, Ramsey ML, Karli DC, Rettig AC. Efficacy of platelet-rich plasma for chronic tennis elbow: a double-blind, prospective, multicenter, randomized controlled trial of 230 patients. Am J Sports Med. 2014;42:463–71.
26. Farrar JT, Young JPJ, LaMoreaux L, Werth JL, Poole RM. Clinical importance of changes in chronic pain intensity measured on an 11-point numerical pain rating scale. Pain. 2001;94:149–58.
27. Wuori JL, Overend TJ, Kramer JF, MacDermid J. Strength and pain measures associated with lateral epicondylitis bracing. Arch Phys Med Rehabil. 1998;79:832–7.
28. Smidt N, Van Der Windt DA, Assendelft WJ, Mourits AJ, Devillé WL, de Winter AF, Bouter LM. Interobserver reproducibility of the assessment of severity of complaints, grip strength, and pressure pain threshold in patients with lateral epicondylitis. Arch Phys Med Rehabil. 2002;83:1145–50.
29. Eygendaal D, Rahussen FT, Diercks RL. Biomechanics of the elbow joint in tennis players and relation to pathology. Br J Sports Med. 2007;41:820–3.
30. Shiri R, Viikari-Juntura E, Varonen H, Heliövaara M. Prevalence and determinants of lateral and medial epicondylitis: a population study. Am J Epidemiol. 2006;164:1065–74.
31. Lumpkin EA, Caterina MJ. Mechanisms of sensory transduction in the skin. Nature. 2007;445:858–65.
32. Koizumi S, Fujishita K, Inoue K, Shigemoto-Mogami Y, Tsuda M, Inoue K. Ca2+ waves in keratinocytes are transmitted to sensory neurons: the involvement of extracellular ATP and P2Y2 receptor activation. Biochem J. 2004;380:329–38.
33. DeLeo JA. Basic science of pain. J Bone Joint Surg Am. 2006;88(Suppl 2):58–62.
34. Hsu YH, Chen WY, Lin HC, Wang WT, Shih YF. The effects of taping on scapular kinematics and muscle performance in baseball players with shoulder impingement syndrome. J Electromyogr Kinesiol. 2009;19:1092–9.
35. Wong OM, Cheung RT, Li RC. Isokinetic knee function in healthy subjects with and without Kinesio taping. Phys Ther Sport. 2012;13:255–8.
36. Yeung SS, Yeung EW, Sakunkaruna Y, Mingsoongnern S, Hung WY, Fan YL, Iao HC. Acute effects of kinesio taping on knee extensor peak torque and electromyographic activity after exhaustive isometric knee extension in healthy young adults. Clin J Sport Med. 2015;25:284–90.
37. Shakeri H, Soleimanifar M, Arab AM, Hamneshin Behbahani S. The effects of KinesioTape on the treatment of lateral epicondylitis. J Hand Ther. 2018;31:35–41.
38. Cai C, P AI, An W, Cheung RT. Facilitatory and inhibitory effects of Kinesio tape: fact or fad? J Sci Med Sport. 2016;19:109–12.
39. Au IPH, Fan PCP, Lee WY, Leong MW, Tang OY, An WW, Cheung RT. Effects of Kinesio tape in individuals with lateral epicondylitis: a deceptive crossover trial. Physiother Theory Pract. 2017;33:914–9.

17

Age-dependent bone loss and recovery during hindlimb unloading and subsequent reloading in rats

Hailey C. Cunningham[1], Daniel W. D. West[2], Leslie M. Baehr[2], Franklin D. Tarke[3], Keith Baar[1,2,4], Sue C. Bodine[2,4] and Blaine A. Christiansen[1,3*]

Abstract

Background: Bone structure and strength are rapidly lost during conditions of decreased mechanical loading, and aged bones have a diminished ability to adapt to increased mechanical loading. This is a concern for older patients that experience periods of limited mobility or bed rest, but the acute effects of disuse on the bones of aged patients have not been thoroughly described. Previous animal studies have primarily examined the effect of mechanical unloading on young animals. Those that have studied aged animals have exclusively focused on bone loss during unloading and not bone recovery during subsequent reloading. In this study, we investigated the effect of decreased mechanical loading and subsequent reloading on bone using a hindlimb unloading model in Adult (9 month old) and Aged (28 month old) male rats.

Methods: Animals from both age groups were subjected to 14 days of hindlimb unloading followed by up to 7 days of reloading. Additional Aged rats were subjected to 7 days of forced treadmill exercise during reloading or a total of 28 days of reloading. Trabecular and cortical bone structure of the femur were quantified using ex vivo micro-computed tomography (μCT), and mechanical properties were quantified with mechanical testing.

Results: We found that Adult rats had substantially decreased trabecular bone volume fraction (BV/TV) following unloading (− 27%) while Aged animals did not exhibit significant bone loss following unloading. However, Aged animals had lower trabecular BV/TV after 3 days of reloading (− 20% compared to baseline), while trabecular BV/TV of Adult rats was not different from baseline values after 3 days of reloading. Trabecular BV/TV of Aged animals remained lower than control animals even with exercise during 7 days of reloading and after 28 days of reloading.

Conclusions: These data suggest that aged bone is less responsive to both increased and decreased mechanical loading, and that acute periods of disuse may leave older subjects with a long-term deficit in trabecular bone mass. These finding indicate the need for therapeutic strategies to improve the skeletal health of elderly patients during periods of disuse.

Keywords: Hindlimb unloading, Reloading, Disuse, Age, Trabecular bone, Micro-computed tomography, Mechanical testing

* Correspondence: bchristiansen@ucdavis.edu
[1]Biomedical Engineering Graduate Group, University of California Davis, Davis, CA, USA
[3]Department of Orthopaedic Surgery, University of California Davis Medical Center, Lawrence J. Ellison Musculoskeletal Research Center, 4635 2nd Avenue, Suite 2000, Sacramento, CA 95817, USA
Full list of author information is available at the end of the article

Background

Bone undergoes a significant and rapid decay in structure and strength in the absence of mechanical loading [1–3]. In addition, bones of aged humans and animals have a diminished ability to adapt to the mechanical loading environment [4, 5], making exercise or increased mechanical loading less effective at building bone mass. This is particularly important for older subjects that commonly experience periods of limited mobility or skeletal disuse during periods of sickness or following an injury or surgery; the ability of these subjects to regain bone mass following a period of unloading may be compromised.

The effect of mechanical unloading on bone has been extensively studied in both humans and animal models. In humans, a prolonged period of unloading significantly decreases bone volume and bone density as illustrated through bed rest and spaceflight studies [2, 6, 7]. For example, women who participated in 60 day bed rest had decreases of 3–4% in bone mineral density (BMD) in the trabecular bone of the femur and tibia [8]. Similarly, astronauts who spent prolonged time in space experienced a 1–2% trabecular BMD loss in the hip and spine per month in space [9]. Similarly, early models of unloading in mice and rats, including spaceflight studies and tail suspension, found that trabecular and cortical bone volume are rapidly lost during periods of disuse [2, 10–13]. Losses of 20–50% of trabecular bone volume in the proximal tibia have been reported after two weeks of hindlimb unloading in adult rats [11, 14]. In addition, longer bouts of unloading (28 days) have resulted in small (~ 5%) decreases in cortical BMD [13, 15]. While the effect of mechanical unloading on bone has been thoroughly investigated, there have been relatively few studies examining the structural recovery of bone during reloading, and the factors that affect this recovery. Some studies examining reloading indicated that full recovery of BMD requires a reloading period of twice the unloading period [13, 16]. In addition it has been observed in rats that while bone volume returns to control levels during reloading, the bones still have fewer osteoblasts and a lower bone formation rate [11].

The effect of mechanical unloading on aged bone is not well established in either humans or animal models. Human spaceflight studies most often involve healthy young males [6, 7], and there are few bed rest studies using older patients, most of which have investigated the effect on muscle rather than bone [17, 18]. In animal models, few studies have investigated the role of age in bone adaptation to unloading [12], and the effect of age on the reloading response has never been investigated. Most rodent studies have used either young skeletally immature animals (5–7 week old rats) [2, 11, 19] or young adult animals (4–6 month old rats) [13, 15, 20]. It has been suggested that bone of aged rats may not respond at all to short bouts of unloading [12], however this is based on a single study, and there has been no examination of aged animals during longer bouts of unloading or reloading to examine longer-term effects. It is therefore unknown whether aged bone is completely unresponsive to mechanical unloading or if there is a delayed adaptive response to mechanical unloading, and to what extent aged bone is able to recover from any unload-induced bone loss during reloading.

In the current study, we used hindlimb unloading and subsequent reloading of skeletally mature Adult (9 month old) and Aged (28 month old) rats to examine the effect of age on bone loss during mechanical unloading and bone recovery during mechanical reloading. Rats underwent hindlimb unloading for 14 days; this unloading duration has been shown to cause a significant loss of trabecular bone in Adult animals [11, 13], and this unloading period was previously used to examine bone loss in Aged rats [12]. Cortical and trabecular bone microstructure were assessed using micro-computed tomography. Three-point bending and trabecular bone compression were used to assess changes in structural and mechanical properties of cortical and trabecular bone. We hypothesized that Adult rats would exhibit considerable bone loss during unloading, while Aged rats would exhibit less or no significant bone loss as was observed in a past study [12]. We further hypothesized that Adult rats would fully recover bone during reloading, while any bone loss observed following unloading in Aged rats would not be fully recovered during the reloading period. The results of this study could inform interventions such as exercise or mechanical loading for bone fragility in older subjects, particularly in the context of periods of mechanical disuse.

Methods

Animals

This study used a total of 63 Fisher 344 x Brown-Norway (FBN-F1) male rats from the National Institute of Aging (NIA) Aged Rodent Colony (Charles River Laboratories, Wilmington, MA). Rats were either 9 months old ("Adult", $n = 23$), or 28 months old ("Aged", $n = 40$). All rats were housed individually. Rats were cared for in accordance with the guidelines set by the National Institutes of Health (NIH) on the care and use of laboratory animals. All procedures were approved by the Institutional Animal Care and Use Committee at UC Davis.

Experimental groups and study design

Eleven experimental groups ($n = 5–6$ rats per group) were used to determine the magnitude of bone loss during hindlimb unloading and bone recovery during reloading (Fig. 1). Baseline animals (5 Adult and 6 Aged)

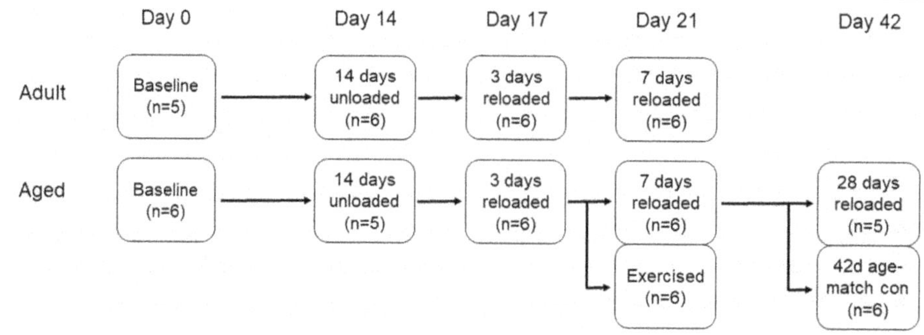

Fig. 1 Experimental Design. Adult (9 month old) and Aged (28 month old) rats ($n = 63$) were used for this study. Baseline rats were euthanized at day 0. Remaining groups underwent 14 days of hindlimb unloading, with a group of rats euthanized immediately following hindlimb unloading. All remaining rats were returned to normal cage activity. Rats from both age groups were euthanized after 3 or 7 days of reloading. An additional group of Aged rats were euthanized after 7 days of reloading with timed treadmill walking. Two additional groups of Aged rats were euthanized after 28 days of reloading or at an equivalent age for age-match control (not subjected to hindlimb unloading)

were euthanized prior to unloading to determine bone structure before intervention. The remaining rats underwent 14 days of hindlimb unloading via tail suspension. Post-unloading, one group of animals (6 Adult and 5 Aged) was euthanized immediately. Remaining rats were removed from hindlimb suspension and allowed to return to normal cage activity for 3 days (6 Adult and 6 Aged) or 7 days (6 Adult and 6 Aged). Additional groups of Aged rats examined the effect of activity level during reloading, and the effect of longer-term reloading. A group of Aged rats ($n = 6$) underwent 14 days of hindlimb unloading followed by 7 days of reloading with daily treadmill walking (an average of 13.8 m/day) to account for a significant decrease in activity observed in this age group during the first 5 days of reloading. Rats were set to walk on the treadmill at a quick walk (73 m/min) until they had covered the decrease in distance between the rats before and after unloading. Another group of Aged rats ($n = 5$) underwent 14 days of hindlimb unloading followed by 28 days of normal cage activity. To account for age-related decrease in bone, an additional group of Aged rats ($n = 6$) that were not subjected to hindlimb unloading were used as an age-match control to the 28 days reloaded group.

Hindlimb unloading via tail suspension

Rats were subjected to hindlimb unloading via tail suspension as originally described by Morey-Holten [1]. Briefly, the skin of the tail was cleaned using an alcohol pad, dried, and then sprayed with a light coating of tincture of benzoin. A tail-wide strip of Skin-Trac was then looped around a metal bar and applied to two sides of the tail. The tail was wrapped with Medi-Rip LF self-adherence bandage and then the animal was suspended by attaching the metal bar to a swivel hook above the suspension cage. The height of the hook was adjusted so that only the front limbs were able to touch the bottom of the cage. The rats were able to freely rotate in all directions within their cage and had free access to food and water. Body weights of the rats were taken prior to suspension and monitored throughout the unloading period. Following unloading or reloading, the rats were euthanized and their hindlimbs collected and stored in 70% ethanol prior to analysis. Previous studies have shown that storing bones in ethanol has little effect on the mechanical properties of the bone if properly rehydrated before testing [21, 22].

Cage activity

Prior to unloading and during reloading, cage activity of Adult and Aged rats was measured using the Home Cage Photobeam Activity System (San Diego Instruments). Each rat was housed individually and activity was tracked throughout the 12-h dark cycle and for the first hour of the light cycle. Data was analyzed using the Photobeam Activity System software.

Micro-computed tomography analysis of trabecular and cortical bone

Femurs were scanned with micro-computed tomography (μCT 35, Brüttisellen, Switzerland) to analyze morphological changes in trabecular and cortical bone during unloading and reloading. Bones were scanned with x-ray tube potential 55 kVp, intensity 114 mA, integration time 900 ms, 15 μm isotropic nominal voxel size. Trabecular bone analysis was performed at the distal femoral metaphysis over a region of 200 slices (3 mm), starting immediately adjacent to the distal femoral growth plate. Trabecular bone volume fraction (BV/TV), trabecular number (Tb.N), trabecular thickness (Tb.Th), trabecular separation (Tb.Sp), and other structural parameters were calculated using the manufacturer's 3D analysis software. Cortical bone was analyzed with 200 slice (3 mm) volumes of interest, centered at 25, 50, and

75% of the length of the diaphysis. Bone area (B.Ar), total cross-sectional area (T.Ar), cortical thickness (C.Th), maximum and minimum moments of inertia (I_{max} and I_{min}), and other structural parameters were calculated using the manufacturer's 3D analysis software.

3-point bending mechanical testing

Following μCT imaging, femurs were mechanically tested in three-point bending using a materials testing system (ELF 3200, TA Instruments, New Castle, Delaware) to determine cortical bone structural and mechanical properties. Femurs were immersed in phosphate-buffered saline for at least 10 min prior to testing to rehydrate the bone tissue in an isotonic solution. The midpoint of each femur was measured and marked, and each sample was placed in the 3-point bending setup such that the midpoint of the bone was directly under the loading platen. The two lower platens were 13 mm apart, and bones were tested with the posterior aspect of the bone in tension. A single monotonic load to fracture was applied at a slow (quasi-static) loading rate of 1 N/sec. Force and displacement data were recorded at 100 Hz. From the resulting force-displacement data, the yield point was visually identified as the point at which the linear portion of the curve ended. Bending stiffness (K), yield force (F_y) and ultimate force (F_{ult}) were determined from this data. Bone geometry determined from the μCT scan was used to calculate bending modulus (E), yield stress, and ultimate stress.

Metaphysis trabecular bone compression

After testing with 3-point bending, trabecular bone of distal femurs was mechanically tested in compression as described by Hogan et al. [23]. Distal femurs were potted in bone cement in a small petri dish to hold the bones stationary. Approximate location of the growth plate (determined from the μCT images) was marked on the outer surface of the femur. A 3 mm thick slice of the femoral metaphysis was then cut from the region adjacent to the growth plate, including both cortical and trabecular bone. Compression testing was performed with a materials testing machine (ELF 3200, TA Instruments, New Castle, DE). Samples were rehydrated in phosphate-buffered saline for at least 10 min prior to mechanical testing. The bone slice was loaded between two circular platens with diameter of 3 mm such that the platens were only in contact with the trabecular bone and not the cortical bone. Following a preload of 1–2 N, a monotonic (quasi-static) load was applied to the slice at a rate of 0.005 mm/sec. Compression continued to a target displacement of 0.2 mm. Force and displacement data was recorded at a rate of 100 Hz for the duration of the test. From this data, yield and ultimate force, yield and ultimate displacement and stiffness were obtained. Effective stress and effective modulus were obtained by normalizing by the surface area of the platens.

Statistical analysis

Differences in body weight and cage activity before and after unloading in Adult and Aged animals were analyzed by paired Student's *t*-test. All other statistical analyses were performed using 2-way analysis of variance (ANOVA) stratified by age and experimental group for main effect, with post-hoc analysis using Tukey's test. Statistical significance was defined as $p < 0.05$. The additional Aged rat group (7 days reloaded with treadmill walking) was analyzed for significance against the Aged baseline group and Aged 7 days reloaded group with a 1-way ANOVA stratified by experimental group with statistical significance defined as $p < 0.05$. The additional Aged rat groups of 28 days reloaded and 28 days age-matched control were analyzed for significance against the baseline group with a 1-way ANOVA stratified by experimental group with statistical significance defined as $p < 0.05$. For the trabecular bone compression test, a linear correlation between trabecular BV/TV and the effective elastic modulus and the correlation coefficient for the correlation was obtained.

Results

Animals

Over 14 days of unloading both age groups of rats experienced a significant decrease in body weight. Adult rats lost 12.2% of their body weight on average and Aged rats lost an average of 14.6% of their body weight. Cage activity measurements indicated a significant decrease in distance traveled of an average of 13.8 m/day in the first 5 days of reloading compared to baseline levels in Aged rats [24]; Adult rats exhibited no decrease in activity during reloading.

Micro-computed tomography analysis of trabecular bone

At baseline, bones from Aged rats had significantly less trabecular bone volume than those from Adult rats (0.169 vs. 0.247 BV/TV). Bones from Aged rats also had significantly lower Tb.N and higher Tb.Sp than Adult rats at baseline (Fig. 2). Trabecular thickness at baseline was not different between the two groups. After 14 days of hindlimb unloading, significant differences from baseline were observed in Adult rats but not Aged rats. Bones from Adult rats had 26.6% lower BV/TV ($p = 0.0493$) after 14 days of unloading compared to baseline. In addition, we observed trends toward decreased Tb.N and increased Tb.Sp at this time point, although these were not statistically significant.

After 3 days of reloading, trabecular bone parameters of Adult rats were not different from baseline values. In contrast, Aged bones had 19.7% lower BV/TV than baseline values (0.136 vs. 0.169), and 12.0% lower Tb.Th ($p = 0.0096$) at this time point. After 7 days of reloading, trabecular bone parameters of Adult bones remained similar to baseline values, while trabecular bone

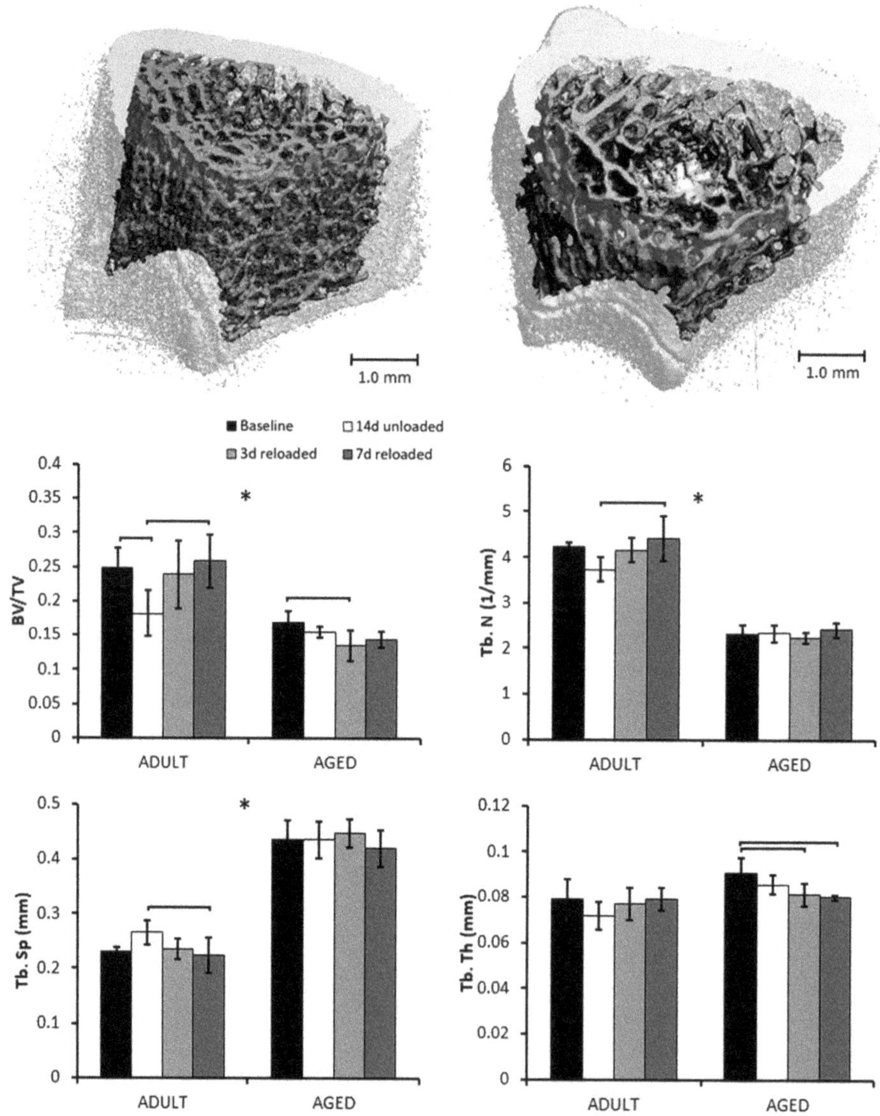

Fig. 2 Distal Femoral Metaphysis μCT results. Representative regions of interest of trabecular bone for Adult (left) and Aged (right) femurs at baseline. Adult rats exhibited greater BV/TV, Tb.N, and reduced Tb.Sp than Aged rats. 14 days of hindlimb unloading resulted in significant loss of trabecular bone in Adult rats, but no significant decrease in Aged rats. By day 3 of reloading, Adult rats had recovered trabecular bone volume, while Aged rats exhibited continued loss of bone. Brackets indicate significant differences between groups ($p < 0.05$). Asterisks (*) indicate a main effect of age in a parameter between Adult and Aged animals ($p < 0.05$)

parameters from Aged rats remained significantly lower than baseline values.

Aged rats subjected to 14 days of unloading followed by 28 days of reloading, had 15.1% lower Tb.Th than baseline ($p = 0.0068$), and 8.2% lower Tb.Th than the age-matched control group, though this difference was not statistically significant (Fig. 3). Trabecular BV/TV was not significantly different from baseline values after 28 days of reloading.

Seven days of treadmill walking during reloading in Aged rats did not considerably increase trabecular bone parameters compared to the 7 days reloaded group. BV/TV was 6.8% higher and Tb.Th was 5.9% higher in the exercised group than in the 7 days reloaded group, but these increases were not statistically significant.

Micro-computed tomography analysis of cortical bone

Significant differences in cortical bone structure were observed between Adult and Aged rats, however no differences were observed for either age group due to unloading or reloading. Aged rats had significantly lower cortical thickness and significantly higher bone area and total area than Adult rats (Fig. 4). I_{max} and I_{min} were also significantly higher in Aged rats than Adult rats. These observations were consistent across all three regions analyzed.

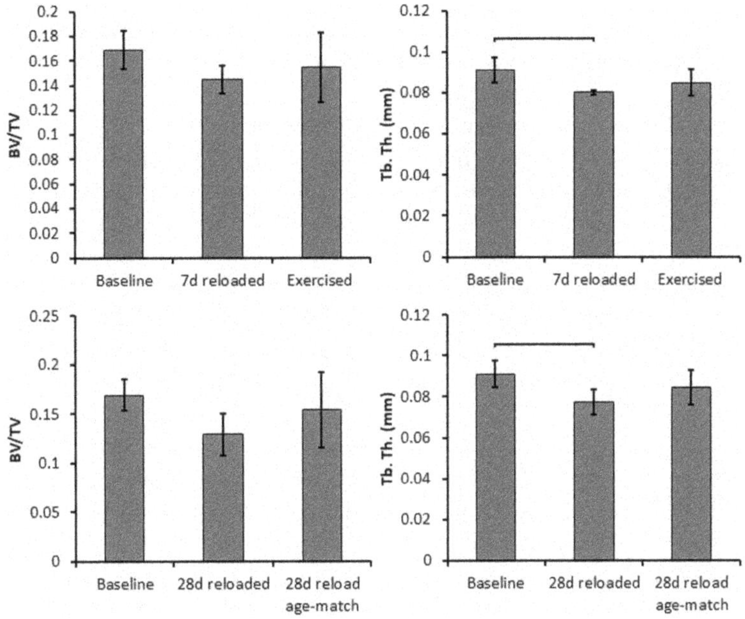

Fig. 3 Metaphyseal trabecular bone structure of Exercised and 28 days reloaded Aged rats. 7 days of treadmill walking during reloading did not significantly increase trabecular bone parameters relative to the 7 days reloaded group. Reloading for 28 days did not restore trabecular bone parameters back to control levels. Brackets indicate significant differences between groups ($p < 0.05$)

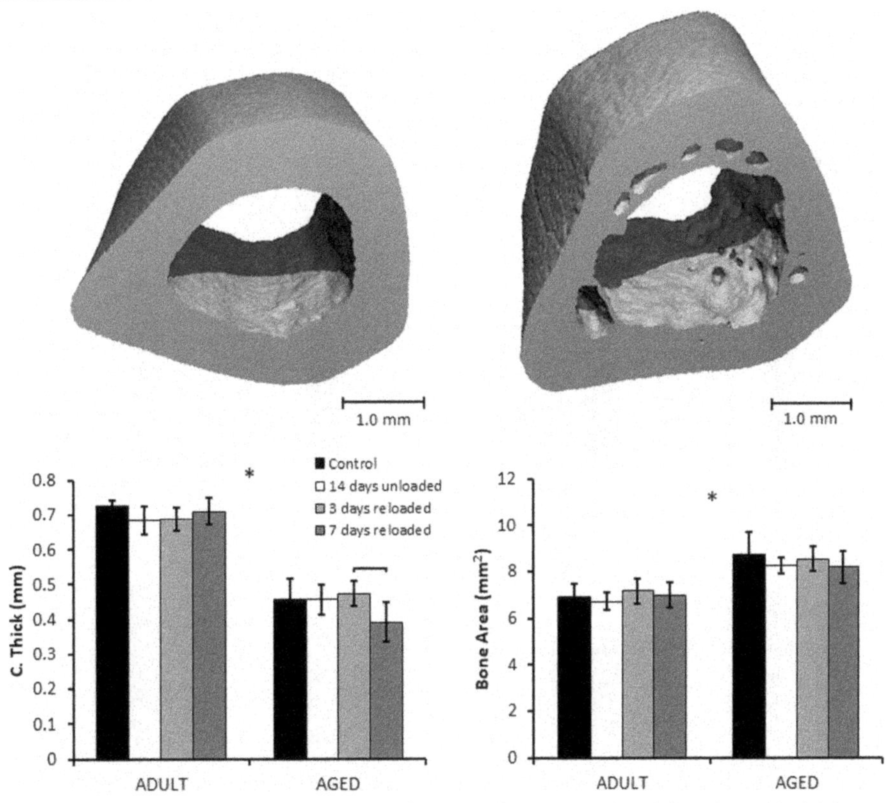

Fig. 4 Mid Femoral Diaphysis μCT Results. Representative samples of regions of interest in Adult (left) and Aged (right) femurs. Aged rats had lower average cortical thickness than Adult rats, but greater bone area and total cross-sectional area. Neither age group exhibited changes in cortical structure due to hindlimb unloading or reloading. Brackets indicate significant differences between groups ($p < 0.05$). Asterisks (*) indicate a main effect of age in a parameter between Adult and Aged animals ($p < 0.05$)

3-point bending mechanical testing

3-point bending yielded similar results to the μCT analysis of cortical bone, with Aged bones generally exhibiting greater structural properties and lower material properties than Adult bones (Fig. 5), but no significant differences in either age group due to hindlimb unloading or reloading. Stiffness and ultimate force were 34.7% higher ($p < 0.0001$) and 11.5% higher ($p < 0.001$) in Aged rats than the Adult rats at baseline, respectively. Yield stress was 39.1% lower ($p < 0.0001$) in Aged rats compared to Adult rats, while ultimate stress similarly was 28.8% lower ($p < 0.0001$) in Aged rats. Elastic modulus was 25.1% lower ($p < 0.0001$) in Aged rats than Adult rats.

Trabecular bone compression

Trabecular bone compression yielded trends similar to results of the trabecular bone μCT analysis. However, only age-related differences achieved statistical significance (Fig. 6). Trabecular bone from Adult rats exhibited significantly higher stiffness (+ 82.5%), effective modulus (+ 82.5%), and effective yield stress (+ 146.5%) than those from Aged rats. In the 14 days unloaded Adult rats, we observed trends towards lower stiffness, effective modulus, and effective yield stress compared to baseline values. However, these differences were not statistically significant due to the high variance in the experimental groups. The correlation between BV/TV and effective modulus yielded a correlation coefficient of 0.758, indicating a high correlation between these variables that was statistically significant ($p < 0.0001$) (Fig. 6).

Discussion

This study investigated difference in bone adaptation to hindlimb unloading and subsequent reloading in Adult and Aged rats. We originally hypothesized that Adult rats would lose more bone compared to Aged animals, and that Aged rats would lose little bone with unloading or even have no apparent bone loss. We also hypothesized that if Aged animals did exhibit bone loss during the unloading period, they would have diminished recovery of bone during reloading. Consistent with this hypothesis, we found that Adult rats showed a marked decrease in trabecular bone volume in response to hindlimb unloading, while Aged rats showed a diminished adaptive response. However, contrary to what has been postulated in previous studies, this does not mean that the Aged rats were necessarily unaffected by unloading. Aged rats did not lose a significant amount of bone volume during the unloading period, but did have lower BV/TV and Tb. Th. than baseline after 3 days and 7 days of reloading. These data suggest that there may be a delay in the adaptation of Aged bone to disuse. Consistent with our initial hypothesis, trabecular bone of Adult rats was not different from baseline levels after 3 days and 7 days of reloading, while bones from Aged rats exhibited deficits in trabecular microstructure even up to

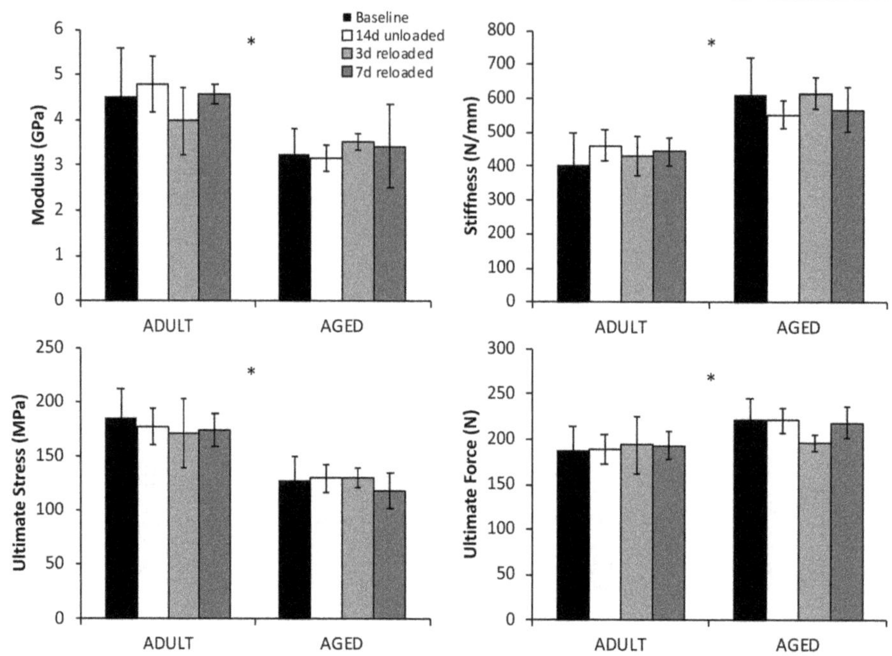

Fig. 5 Three-Point Bending Results. Bones from Aged rats exhibited greater stiffness and ultimate force, but lower bending modulus and ultimate stress compared to bones from Adult rats. No significant differences were observed as a result of hindlimb unloading or reloading. Asterisks (*) indicate a main effect of age in a parameter between Adult and Aged animals ($p < 0.05$)

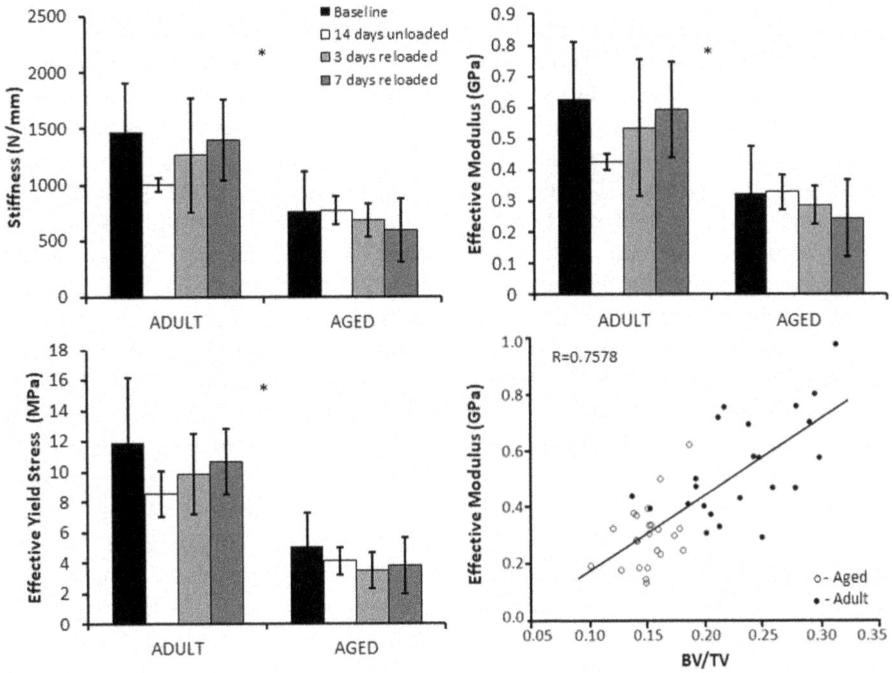

Fig. 6 Trabecular Bone Compression Results. Bones from Adult rats exhibited significantly greater stiffness, effective modulus, and effective yield stress than bones from Aged rats. However, there were no significant differences observed as a result of hindlimb unloading or reloading. Effective modulus showed a strong correlation to BV/TV. Asterisks (*) indicate a main effect of age in a parameter between Adult and Aged animals ($p < 0.05$)

28 days of reloading. These results may suggest that the Aged bones are overall less able to adapt to both unloading and reloading, and that the adaptive response may be temporally delayed. These results may also be a reflection of age-related changes in bone turnover rates and/or bone cellularity, which could lead to different responses to the same periods of unloading and reloading.

The magnitude of trabecular bone loss we observed in Adult rats during hindlimb unloading was similar to previous studies [13, 15]. Decreases in bone formation biomarkers and increases in bone absorption biomarkers have been observed in bed rest studies [25, 26] while in adult rats, bone formation in the hindlimbs has been shown to slow and ultimately cease after one week of tail suspension [27]. In addition, unloading leads to decreased vascularization in the bone, which could impair remodeling and slow recovery during reloading [28]. These are all possible mechanisms for trabecular bone loss observed during unloading in this study, though further studies are needed to confirm these mechanisms.

Few studies have examined the effect of tail suspension on aged animals, and those that have focused solely on unloading with no examination of bone recovery during reloading. One such study found that aged rats are less responsive to unloading and do not lose a significant amount of bone during 14 days of unloading [12]. This is consistent with our observations in this study, in which there was no significant loss of trabecular bone volume during unloading of Aged rats, though a non-significant trend toward bone loss was observed. However, this previous study suggested that aged bone may not respond at all to decreased mechanical stimulation [12]; our current data somewhat contradict these conclusions. While it is true that Aged bones showed no significant decreases in trabecular bone microstructure following the unloading period of our study (14 days), we observed a significant decrease from baseline values in trabecular BV/TV after 3 days of reloading and significant decreases in Tb.Th after 3 and 7 days of reloading. This implies that rather than aged bones being unresponsive to disuse, they may instead experience a delayed reaction to unloading.

It is possible that the gradual loss of trabecular bone in Aged rats could be partially due to normal age-related decreases in bone mass or diminished activity by Aged rats during the reloading period. To address these potential factors, we included a group of Aged rats that were age-matched for the 28 days reloaded group, and a group that was subjected to 7 days of treadmill walking during reloading to restore normal activity levels. We discovered that forcing Aged rats to resume a moderate activity level did appear to lessen some of the bone loss at 7 days of reloading, but did not account for the entire magnitude of bone loss. This implies that a return to a moderate exercise level following periods of disuse could be beneficial in mitigating bone's delayed reaction to unloading.

In Aged rats there was evidence that some bone recovery eventually occurs during reloading. The 28 days reloaded group had no significant differences in BV/TV from baseline. However, Tb.Th was still lower than baseline after 28 days of reloading in Aged rats. This decrease may be in part due to natural loss of bone due to aging but cannot fully be explained by this since the age-matched control group had trabecular bone parameters that were not significantly different from either the baseline or the 28 days reloading. These data suggest that even after a long reloading period, Aged rats may still have residual deficits in trabecular bone microstructure.

A previous study by Shirazi-Fard et al. showed that over a long period of reloading (28 days or more) in young adult rats, trabecular bone mineral content eventually returns to baseline levels, with recovery requiring twice the unloading time [16]. This is in contrast to what we observed in our study, wherein Adult rats exhibited recovery of trabecular bone volume in a much shorter time frame (3–7 days). It is unclear why these different outcomes were observed. Rats in our study were hindlimb unloaded for 14 days, while the study by Shirazi-Fard used 28 days of hindlimb unloading. This longer period of unloading may have caused biological changes that made it more difficult for trabecular bone to recover during reloading. For example, it has been observed that while bone volume may return to control levels, reloaded bones still have fewer osteoblasts and a lower bone formation rate than control bones [11], indicating that there are important long-term biological effects of unloading. Our current study did not examine changes in cellular activity in these bones, therefore we cannot determine if osteoblast number or activity were altered. Importantly, our study used a cross-sectional study design, so longitudinal changes are inferred using different groups of rats, rather than tracking the same group of rats over time. In contrast, the study by Shirazi-Fard [16] used both longitudinal assessment of bone structure and cross-sectional bone imaging and mechanical testing. It is difficult to say how accurately the inferred longitudinal changes in our study represent the true magnitudes and timeline of adaptive bone changes.

In this study, we observed that cortical and trabecular bone adapted very differently to changes in the mechanical loading environment. Differences in trabecular bone microstructure were easily detected in Adult rats immediately following unloading and at early time points during reloading, while Aged rats exhibited differences in trabecular microstructure at later time points. In contrast, cortical bone did not exhibit any adaptation to changes in loading at any time points. This is consistent with previous studies that have found that hindlimb unloading in rats and mice has an effect on cortical bone only for unloading bouts of longer than 14 days [15]. Considering the lack of cortical bone adaptation determined by μCT, it was not surprising that three-point bending showed no changes in mechanical properties as a function of unloading and reloading. In trabecular bone mechanical testing, we anticipated a similar trend to the changes in trabecular bone structural parameters from the μCT analysis. The high variances in the test resulted in no significant differences between experimental groups, however we were able to demonstrate that the mechanical properties of the trabecular bone were highly correlated to the structural properties found in μCT analysis. In this study we observed significant age-related differences in structural and material properties between Adult and Aged rats. The structural differences we observed, such as lower Ct.Th and larger I_{min}, and I_{max} in Aged rat bones, are consistent with previous studies in which bones from older animals had larger diameters but thinner cortical shells [29, 30]. We also observed that stiffness was higher in Aged animals while modulus and ultimate stress were lower; these data are also consistent with previous studies [29, 31].

The findings of this study have significant implications for aged patients. During sickness, or following an injury or surgery, older patients may spend a prolonged period in bed rest or with limited movement. Such a period of disuse could result in a loss of bone mass, which has previously been confirmed in human studies [8, 25]. Our data suggests that there may be a delay in the skeletal response to a decrease in mechanical loading, and bone loss may continue even during reloading. Clinically, this delay would be concerning as elderly patients who are remobilizing after bed rest may be more vulnerable to subsequent fracture. Our findings may motivate a rethinking of how elderly patients are treated during bed rest or limited mobility, and may imply that simply a return to normal activity levels following a period of disuse may not be enough to fully regain skeletal health.

While this study makes strong conclusions about differences between aged and adult bone in response to unloading and reloading, there are a number of limitations that must be addressed. First, this was a cross-sectional study, and did not examine the same animals at baseline, following unloading, and during reloading. Therefore, longitudinal changes due to unloading and reloading must be inferred based on cross-sectional data from different experimental groups. Second, we did not directly analyze bone formation or bone resorption rates, or other measures of cellular activity in these rats. Even with this limitation, we were able to determine significant differences in trabecular bone as a function of unloading and reloading, and differences in both cortical bone and trabecular bone as a function of age. Third, the group sizes (5–6 animals per group) were small. As a result of the small group sizes, several biologically meaningful measures did not yield statistically significant results. However, even with limited sample size, we were able to demonstrate differences between how aged and adult bones respond during the unloading-reloading timeline. Finally, this study did not examine other factors that could contribute to bone remodeling during unloading and reloading such as changes in food and water consumption, changes in gait, or effects of muscle atrophy on loads applied to the bones by muscles.

Conclusions

This study is one of few studies to examine the effect of age on bone adaptation to mechanical unloading, and the first to examine bone adaptation during subsequent reloading as a function of age. We demonstrate that bones from Aged animals have a delayed and diminished adaptive response to mechanical unloading, and an impaired capacity to recover bone during reloading. The delayed response of Aged bone could have meaningful consequences with respect to fracture risk and skeletal health of elderly patients, and should be considered for therapies aimed at preserving bone health during periods of disuse and subsequent remobilization.

Abbreviations

B.Ar: Bone area; BMD: Bone mineral density; BV/TV: Trabecular bone volume fraction; C.Th: Cortical thickness; F_{ult}: Ultimate force; F_y: Yield force; I_{max}: Maximum moment of inertia; I_{min}: Minimum moment of inertia; T.Ar: Total cross-sectional area; Tb.N: Trabecular number; Tb.Sp: Trabecular separation; Tb.Th: Trabecular thickness; μCT: Micro-computed tomography

Funding

Research reported in this publication was supported by the National Institute of Arthritis and Musculoskeletal and Skin Diseases under Award Number AG045375, and by the Department of Veterans Affairs under Award Number RX000673. The content is solely the responsibility of the authors and does not necessarily represent the official views of the funding bodies. The funding body was not involved with design, collection, analysis, or interpretation of data, or in the writing of the manuscript.

Authors' contributions

HCC performed data collection and analysis, statistical analysis, wrote the first draft of the manuscript, constructed all figures and tables. DWDW performed animal procedures and materials collection, contributed to study design. LMB performed animal procedures and materials collection, contributed to study design. FDT assisted with data collection and analysis. KB contributed to study design, oversaw experimental procedures, contributed to data interpretation. SCB contributed to study design, oversaw experimental procedures, contributed to data interpretation. BAC oversaw data collection and analysis, statistical analysis, contributed to drafting the manuscript and constructing figures and tables. All authors approved the final version of the manuscript and take responsibility for the integrity of the data analysis.

Consent for publication

Not applicable.

Competing interests

The authors declare that they have no competing interests.

Author details

[1]Biomedical Engineering Graduate Group, University of California Davis, Davis, CA, USA. [2]Department of Physiology & Membrane Biology, University of California Davis, Davis, CA, USA. [3]Department of Orthopaedic Surgery, University of California Davis Medical Center, Lawrence J. Ellison Musculoskeletal Research Center, 4635 2nd Avenue, Suite 2000, Sacramento, CA 95817, USA. [4]Department of Neurobiology, Physiology, and Behavior, University of California Davis, Davis, CA, USA.

References

1. Morey-Holton ER, Globus RK. Hindlimb unloading of growing rats: a model for predicting skeletal changes during space flight. Bone. 1998;22:83S–8S.
2. Bikle DD, Halloran PB. The response of bone to unloading. J Bone Miner Metab. 1999;17:233–44.
3. Burr DB. Muscle strength, bone mass, and age-related bone loss. J Bone Miner Res. 1997;12:1547–51.
4. Holguin N, Brodt MD, Sanchez ME, Silva MJ. Aging diminishes lamellar and woven bone formation induced by tibial compression in adult C57BL/6. Bone. 2014;65:83–91.
5. Rubin CT, Bain SD, McLeod KJ. Suppression of the osteogenic response in the aging skeleton. Calcif Tissue Int. 1992;50:306–13.
6. Collet P, Uebelhart D, Vico L, Moro L, Hartmann D, Roth M, Alexandre C. Effects of 1- and 6-month spaceflight on bone mass and biochemistry in two humans. Bone. 1997;20:547–51.
7. Vico L, Collet P, Guignandon A, Lafage-Proust MH, Thomas T, Rehaillia M, Alexandre C. Effects of long-term microgravity exposure on cancellous and cortical weight-bearing bones of cosmonauts. Lancet. 2000;355:1607–11.
8. Beller G, Belavy DL, Sun L, Armbrecht G, Alexandre C, Felsenberg D. WISE-2005: bed-rest induced changes in bone mineral density in women during 60 days simulated microgravity. Bone. 2011;49:858–66.
9. Lang T, LeBlanc A, Evans H, Lu Y, Genant H, Yu A. Cortical and trabecular bone mineral loss from the spine and hip in long-duration spaceflight. J Bone Miner Res. 2004;19:1006–12.
10. Jee WS, Wronski TJ, Morey ER, Kimmel DB. Effects of spaceflight on trabecular bone in rats. Am J Physiol Regul Integr Comp Physiol. 1983;244: R310–4.
11. Basso N, Jia Y, Bellows CG, Heersche JN. The effect of reloading on bone volume, osteoblast number, and osteoprogenitor characteristics: studies in hind limb unloaded rats. Bone. 2005;37:370–8.
12. Perrien DS, Akel NS, Dupont-Versteegden EE, Skinner RA, Siegel ER, Suva LJ, Gaddy D. Aging alters the skeletal response to disuse in the rat. Am J Physiol Regul Integr Comp Physiol. 2007;292:R988–96.
13. Shirazi-Fard Y, Anthony RA, Kwaczala AT, Judex S, Bloomfield SA, Hogan HA. Previous exposure to simulated microgravity does not exacerbate bone loss during subsequent exposure in the proximal tibia of adult rats. Bone. 2013; 56:461–73.
14. David V, Lafage-Proust MH, Laroche N, Christian A, Ruegsegger P, Vico L. Two-week longitudinal survey of bone architecture alteration in the hindlimb-unloaded rat model of bone loss: sex differences. Am J Physiol Endocrinol Metab. 2006;290:E440–7.
15. Bloomfield SA, Allen MR, Hogan HA, Delp MD. Site- and compartment-specific changes in bone with hindlimb unloading in mature adult rats. Bone. 2002;31:149–57.
16. Shirazi-Fard Y, Kupke JS, Bloomfield SA, Hogan HA. Discordant recovery of bone mass and mechanical properties during prolonged recovery from disuse. Bone. 2013;52:433–43.
17. English KL, Paddon-Jones D. Protecting muscle mass and function in older adults during bed rest. Current opinion in clinical nutrition and metabolic care. 2010;13:34.
18. Kortebein P, Ferrando A, Lombeida J, Wolfe R, Evans WJ. EFfect of 10 days of bed rest on skeletal muscle in healthy older adults. JAMA. 2007;297:1769–74.
19. Weinreb M, Rodan GA, Thompson DD. Osteopenia in the immobilized rat hind limb is associated with increased bone resorption and decreased bone formation. Bone. 1989;10:187–94.

20. Maeda H, Kimmel DB, Raab DM, Lane NE. Musculoskeletal recovery following hindlimb immobilization in adult female rats. Bone. 1993;14:153–9.
21. Linde F, Sørensen HCF. The effect of different storage methods on the mechanical properties of trabecular bone. J Biomech. 1993;26:(10):1249–52.
22. Beaupied H, Dupuis A, Arlettaz A, Brunet-Imbault B, Bonnet N, Jaffré C, Benhamou C-L, Courteix D. The mode of bone conservation does not affect the architecture and the tensile properties of rat femurs. Biomed Mater Eng. 2006;16:253–9.
23. Hogan HA, Ruhmann SP, Sampson HW. The mechanical properties of cancellous bone in the proximal tibia of ovariectomized rats. J Bone Miner Res. 2000;15:284–92.
24. Baehr LM, West DW, Marcotte G, Marshall AG, De Sousa LG, Baar K, Bodine SC. Age-related deficits in skeletal muscle recovery following disuse are associated with neuromuscular junction instability and ER stress, not impaired protein synthesis. Aging (Albany NY). 2016;8:127–46.
25. Zerwekh JE, Ruml LA, Gottschalk F, Pak CYC. The effects of twelve weeks of bed rest on bone histology, biochemical markers of bone turnover, and calcium homeostasis in eleven normal subjects. J Bone Miner Res. 1998;13: 1594–601.
26. Inoue M, Tanaka H, Moriwake T, Oka M, Sekiguchi C, Seino Y. Altered biochemical markers of bone turnover in humans during 120 days of bed rest. Bone. 2000;26:(3):281–6.
27. Globus RK, Bikle DD, Morey-Holton E. The temporal response of bone to unloading. Endocrinology. 1986;118:733–42.
28. Stabely JD, RDP BJB, Delp MD. Chronic skeletal unloading of the rat femur: mechanisms and functional consequences of vascular remodeling. Bone. 2013;57:355–60.
29. Danielsen CC, Mosekilde L, Svenstrup B. Cortical bone mass, composition, and mechanical properties in female rats in relation to age, long-term ovariectomy, and estrogen substitution. Calcif Tissue Int. 1993;52:26–33.
30. Akkus O, Adar F, Schaffler MB. Age-related changes in physicochemical properties of mineral crystals are related to impaired mechanical function of cortical bone. Bone. 2004;34:(3):443–53.
31. Turner CH. Bone strength: current concepts. Ann N Y Acad Sci. 2006;1068: 429–46.

18

Triamcinolone Acetonide affects TGF-β signaling regulation of fibrosis in idiopathic carpal tunnel syndrome

Tai-Hua Yang[1], Anne Gingery[1], Andrew R. Thoreson[1], Dirk R. Larson[2], Chunfeng Zhao[1] and Peter C. Amadio[1,3*]

Abstract

Background: Fibroblast behavior and cell-matrix interactions of cells from normal and idiopathic carpal tunnel syndrome (CTS) subsynovial connective tissue (SSCT) with and without Triamcinolone Acetonide (TA) were compared in this study. A cell-seeded gel contraction model was applied to investigate the effect of steroid treatment on SSCT fibroblast gene expression and function.

Methods: SSCT cells were obtained from CTS patients and fresh cadavers. Cells were isolated by mechanical and collagenase digestion. Collagen gels (1 mg/ml) were prepared with SSCT cells (1×10^6/mL). A sterile Petri dish with a cloning ring in the center was prepared. The area between the ring and outer dish was filled with cell-seeded collagen solution and gelled for 1 h. The gel was released from the outer way of the petri dish to allow gel contraction. Cell seeded gels were treated with 10 M triamcinolone acetonide (TA) or vehicle (DMSO) in modified MEM. Every 4 h for 3 days the contracting gels were photographed and areas calculated. Duplicate contraction tests were performed with each specimen, and the averages were used in the analyses, which were conducted using two-factor analysis of variance in a generalized linear model framework utilizing generalized estimating equations (GEE) to account for the correlation between samples. The contraction rate was determined by the area change over time, and the decay time constant was calculated. A customized mechanical test system was used to determine gel stiffness and tensile strength. Gene expression was assessed using Human Fibrosis and Cell Motility PCR arrays.

Results: TA-treated gels had a significantly higher contraction rate, tensile strength and stiffness than the untreated gels. Proteinases involved in remodeling had increased expression in TA-treated gels of the patient group. Pro-fibrotic genes and ECM regulators, such as TGF-β, collagens and integrins, were down-regulated by TA, indicating that TA may work in part by decreasing fibrotic gene expression.

Conclusions: This study showed that TA affects cell-matrix interaction and suppresses fibrotic gene expression in the SSCT cells of CTS patients.

Keywords: Carpal tunnel syndrome, Collagen gel contraction, Fibrosis, Subsynovial connective tissue, Triamcinolone Acetonide

* Correspondence: pamadio@mayo.edu
[1]Biomechanics & Tendon and Soft Tissue Biology Laboratory, Division of Orthopedic Research, Rochester, USA
[3]Tendon and Soft Tissue Biology Laboratory, Division of Orthopedic Research, Mayo Clinic, 200 First Street SW, Rochester, MN 55905, USA
Full list of author information is available at the end of the article

Background

In the United States, hundreds of thousands of carpal tunnel release (CTR) procedures are performed each year [1, 2]. Although most cases of carpal tunnel syndrome (CTS) are idiopathic [3, 4], other causes have been reported, such as repetitive motion, congenital anomalies, autoimmune disorders, arthritis and trauma [5–7]. Subsynovial connective tissue (SSCT) fibrosis and vascular proliferation have been reported as significant factors in CTS development [8, 9]. This fibrosis impedes the normal ulnodorsal motion of the median nerve when the hand is pinching and gripping while the wrist is flexed and may therefore result in nerve compression between the flexor tendons and flexor retinaculum [10–12].

Surgical decompression is the most common treatment of moderate to severe CTS [13]. However, non-surgical treatments, such as anti-inflammatory medication, corticosteroid injection, immobilization and physical therapy, are often used in milder cases [14–16]. Steroid injection was first described by Kendrick in 1957 [17]. Subsequent studies have reported a wide range of success rates, from 50 to 90% at 4–12 weeks and less at longer time points [14, 15].

One concern about the effectiveness of corticosteroid therapy for CTS is that these drugs are normally used for their anti-inflammatory effect, whereas the fibrosis in CTS is typically non-inflammatory [8, 11]. Therefore, the mechanism by which local steroid injection affects CTS remains unknown.

In this study, our hypothesis was that steroid treatment reduces TGF-β–related fibrosis activation and SSCT fibroblast activity. Both mechanical and molecular biology approaches were used to examine differences in SSCT fibroblast behavior and collagen interactions between cells from normal tissue and cells from idiopathic CTS tissue, with and without steroid, i.e., Triamcinolone Acetonide (TA), treatment. We chose TA because it is commonly injected clinically to treat CTS [16, 18].

Methods

Study design

We used a gel contraction model as a measure of SSCT fibroblast activation, based on the rate of collagen gel contraction and the change of the contracted gel's mechanical and temporal contraction properties as previously described [19]. Molecular assays of gene expression and an assay of collagen degradation products in the conditioned media were used to investigate the molecular response to TA treatment on TGF-β regulation and various molecular markers associated with CTS.

SSCT fibroblast preparation

SSCT tissue was harvested with our Institutional Review Board's approval. Tissues were harvested from the operated hands of 5 patients with idiopathic CTS, 3 female and 2 male, with a mean age of 58.4 (SD 4.8) years. Tissue was also harvested from the hands of same number fresh cadavers (within 12 h post mortem) of individuals with no history of CTS, with a mean age of 58.6 (SD 6.9). Patients and cadavers were excluded if they had a history of major trauma, prior steroid injection or surgery for CTS, or hand/wrist pathology, including known tumors/deformities, arthritis or metabolic disorders.

The tissue was harvested with 10x5x1 mm in size as needed from patients undergoing open carpal tunnel release and minced in minimal essential medium (MEM) with Earle's salts (GIBCO, Grand Island, NY) modified with 10% fetal bovine serum (GIBCO) and 1% Antibiotic-Antimycotic (GIBCO). Cells were cultured in 10-cm–diameter culture dishes and grown in the same media and supplements at 37 °C, in a 5% CO_2 humidified atmosphere, with the media changed every 3 days. The SSCT cells were passaged at 90% confluence, and passage 4 cells were used in all experiments.

Cell-seeded collagen gel preparation

Collagen gels were prepared as previously reported [19]. Briefly, a 1.0 mg/ml collagen/modified MEM sterile solution was made from 1.88 ml Vitrogen type I bovine dermal collagen (Cohesion Technologies, Palo Alto, CA), 1.2 ml 5X-modified MEM and 2.92 ml distilled water and maintained at pH 7.4 ± 0.2 on ice. SSCT cells were seeded at 1.0×10^6 cells/ml in a 0.5 mg/ml collagen/modified MEM solution and mixed into the collagen solution at room temperature. A small sterile cloning ring (8-mm outer diameter, 8-mm height) was attached to the center of each of four 3.5-cm Petri dishes with sterile vacuum grease (Dow Corning Corporation, Midland, MI). Then, the area between the ring and the outer part of each dish was filled with a 2-ml cell-seeded collagen solution and was gelled at 37 °C in a 5% CO_2 humidified incubator for 1 h. During gelation, two media with modified MEM were prepared: one was supplemented with 10 μM TA (Sigma-Aldrich, St. Louis, MO), and the other was a dimethyl sulfoxide (Sigma-Aldrich) vehicle media. To facilitate gel contraction, a scalpel was used to release the gelled solution from the dish's wall after 1 h of gelation. For each sample, four plates were prepared with 2 ml of media, two with TA-supplemented and two with vehicle media. All experiments were cultured at 37 °C in a 5% CO_2 humidified incubator with the media changed every 48 h as per treatment protocol.

Quantification and mechanical testing

Every 4 h for 3 days, the contracting gels were photographed and the areas calculated following previously described procedures [19, 20]. The gel contraction rate was determined by the change over time of the gel contraction percentage (the ratio of the current gel surface area over the initial area). Complete gel contraction was determined when gel contracted to less than 5% of original size. The decay time constant (*B*), which is directly proportional to the gel contraction rate, was calculated following an established equation (Eq. 1) [19], in which the area data at each time point were modeled with linear regression and optimization to fit an exponential decay function of time. A_0 is the initial area ($t = 0$); B is the decay time constant; and C is the non-zero asymptote as $t \rightarrow \infty$.

$$A(t) = A_0 e^{-Bt} + C \tag{1}$$

At the end of day 3, the fully contracted gel ring was taken from the dish. A customized mechanical testing system [19] was used to perform a uniaxial tensile test under displacement control at a 0.5 mm/sec distraction rate to determine stiffness and maximal tensile strength. The contracted gel ring was looped around a set of two hooks on the testing machine, which recorded force and displacement data at a sample rate of 10 Hz. The ring was submerged in a room-temperature phosphate-buffered saline (GIBCO) solution to keep the ring moist throughout the test.

PCR Array analyses

The contracted gel was homogenized with 1 mL of Trizol reagent (Invitrogen Life Technologies, Grand Island, NY). Total RNA was isolated as previously reported [21]. cDNA was synthesized from equal quantities of total RNA with an iScriptTM cDNA Synthesis Kit (Bio-Rad Laboratories, Inc., Hercules, CA). Gene expressions was measured using Human Fibrosis PCR arrays and Cell Motility PCR arrays (PAHS-120Z and PAHS-128Z, respectively, of SA Biosciences, Frederick, MD) according to the manufacturer's instructions. Fold changes were calculated with a log 2 scale between patient and control tissue, with and without TA treatment. Gene expression analysis was completed using SA Biosciences RT^2 Profiler™ PCR Array Data Analysis software from The GeneGlobe Data Analysis Center of QIAGEN (https://www.qiagen.com/us/geneglobe).

Quantitative real-time PCR

In order to confirm array results, select regulated genes from the arrays were analyzed with qRT-PCR (Table 1). Genes were analyzed in triplicate using the original cDNA, as previously described [22], and values were normalized with TATA binding protein (TBP) as a housekeeping gene. Primers were designed using Primer3web version 4.0.0 software (http://bioinfo.ut.ee/primer3) and purchased from Integrated DNA Technologies (Coralville, IA).

Collagen degradation assessment

Conditioned media was collected after the first 48 h and centrifuged at 1500 RPM for 5 min, and the supernatant was collected and stored at − 80 °C. Conditioned media was warmed to room temperature, and CrossLaps® for Culture ELISA (Immunodiagnostic Systems, Inc., Fountain Hills, AZ) was used to determine the degradation marker, C-terminal telopeptide of type I collagen, from the breakdown of the contracted cell-seeded gel according to the manufacturer's instructions. Briefly, preparation a two-fold dilution row of the standards, pre-dilution of test specimens with standard diluent and preparation of antibody solution were performed before the test. Then each of standards, control and samples were pipetted into appropriate wells to mix with antibody solution and incubated at room temperature for 2 h. Wash with diluted washing buffer for 5 washing cycles followed by adding substrate solution into each well and incubating for 15 min at room temperature in the dark on the mixing apparatus. Finally, add stopping solution into each well followed by measuring the absorbance at 450 nm in an absorbance microplate reader.

Statistical considerations

The effect of cell type (patient cells or control cells) and treatment type (with TA-supplemented or vehicle media) on the outcomes of decay time constant, tensile strength, stiffness and collagen degradation concentration was analyzed. A total of 10 samples were created from patient and control cells individually (five with TA-supplemented and five with vehicle media for each cell type). Duplicate contraction tests were performed with each specimen, and the averages were used in the analyses, which were conducted using two-factor analysis of variance in a generalized linear model framework utilizing generalized estimating equations (GEE) to account for the correlation between samples. Because significant interactions were observed between cell type and treatment type in the main

Table 1 Primers used in RT-PCR

Gene	Reference	Forward	Reverse
TGF-β1	NM_000660	GTGGAAACCCACAACGAAAT	CGGAGCTCTGATGTGTTGAA
COL1A2	NM_000089	TCCAAAGGAGAGAGCGGTAA	CAGATCCAGCTTCCCCATTA
COL3A1	NM_000090	CCAGGAGCTAACGGTCTCAG	CAGGGTTTCCATCTCTTCCA
VEGFA	NM_003376	AGGCCAGCACATAGGAGAGA	TTTCTTGCGCTTTCGTTTTT
TBP	NM_003194	GGTTTGCTGCGGTAATCATGA	CTCCTGTGCACACCATTTTCC

analysis, additional analyses were performed by generating separate one-factor models to analyze TA's effect separately for patient and control cells. All statistical tests were two-sided and p-values less than 0.05 were considered significant.

Results

Mechanical testing of gel contraction

Morphologically, in both the control and patient cell types, gels with TA-supplemented media had rough margins after full contraction (Fig. 1). The outcomes organized by factor and by group are shown in Tables 2 and 3, respectively. Regarding the main effects by factor, gels with TA-supplemented media had a significantly higher contraction rate, tensile strength and stiffness than those with vehicle media. Gels seeded with patient cells had a higher contraction rate and stiffness than those seeded with control cells, but no significant difference was observed respecting tensile strength.

Additionally, in individual group comparisons, the gels of control cells with TA-supplemented media had a higher mean contraction rate and mean tensile strength than those with vehicle media. The gels of patient cells with TA-supplemented media also had a higher mean contraction rate and mean tensile strength than those with vehicle media, but the difference was not statistically significant (Fig. 2a and b). The stiffness of the gels with TA-supplemented media was significantly higher than those with vehicle media regardless of cell type (Fig. 2c).

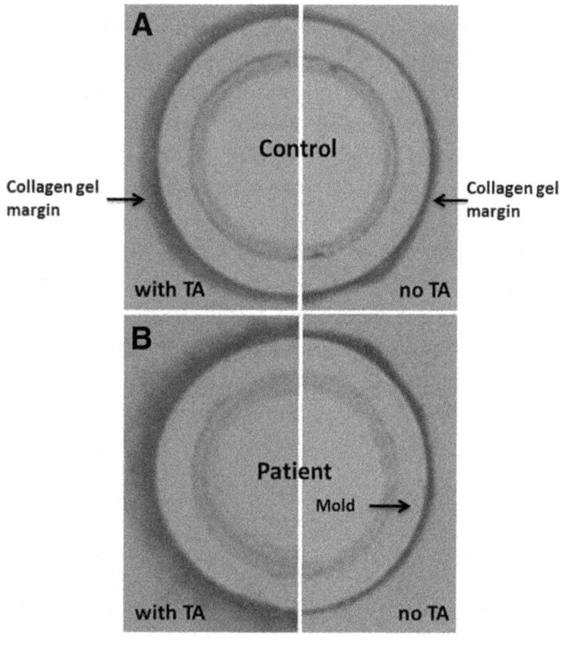

Fig. 1 TA treatment resulted in poorly defined margin formation regardless of cell type. **a** control, **b** patient

PCR Array analyses of fully contracted gels

In all comparisons, only a twofold or greater up- or down-regulation was considered to represent a changed gene expression. For the Human Fibrosis array (Additional file 1: Table S1), in the gels of patient cells with vehicle media compared to those of control cells with vehicle media, 3 genes were upregulated, e.g., collagen (COL) 3A1, and thrombospondins (THBS) 1 and 2, and 17 were down-regulated, e.g., platelet-derived growth factor (PDGF), vascular endothelial growth factor (VEGF), integrins (ITG) A3 and B6, and matrix metallopeptidase (MMP) 1 (Fig. 3a). In the Cell Motility array (Additional file 2: Table S2), 2 genes were upregulated in the gels of patient cells with vehicle media compared to those of control cells with vehicle media (Fig. 3b). But no down-regulated genes were found.

Regarding TA's effect on gel contraction, in the gels of patient cells with TA-supplemented compared to those with vehicle media, 9 genes in the Human Fibrosis array were upregulated, e.g., tissue inhibitors of metalloproteinase (TIMP) 4, MMP 3 and THBS 1, and 11 were down-regulated, e.g., TGF-β 2 and 3, ITG B1 and B3, COL 3A1 and 1A2, and MMP 1 and 9 (Additional file 3: Table S3 and Fig. 4a). In the Cell Motility array (Additional file 4: Table S4), 1 gene was upregulated in the gels of patient cells with TA-supplemented compared to patient cells with vehicle media, and 20 were down-regulated (Fig. 4b).

Quantitative real-time PCR

To confirm the microarray data, select genes that expressed twofold or greater changes in the arrays and were related to the TGF-β signaling were analyzed with quantitative Real-Time PCR (RT-PCR). All gene expressions were consistent with array results. In the comparison of patient and control cells in vehicle media, TGF-β1, COL1A2 and COL3A1 were all significantly upregulated, and VEGFA was down-regulated (Fig. 5a). Similarly, patient cells treated with TA all showed significant decreases in TGF-β1, COL1A2, COL3A1 and VEGFA as was found in the arrays (Fig. 5b).

Collagen degradation assessment by immunoassay (ELISA)

No significant difference in collagen fragment concentration was observed between treatment types or cell types, or in individual group comparisons.

Discussion

CTS is typified by non-inflammatory SSCT fibrosis with median nerve compression [8, 9]. Surgical decompression is the most effective therapy, but steroid injection has been the main non-operative therapy. TA and other anti-inflammatory steroids are used to treat orthopedic conditions such as tendinopathy, neuropathy, repetitive

Table 2 Summary of the analysis of the main effects on mechanical testing

Outcome	Factor	Level	Mean (SD)	*p*-value
Decay Time Constant (days-1)	Treatment Type	TA	2.9 (1.0)	< 0.001*
		No TA	2.2 (0.7)	
	Cell Type	Cadaver (control)	2.5 (1.1)	< 0.001*
		CTS patient	2.6 (0.7)	
Tensile Strength (mN)	Treatment Type	TA	7.0 (1.2)	< 0.001*
		No TA	5.8 (1.3)	
	Cell Type	Cadaver (control)	6.6 (1.4)	0.921
		CTS patient	6.1 (1.3)	
Stiffness (mN/mm)	Treatment Type	TA	1.1 (0.4)	< 0.001*
		No TA	0.7 (0.3)	
	Cell Type	Cadaver (control)	0.8 (0.3)	0.004*
		CTS patient	1.0 (0.4)	

* = Statistically significant

motion injuries and inflammatory symptoms and reduce pain, inflammation and limitations in mobility [23, 24]. However, the mechanism of steroid therapy is not yet completely understood. Cell-seeded gel contraction—the transformation of a collagen lattice caused by cellular action—is a useful quantitative model and has been used to study fibroblast proliferation and reorganization of structural proteins in the extracellular matrix (ECM) and the effects of TGF-β signaling on these processes [25, 26]. In this study, we sought to characterize changes in both SSCT fibroblast behavior and fibroblasts' interaction with collagen seeded with cells from normal tissue and idiopathic CTS tissue individually, with and without TA treatment, to investigate the effect of steroid treatment on SSCT fibroblast gene expression and function in a gel ring contraction model.

The results of the mechanical property test of gels with vehicle media (Fig. 2) support those of our previous study comparing patient and control cells, although the difference in tensile strength was not significant [19]. Regarding TA treatment, the effect of blurring the margins was greater in gels seeded with patient cells (Fig. 1), suggesting that TA had a greater effect on these cells and may have impeded their ability to contract the gel. While the mechanism of action of TA when injected to treat CTS is unknown, this finding suggests that TA may somehow interfere with the progress of synovial fibrosis that is commonly seen in CTS patients. Additionally, TA treatment significantly increased gel contraction rate, tensile strength and stiffness in control cells but only stiffness in patient cells (Fig. 2), suggesting that TA has a different effect in normal and CTS-affected cells. Specifically, TA treatment seems to involve impeding collagen synthesis and reorganizing molecular cross-linking in collagen, resulting in increased tissue stiffness and tensile strength, which is consistent with previous studies [17, 27, 28].

In this study, the changes in fibrotic and ECM gene expression in gels seeded with patient cells compared to

Table 3 Summary of analysis of the effect of TA, separately by gel type

Outcome	Cell Type	TA	Mean (SD)	*p*-value
Decay Time Constant (days^{-1})	Cadaver (control)	No TA	1.9 (0.8)	< 0.001*
		TA	3.0(1.2)	
	CTS patient	No TA	2.5 (0.6)	0.225
		TA	2.7 (0.8)	
Tensile Strength (mN)	Cadaver (control)	No TA	5.8 (1.3)	< 0.001*
		TA	7.4 (1.0)	
	CTS patient	No TA	5.8 (1.4)	0.157
		TA	6.5 (1.2)	
Stiffness (mN/mm)	Cadaver (control)	No TA	0.6 (0.1)	< 0.001*
		TA	1.0 (0.3)	
	CTS patient	No TA	0.9 (0.3)	0.042*
		TA	1.2 (0.4)	

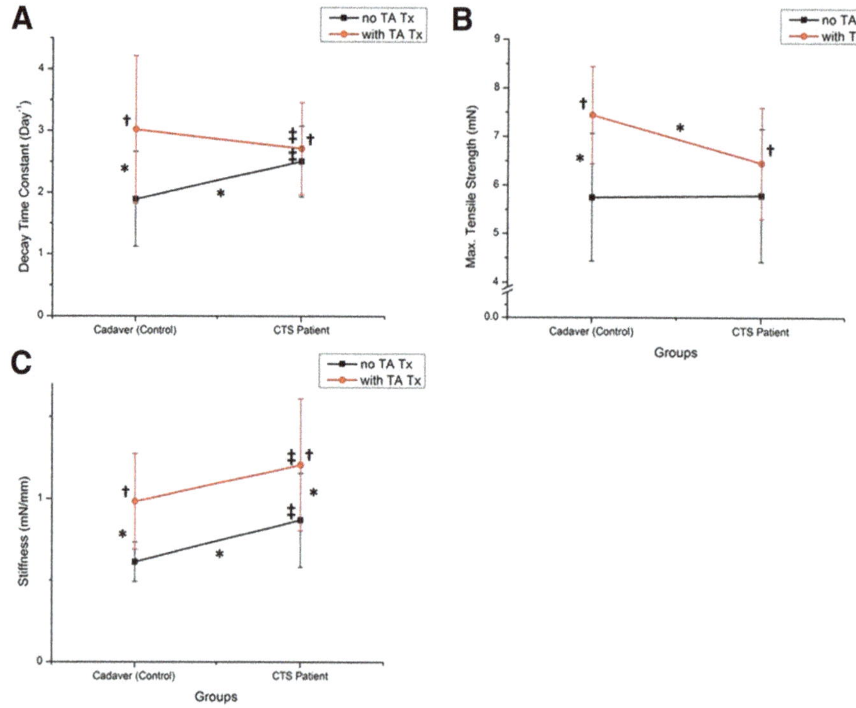

Fig. 2 a Decay time constant means, **b** Tensile strength means and **c** Stiffness means for the cell type and treatment type. Bars denote mean ± SD. Two-way ANOVA showed significant effects of cell type and treatment type. †$p < 0.05$, TA treatment overall compared with vehicle control; ‡$p < 0.05$, patient overall compared with control; *$p < 0.05$, significant difference between groups in individual factors

those seeded with control cells (Fig. 3) were consistent with those in previous studies, indicating that fibrotic pathways are important mediators in this model and supporting the common histopathological observation that the fibrosis seen in CTS is not associated with inflammation [8, 9, 21].

Regarding TA treatment of gels seeded with patient cells (Fig. 4), TA inhibited the expression of TGF-β–related fibrotic and ECM genes, such as collagens, TGF-βs and MMPs, and promoted expression of remodeling proteinase genes, including TIMP and thrombospondin. These results were consistent with those of previous studies, which showed that TA modulates TGF-β's transcription and translation and in turn ECM composition [27, 29]. One mechanism of action is the steroids' inhibition of MMP transcription, which may negatively impact collagen synthesis by suppressing protein binding activity [30, 31]. In this study, some integrins (Additional file 1: Table S1), such as ITGB1 and ITGB3, were upregulated in the gels of patient cells with vehicle media compared to those of control cells with vehicle media, although the change was less than twofold. However, in the patient cells with TA treatment, integrins were down-regulated twofold compared to those with vehicle

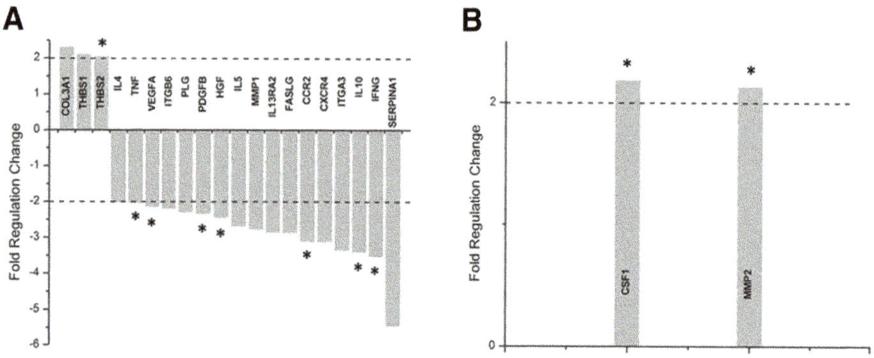

Fig. 3 a Human fibrosis array and **b** Cell motility array relative fold change in genes from the patient group without TA treatment compared to the control group without TA treatment. (* indicates significant differences, $p < 0.05$)

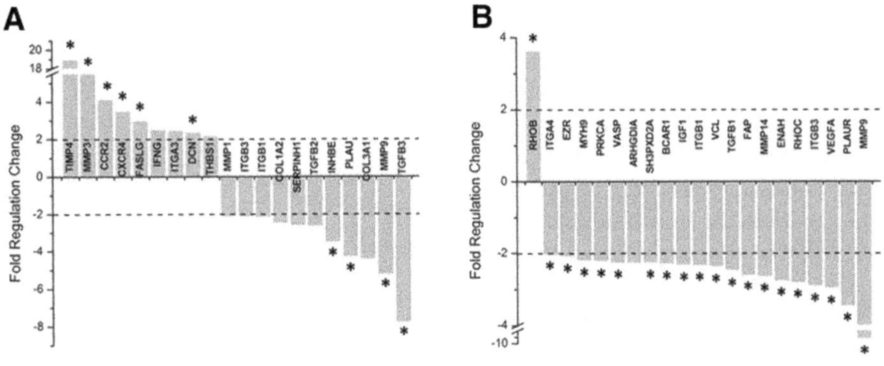

Fig. 4 a Human fibrosis array and **b** Cell motility array relative fold change in genes from the patient group with TA treatment compared to the patient group without TA treatment. (* indicates significant differences, $p < 0.05$)

media (Fig. 4). These results are consistent with those of previous studies, in which dexamethasone treatment of human-derived tendon cells decreased β1-integrin synthesis and reduced type I collagen production [32]. Integrins mediate translational signaling from the adjacent ECM to change cell behaviors such as adhesion, migration and proliferation to modulate cell-ECM and cell-cell adhesion, resulting in fibrosis [32, 33]. Integrins can regulate canonical and non-canonical TGF-β fibrotic signaling processes (such as systemic sclerosis, pulmonary fibrosis and cancer). Additionally, TGF-β regulates integrins to modulate cell behaviors, such as migration and adhesion [34, 35]. The cytokines VEGF and PDGF are additional known mediators of fibrosis both separately and in conjunction with TGF-β. However, in our study, PDGF and VEGF expressions were suppressed in the patient groups regardless of treatment type (Figs. 3 and 4). Thus, TA does not seem to affect these pro-fibrotic pathways. Reducing fibrosis via these other pathways may be a promising avenue for further research into medical treatments of CTS.

To understand how the untreated and TA-treated fibroblasts modulate and regulate the adjacent ECM in our gel contraction model, we examined whether collagen breakdown was a mechanism involved in the gel contraction in both control and treated conditions. Many studies have demonstrated that collagen breakdown is normally a part of tissue regeneration and that corticosteroids inhibit the degradation of mature collagen by suppressing the collagen breakdown [36, 37]. There was no significant difference in the products of collagen breakdown between gel types or treatment types, indicating that collagen breakdown is not the likely mechanism of this cell-seeded gel contraction model.

There are some limitations in this study. First, despite the gender and age match between the patient and control cells, the sample size was small. However, we were able to see significant cell and treatment interactions. Second, the phenomenon of the rough edge (margin) of contracted gel was found in all TA treatment groups regardless of cell type. In order to quantify and compare the rough edge we measured a solidly visible edge as the

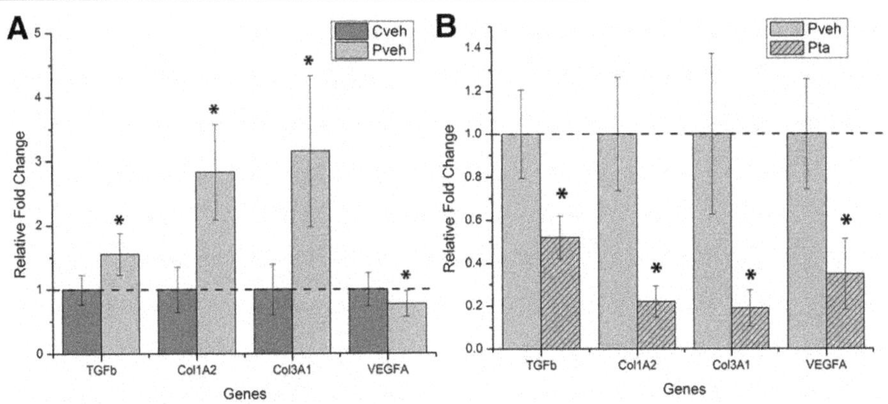

Fig. 5 Confirmation of the arrays' gene expressions was analyzed by quantitative RT-PCR between **a** the untreated patient group (Cveh) and the untreated control group (Pveh) (results are normalized to the untreated control group); **b** the treated patient group (Pta) and the untreated patient group (results are normalized to the untreated patient group). (* indicates significant differences, $p < 0.05$)

contraction edge to quantify the contraction rate. Third, we investigated only canonical TGF-β fibrotic signaling processes. In the future, we plan to investigate and compare the quality and arrangement, and the changes of inter−/intra-collagen fibers after contraction between treated and non-treated groups using confocal microscope and scanning electron microscope respectively. Moreover, we plan to study other possible signaling processes related to fibrosis. However, researchers may be able to use the current model to understand the dynamics of SSCT pathogenesis and treatment more clearly find ways to block signaling pathways or test new therapies.

Conclusion

In conclusion, our results in collagen gel contraction were consistent with those of previous studies: there was an increased cell-seeded gel contraction rate, stiffness and tensile strength in gels with media of patient cells compared to those of control cells. We also found that the TA-treated groups had poorly defined margins after contraction in both cell types (though this was more pronounced in the patient groups), which suggests that TA affected gel structural integrity. Fibrotic genes and ECM regulators, such as TGF-β, collagens and integrins, were upregulated in the gels of patient cells with vehicle media compared to the gels of control cells with vehicle media. Additionally, in gels with TA-supplemented cells, the patient cell groups had increased expression of remodeling proteinases compared to the control cell groups, indicating that TA modulates TGF-β signaling and affects ECM composition. Furthermore, with TA treatment, patient cells' fibrotic genes and ECM regulators, such as TGF-β, collagens and integrins, were down-regulated, indicating that TA may be working in part by decreasing an overall fibrotic gene expression. This study shows that steroids affect cell regulation on gel structural integrity and regulate fibrotic gene expression in patient cells and may affect CTS by modulating cellular function. This may explain the reported decreases in CTS symptoms for some patients treated with steroids. Further study of these identified genes and pathways may help researchers discover new and more effective therapeutic targets for CTS treatment.

Additional files

Additional file 1: Table S1. Gene fold changes of the CTS group without TA treatment compared to the control group without TA treatment in Human Fibrosis Array

Additional file 2: Table S2. Gene fold changes of the CTS group without TA treatment compared to the control group without TA treatment in Cell Motility Array.

Additional file 3: Table S3. Gene fold changes of the CTS group with TA treatment compared to the CTS group without TA treatment in Human fibrosis array.

Additional file 4: Table S4. Gene fold changes of the CTS group with TA treatment compared to the CTS group without TA treatment in Cell Motility Array.

Acknowledgements
No one else contributed towards the article except for the authors.

Funding
This study was supported by NIH/NIAMSAR49823, NIH/NIAMS F32 AR063596 and a 2013 American Society for Surgery of the Hand Basic Science Grant.

Authors' contributions
Substantial contributions to research design, or the acquisition, analysis or interpretation of data: THY; AG; ART; DRL; CZ; PCA; Drafting the paper or revising it critically: THY; AG; DRL; PCA. All authors read and approved the final manuscript.

Consent for publication
Not applicable.

Competing interests
Authors Anne Gingery and Andrew Thoreson are editorial board members of BMC Musculoskeletal Disorders.

Author details
[1]Biomechanics & Tendon and Soft Tissue Biology Laboratory, Division of Orthopedic Research, Rochester, USA. [2]Division of Biomedical Statistics and Informatics, Department of Health Science Research, Mayo Clinic, Rochester, MN 55905, USA. [3]Tendon and Soft Tissue Biology Laboratory, Division of Orthopedic Research, Mayo Clinic, 200 First Street SW, Rochester, MN 55905, USA.

References

1. Gelfman R, Melton LJ 3rd, Yawn BP, Wollan PC, Amadio PC, Stevens JC. Long-term trends in carpal tunnel syndrome. Neurology. 2009;72(1):33–41.
2. Palmer DH, Hanrahan LP. Social and economic costs of carpal tunnel surgery. Instr Course Lect. 1995;44:167–72.
3. Atroshi I, Gummesson C, Johnssson R, Ornstein E, Ranstam J, Rosen I. Prevalence of carpal tunnel syndrome in a general population. JAMA. 1999; 282(2):153–8.
4. Szabo RM, Madison M. Carpal tunnel syndrome. Orthop Clin North Am. 1992;23(1):103–9.
5. Armstrong TJ. Ergonomics and cumulative trauma disorders. Hand Clin. 1986;2(3):553–65.
6. Blanc PD, Faucett J, Kennedy JJ, Cisternas M, Yelin E. Self-reported carpal tunnel syndrome: predictors of work disability from the National Health Interview Survey Occupational Health Supplement. Am J Ind Med. 1996; 30(3):362–8.
7. Leclerc A, Franchi P, Cristofari MF, Delemotte B, Mereau P, Teyssier-Cotte C, Touranchet A. Carpal tunnel syndrome and work organisation in repetitive work: a cross sectional study in France. Study group on repetitive work. Occup Environ Med. 1998;55(3):180–7.
8. Donato G, Galasso O, Valentino P, Conforti F, Zuccala V, Russo E, Maltese L, Perrotta I, Tripepi S, Amorosi A. Pathological findings in subsynovial connective tissue in idiopathic carpal tunnel syndrome. Clin Neuropathol. 2009;28(2):129–35.
9. Schuind F, Ventura M, Pasteels JL. Idiopathic carpal tunnel syndrome: histologic study of flexor tendon synovium. J Hand Surg Am. 1990;15(3): 497–503.

10. Zhao C, Ettema AM, Berglund LJ, An KN, Amadio PC. Gliding resistance of flexor tendon associated with carpal tunnel pressure: a biomechanical cadaver study. J Orthop Res. 2011;29(1):58–61.
11. Ettema AM, Zhao C, Amadio PC, O'Byrne MM, An KN. Gliding characteristics of flexor tendon and tenosynovium in carpal tunnel syndrome: a pilot study. Clin Anat. 2007;20(3):292–9.
12. Yoshii Y, Zhao C, Zhao KD, Zobitz ME, An KN, Amadio PC. The effect of wrist position on the relative motion of tendon, nerve, and subsynovial connective tissue within the carpal tunnel in a human cadaver model. J Orthop Res. 2008;26(8):1153–8.
13. Keith MW, Masear V, Chung KC, Amadio PC, Andary M, Barth RW, Maupin K, Graham B, Watters WC 3rd, Turkelson CM, et al. American Academy of Orthopaedic surgeons clinical practice guideline on the treatment of carpal tunnel syndrome. J Bone Joint Surg Am. 2010;92(1):218–9.
14. Plotkin MB, Foss ML, Goldin B, Ellis DG. Dose response effects of anti inflammatory steroid injections on mechanical properties of rat tail tendons. Med Sci Sports Exerc. 1976;8(4):230–4.
15. Zeisig E. Natural course in tennis elbow-lateral epicondylitis after all? Knee Surg Sport Tr A. 2012;20(12):2549–52.
16. Karadas O, Tok F, Akarsu S, Tekin L, Balaban B. Triamcinolone Acetonide vs procaine hydrochloride injection in the Management of Carpal Tunnel Syndrome: randomized placebo-controlled trial. J Rehabil Med. 2012;44(7):601–4.
17. Mackie JW, Goldin B, Foss ML, Cockrell JL. Mechanical properties of rabbit tendons after repeated antiinflammatory steroid injections. Med Sci Sports Exerc. 1974;6(3):198–202.
18. Cartwright MS, White DL, Demar S, Wiesler ER, Sarlikiotis T, Chloros GD, Yoon JS, Won SJ, Molnar JA, Defranzo AJ, et al. Median nerve changes following steroid injection for carpal tunnel syndrome. Muscle Nerve. 2011;44(1):25–9.
19. Yang T-H, Thoreson AR, Gingery A, An K-N, Larson DR, Zhao C, Amadio PC. Collagen gel contraction as a measure of fibroblast function in carpal tunnel syndrome. J Biomed Mater Res A. 2015;103(2):574–80.
20. Chen H-C, Yang T-H, Thoreson AR, Zhao C, Amadio PC, Sun Y-N, Su F-C, An K-N. Automatic and quantitative measurement of collagen gel contraction using model-guided segmentation. Meas Sci Technol. 2013;24(8):085702.
21. Gingery A, Yang TH, Passe SM, An KN, Zhao C, Amadio PC. TGF-β signaling regulates fibrotic expression and activity in carpal tunnel syndrome. J Orthop Res. 2014;32(11):1444–50.
22. Hawse JR, Cicek M, Grygo SB, Bruinsma ES, Rajamannan NM, van Wijnen AJ, Lian JB, Stein GS, Oursler MJ, Subramaniam M, et al. TIEG1/KLF10 modulates Runx2 expression and activity in osteoblasts. PLoS One. 2011;6(4):e19429.
23. Hollander JL. Intra-articular hydrocortisone in arthritis and allied conditions; a summary of two years' clinical experience. J Bone Joint Surg Am. 1953;35-A(4):983–90.
24. Stephens MB, Beutler AI, O'Connor FG. Musculoskeletal injections: a review of the evidence. Am Fam Physician. 2008;78(8):971–6.
25. Chieh HF, Sun YL, Liao JD, Su FC, Zhao CF, Amadio PC, An KN. Effects of cell concentration and collagen concentration on contraction kinetics and mechanical properties in a bone marrow stromal cell-collagen construct. J Biomed Mater Res A. 2010;93A(3):1132–9.
26. Bell E, Ivarsson B, Merrill C. Production of a tissue-like structure by contraction of collagen lattices by human fibroblasts of different proliferative potential in vitro. Proc Natl Acad Sci U S A. 1979;76(3):1274–8.
27. McCoy BJ, Diegelmann RF, Cohen IK. In vitro inhibition of cell growth, collagen synthesis, and prolyl hydroxylase activity by triamcinolone acetonide. Proc Soc Exp Biol Med. 1980;163(2):216–22.
28. Vogel HG. Influence of age, treatment with corticosteroids and strain rate on mechanical properties of rat skin. Biochim Biophys Acta. 1972;286(1):79–83.
29. Carroll LA, Hanasono MM, Mikulec AA, Kita M, Koch RJ. Triamcinolone stimulates bFGF production and inhibits TGF-β1 production by human dermal fibroblasts. Dermatol Sur. 2002;28(8):704–9.
30. Aljada A, Ghanim H, Mohanty P, Hofmeyer D, Tripathy D, Dandona P. Hydrocortisone suppresses intranuclear activator-protein-1 (AP-1) binding activity in mononuclear cells and plasma matrix metalloproteinase 2 and 9 (MMP-2 and MMP-9). J Clin Endocr Metab. 2001;86(12):5988–91.
31. LeBert DC, Squirrell JM, Rindy J, Broadbridge E, Lui Y, Zakrzewska A, Eliceiri KW, Meijer AH, Huttenlocher A. Matrix metalloproteinase 9 modulates collagen matrices and wound repair. Development. 2015;142(12):2136–46.
32. Sendzik J, Shakibaei M, Schafer-Korting M, Lode H, Stahlmann R. Synergistic effects of dexamethasone and quinolones on human-derived tendon cells. Int J Antimicrob Agents. 2010;35(4):366–74.
33. van der Flier A, Sonnenberg A. Function and interactions of integrins. Cell Tissue Res. 2001;305(3):285–98.
34. Margadant C, Sonnenberg A. Integrin-TGF-beta crosstalk in fibrosis, cancer and wound healing. EMBO Rep. 2010;11(2):97–105.
35. Henderson NC, Sheppard D. Integrin-mediated regulation of TGFβ in fibrosis. Biochim Biophys Acta. 2013;1832(7):891–6.
36. Nimni ME, Bavetta LA. Collagen synthesis and turnover in the growing rat under the influence of methyl prednisolone. Proc Soc Exp Biol Med. 1964; 117:618–23.
37. Koob TJ, Jeffrey JJ, Eisen AZ. Regulation of human skin collagenase activity by hydrocortisone and dexamethasone in organ culture. Biochem Biophys Res Commun. 1974;61(3):1083–8.

19

Global postural re-education in pediatric idiopathic scoliosis: a biomechanical modeling and analysis of curve reduction during active and assisted self-correction

Sarah Dupuis[1,2], Carole Fortin[2,3], Christiane Caouette[1,2], Isabelle Leclair[2,3] and Carl-Éric Aubin[1,2,3*]

Abstract

Background: Global postural re-education (GPR) is a physiotherapy treatment approach for pediatric idiopathic scoliosis (IS), where the physiotherapist qualitatively assesses scoliotic curvature reduction potential (with a manual correction) and patient's ability to self-correct (self-correction). To the author's knowledge, there are no studies regarding GPR applied to IS, hence there is a need to better understand the biomechanics of GPR curve reduction postures. The objective was to biomechanically and quantitatively evaluate those two re-education corrections using a computer model combined with experimental testing.

Methods: Finite elements models of 16 patients with IS (10.5–15.4 years old, average Cobb angle of 33°) where built from surface scans and 3D radiographic reconstructions taken in normal standing and self-corrected postures. The forces applied with the therapist's hands over the trunk during manual correction were recorded and used in the FEM to simulate this posture. Self-correction was simulated by moving the thoracic and lumbar apical vertebrae from their presenting position to their self-corrected position as seen on radiographs. A stiffness index was defined for each posture as the global force required to stay in the posture divided by the thoracic curve reduction (force/ Cobb angle reduction).

Results: The average force applied by the therapist during manual correction was 31 N and resulted in a simulated average reduction of 26% ($p < 0.05$), while kyphosis slightly increased and lordosis remained unchanged. The actual self-correction reduced the thoracic curve by an average of 33% ($p < 0.05$), while the lumbar curve remained unchanged. The thoracic kyphosis and lumbar lordosis were reduced on average by 6° and 5° ($p < 0.05$). Self-correction simulations correlated with actual self-correction ($r = 0.9$).

Conclusions: This study allowed quantification of thoracic curve reducibility obtained by external forces applications as well as patient's capacity to self-correct their posture, two corrections commonly used in the GPR approach.

Keywords: Scoliosis, Global postural re-education, Biomechanical modeling, Finite element model

* Correspondence: carl-eric.aubin@polymtl.ca
[1]Department of Mechanical Engineering, École Polytechnique de Montréal, P.O. Box 6097, Downtown Station, Station "Centre-ville", Montreal, Quebec H3C 3A7, Canada
[2]Research Centre, Sainte-Justine University Hospital Centre, 3175 chemin de la Côte-Sainte-Catherine, Montreal, Quebec H3T 1C5, Canada
Full list of author information is available at the end of the article

Background

Idiopathic scoliosis (IS) is a tridimensional (3D) spine deformity of unknown cause that alters body posture and affects perception of self-image and psychological confidence [1]. The deformation severity is conventionally evaluated with Cobb angle measurement on the coronal radiographs. Conservative treatments are recommended for small (10°–20°) and moderate deformities (20°–45°), which in North America traditionally consist of bracing and/or observation [1].

Since 2011, the international society on Scoliosis Orthopaedic and Rehabilitation Treatment (SOSORT) recognizes physiotherapy specific scoliosis exercises (PSSE) as a complementary or alternative conservative management to bracing [2]. More recently, the 2016 SOSORT guidelines have shown a higher strength of evidence regarding the efficacy of PSSE to prevent curve progression in IS [3]. Among them, Global Postural Re-education (GPR) aims to reduce postural impairments, regain back muscle symmetry and adequate posture through active muscular stretching postures, motor control and sensory integration exercises [4, 5]. The selection of the appropriate exercises is based on a 3-steps comprehensive evaluation focusing on 1) body morphology and symptomatology, 2) examination of muscle retractions associated with posture alterations [6] and 3) re-equilibration tests to assess back muscle flexibility and spine deformity correction (curve reducibility) [6, 7].

Like other PSSE, GPR treatment is personalized to the patient condition [8], and curve reducibility potential assessment orients the treatment planning, in a way similar to flexibility tests for surgical planning. Manual correction and self-correction are two re-equilibration tests that aims to achieve a passive and active momentary correction used in GPR for curve reducibility assessment [9]. Self-correction is also an integration exercise used at the end of a treatment session in order to progressively integrate changes in posture [9]. Manual correction involves the physiotherapist applying targeted force with his hands to the patient's trunk to reduce scoliosis. This re-equilibration test aims to reach a posture that reduces momentarily the scoliotic deformation and to qualitatively assess trunk muscles stiffness as well as posture compensations. Self-correction is an active recruitment of trunk muscles by the patient in order to reduce the spine deformity, ideally in 3D. Self-correction also aims to assess the patient's ability to integrate the correction, in real time and is an exercise common to many other PSSE programs [10].

Recent studies have shown a beneficial outcome from PSSE on scoliosis stabilisation and quality of life [11–13], although there is still a need for quantitative studies to confirm their effectiveness and further understand the biomechanical mechanisms [10, 14, 15]. There are very few studies regarding GPR applied to IS [6, 7, 11], hence there is also a need to quantify and better understand the biomechanics of GPR curve reduction postures.

Finite element models (FEM) are often used to biomechanically assess IS and brace treatments [16–21]. A personalized FEM was developed to simulate and optimize brace design for adolescent IS [22–25]. This model has the potential to be adapted for other conservative treatment simulations such as physiotherapist's treatment.

The objective of this study was to biomechanically and quantitatively evaluate two re-education corrections (manual correction and self-correction) in pediatric idiopathic scoliosis using FEM combined with experimental testing.

Methods

Experimental study design

Patients

A total of 17 patients diagnosed with pediatric IS, aged 10.5 to 15.4 (one boy, 16 girls) and Risser sign 0 to 4, were recruited during their routine visit at our orthopedic clinic over a three months period. They all had a right thoracic major curve or a double major curve with right thoracic component, with a thoracic Cobb angle ranging from 11° to 45° (average 33° ± 9°), analytically measured between the perpendicular to the spine curve at its side change point near the end vertebrae. Their apical thoracic vertebral rotation ranged from 22° to − 6° (average 11° ± 9°), analytically measured using a 3D reconstruction method using pedicles and vertebral body orientation. One patient was excluded because the thoracic curve was less than 10°. Among the patients, seven were wearing thoraco-lombo-sacral orthosis (TLSO) and four were wearing nighttime braces. Two patients had done physical therapy in the past and six were still following PSSE or GPR treatment alone or in complement with their brace treatment. Patients filled a pain questionnaire (Numeric Pain Rating Scale NPRS-11) to ensure they had no physical contraindication to participate to the study. The study protocol was approved by the Institutional Ethics Committee of Sainte-Justine university hospital centre, and each patient and their parents signed a consent form.

Experimental protocol

The recruited patients had their routine surface topography (InSpeck 3D Capturor, Creaform inc., Québec, Canada) and low dose biplanar radiographs (EOS™, EOS Imaging, Paris, France) taken in the presenting standing (reference) posture. A therapist who was trained specifically for this study (co-author IL) by a certified GPR physiotherapist (co-author CF) then performed the manual correction. To do so, the therapist stood behind the patient and applied a force with her right hand slightly under the right thoracic apex until a satisfying spine correction was obtained, while the left hand was positioned over the left iliac crest to stabilize the pelvis and overall posture (Fig. 1). The therapist wore gloves with force sensors (FlexiForce™ A301, sensitivity 5%, TekScan, Boston, MA, USA) to record the applied forces on the trunk surface. The sensors were sensitive to the normal force but not to shear forces. The posture was held for 10 s and repeated three times to obtain an average force value applied over time.

Then the self-correction posture was taught to the patient. When the posture was well understood and properly integrated, surface topography and biplanar radiographs were successively taken in this posture.

Simulation methodology

The two GPR immediate corrections were simulated using a personalized FEM and compared to the clinical data collected for model verification purposes. For each patient, the personalized FEM was built in the reference standing posture and in the self-correction posture combining the surface topography and radiographs using Ansys 14.5 package (Ansys Inc., Canonsburg, PA, USA). The reconstruction method and FEM were initially developed and validated for brace wearing simulations [22, 23]. The model included the pelvis, sacrum, lumbar and thoracic vertebrae, ribs, costal cartilages, sternum, intervertebral disks and soft tissues. The mechanical properties were taken from previous published data and cadaveric studies [18, 26]. The model also included gravitational loads [27]. The model trunk rigidity can be personalized to the patient if an adequate radiograph is available (suspension, supine in traction, bending, etc.). However, ethical considerations precluded the obtention of these additional radiographs.

The manual correction was simulated by inputting the mean recorded force of the therapist's right hand into the reference standing posture FEM. The pelvis was fixed in space to reproduce the therapist's left hand action (Fig. 1). The first thoracic (T1) vertebra was allowed to move along the vertical axis, but was fixed in the sagittal plane at its reference standing position and was aligned with the Central Sacral Vertical Line (CSVL) in the coronal plane. These boundary conditions on T1 replace muscular forces generated by the patient to maintain his or her coronal alignment (righting reflex). The simulation allowed to calculate the curve reduction resulting from the external force exerted by the therapist.

To simulate the self-correction posture, the position of T1 and of the thoracic and lumbar apical vertebrae as measured in the sagittal and coronal radiographs were then applied to the reference FEM. The pelvis was fixed in space and the spine could move vertically (Fig. 2). The simulation allowed to calculate the thoracic curve correction and the reaction force at the thoracic apical vertebra required to achieve such correction. Self-correction simulation results were compared to the actual self-correction as documented with the acquired radiographs.

Indices were computed to quantify the patient's ability to achieve scoliosis curve reduction during GPRs postures. For the manual correction, a stiffness index was defined as the ratio of the force applied at thoracic apex over the Cobb angle reduction (force/Δ Cobb angle). For the self-correction, the stiffness index was defined as the reaction force computed at thoracic apex over the thoracic curve reduction (force/Δ Cobb angle).

An ANOVA analysis with post-hoc Tukey test with 95% confidence interval was performed to compare the resulting Cobb angles using GraphPad Prism (GraphPad,

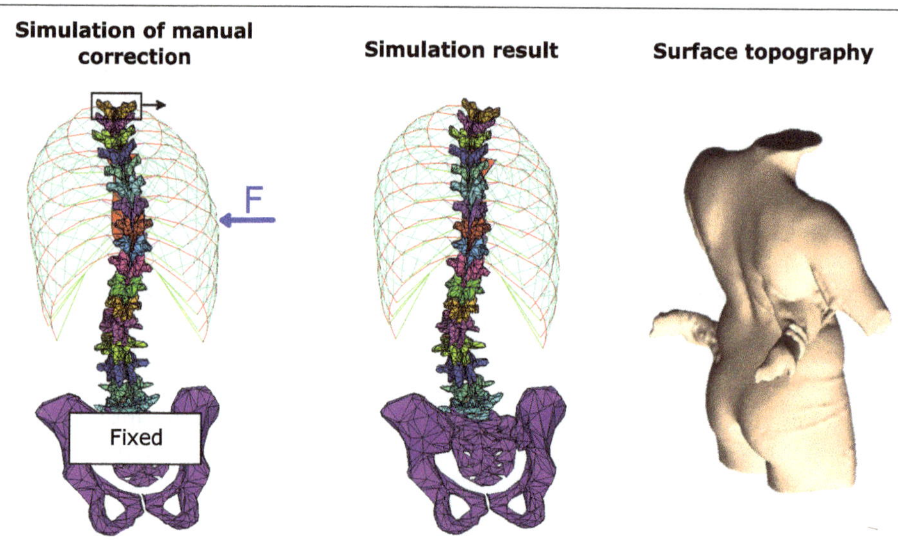

Fig. 1 Manual correction simulation and measurement methodology

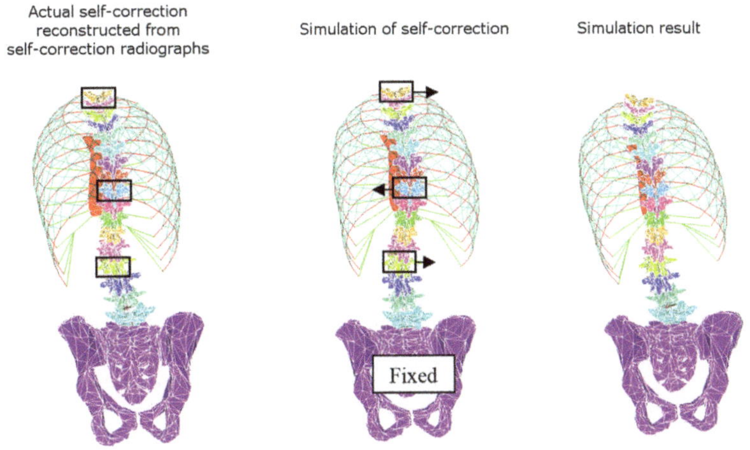

Fig. 2 Self-correction was simulated by moving the position of T1 and of the thoracic and lumbar apical vertebrae of the reference FEM to their self-correction position as measured in the self-correction reconstruction from radiographs

La Jolla, CA, USA). Pearson coefficients were calculated to establish correlation between the different results. Differences and correlation with a p value < 0.05 were considered statistically significant.

Results

Thoracic Cobb angles reduction and forces involved are summarized in Tables 1 and 2. The average equivalent force applied by the therapist during manual corrections over the thoracic curve was 31 ± 6 [23–55] N. The sensor under the main application point recorded an average pressure of 30.9 ± 14.1 [19.3–77.7] kPa. Manual correction simulations reduced the coronal thoracic curve on average by 26% [7–64%] (average Cobb angle correction of 8° [3°–19°], $p < 0.05$), while the coronal lumbar curve slightly increased compared to the reference standing posture (average of 27° [13°–42°] in reference standing posture vs. 29° [16°–43°] with the manual correction, $p < 0.05$). Thoracic kyphosis slightly increased while lumbar lordosis remained unchanged (kyphosis average of 30° [10°–47°] in the reference standing posture vs. 33° [11°–50°] with the manual correction

Table 1 Manual correction's thoracic Cobb angle simulation results compared to reference standing posture and associated stiffness indices

Patient	Presenting deformity (standing posture)	Simulation of manual correction (% reduction)	Mean force applied by therapist over thoracic apex	Manual correction's stiffness index
	deg	deg (%)	N	N / deg
P1	45	42 (7)	31	10
P2	25	21 (14)	33	10
P3	40	27 (31)	31	3
P4	33	25 (23)	28	4
P5	36	32 (13)	28	6
P6	23	16 (31)	23	3
P7	42	35 (17)	25	4
P8	36	27 (26)	25	3
P9	39	37 (7)	26	10
P10	28	10 (64)	55	3
P11	25	13 (48)	29	2
P12	37	31 (18)	33	5
P13	45	26 (43)	42	2
P14	11	5 (53)	31	5
P15	30	26 (13)	34	9
P16	31	27 (13)	28	7
Mean ± sd [min - max]	33 ± 9 [11–45]	25 ± 10 [5–42]	31 ± 8 [23–55]	5 ± 3 [2–10]

Table 2 Actual and simulated self-correction results of thoracic Cobb angle compared to reference standing posture and associated stiffness indices

Patient	Presenting deformity (standing posture)	Actual self-correction (% correction)	Self-correction simulation (% correction)	Reaction force at thoracic apex	Self-correction's stiffness index
	deg	deg (%)	deg (%)	N	N/deg
P1	45	30 (33)	35 (22)	68	7
P2	25	19 (24)	21 (17)	27	6
P3	40	25 (37)	27 (33)	29	2
P4	33	23 (29)	24 (27)	22	2
P5	36	23 (35)	31 (15)	64	12
P6	23	16 (29)	12 (47)	8	1
P7	42	39 (7)	42 (2)	16	21
P8	36	17 (53)	27 (27)	52	5
P9	39	26 (34)	32 (19)	77	10
P10	28	22 (19)	25 (11)	24	8
P11	25	28 (−15)	28 (−13)	1	−0,40
P12	37	27 (29)	30 (19)	39	5
P13	45	29 (36)	30 (33)	79	5
P14	11	4 (61)	4 (66)	27	4
P15	30	9 (69)	15 (50)	100	7
P16	31	15 (53)	24 (25)	80	10
Mean ± sd [min - max]	33 ± 9 [11–45]	22 ± 9 [4–39]	25 ± 9 [4–42]	45 ± 30 [1–100]	7 ± 5 [0–21]

($p < 0.05$), lordosis average of 70° [57°–85°] in the reference standing posture vs. 71° [58°–85°] with the manual correction). The stiffness index ranged between 2 and 10 N/°. There was a significant correlation between the pressure applied by the therapist and the curve reduction obtained ($r = 0.6$, $p < 0.05$).

The actual self-correction reduced the thoracic curve deformity on average by 33% [from 69% reduction to 15% augmentation] (Cobb angle correction of 11° [- 4°–21°], $p < 0.05$), while the lumbar curve remained constant (average of 27° [13°–42°] in reference standing posture vs. 26° [14°–42°] with the self-correction posture). All patients except two reduced their thoracic curve by 19% or more; the two other patients had a smaller reduction of 3° (P7) or a slight increase of 4° (P12). The thoracic kyphosis and lumbar lordosis were reduced on average by 6° [from 17° reduction to 5° augmentation] and 5° [from 13° reduction to 6° augmentation] respectively ($p < 0.05$). Apical thoracic vertebral rotation ranged from 21° to - 13° (average 7° ± 11°). Self-correction simulations reduced the thoracic curve on average by 25% [from 66% reduction to 13% augmentation] (Cobb angle correction of 8° [- 3°–15°], $p < 0.05$)), while the lumbar curve remained constant. The thoracic kyphosis and lumbar lordosis were reduced on average by 7° [from 18° reduction to 5° augmentation] and 5° [from 12° reduction to 7° augmentation] respectively ($p < 0.05$)). There was a good correlation between the actual and simulated thoracic curve reduction with the self-correction ($r = 0.9$, $p < 0.05$). Simulated reaction force at thoracic apical vertebra was 45 N on average, resulting in a stiffness index between 0 and 21 N/°.

There was no correlation between the Cobb angle correction with the simulated self-correction and manual-correction ($r = 0.1$, $p > 0.05$).

Discussion

This study allowed to quantify trunk stiffness in relation with thoracic curve reducibility as well as patient's capacity to self-correct their posture through a clinical study and the use of a personalized FEM. Two different immediate correction mechanisms were analyzed to obtain a curve reduction depending on whether external force (manual correction) or active muscle recruitment solely (self-correction) are involved.

Manual correction

To our knowledge this is the first study to report the forces applied by the physiotherapist over the trunk to manually correct the scoliotic deformities as part of a GPR approach. With no other existing adequate references, force and pressure ranges applied by the therapist's right hand at thoracic apical vertebra were compared to reported values of force or pressure measured under thoracic pads of similar patients treated conservatively with orthopedic braces. Our results of force and pressure ranges are in agreement with studies on brace fitting [28–31]. Romano reported similar values of 25.9 [18.7–42.8] kPa with fiberglass braces in the sitting position with 17 patients [30], but Pham reported smaller pressure values with the Chêneau brace (average 8 kPa, 32 patients) [31], versus 30.9 kPa in the current study. Both Van den Hout ([4–209] N, 16 patients) and Périé ([0–113] N, 12 patients) studied Boston brace and reported a wide range of forces [28, 29], versus [23–55] N in the current study.

The stiffness index calculated allowed the development of a relative ranking according to the measured and simulated patient spine stiffness. We found a significant but moderate correlation between the force applied by the therapist and thoracic Cobb reduction ($r = 0.6$, $p < 0.05$) calculated in the FEM. Our findings are similar to a similar study of brace correction and measured pressures under brace pads ($r = 0.9$) (Wong (2000)) [32], but differ from the brace studies of Van den Hout (2002) (thoracic $r = 0.5$, lumbar $r = 0.3$) and Pham (2008) ($r = -0.08$) [29, 31] that found smaller correlations. The cohort of Wong (2000) had flexible and correctable spines as documented by a supine lateral bending test, whereas this aspect was not specified in the two other studies. Because trunk rigidity is directly related to the slope of the correlation line, a moderate or low correlation could be explained by the variability in trunk rigidity between the cases that was not adjusted in the FEM. A two-factor correlation involving both the applied force and trunk stiffness related to thoracic correction would be interesting to calculate.

Manual correction simulation is coherent with the therapist's empirical experience since it allowed to reduce momentarily the main curve deformity concurrently with a non-clinically significant 2° increase of the lumbar curve, under the recognized measuring error of 5° [33]. The lack of change of the lumbar curve was on purpose, because the main focus was to achieve the best correction possible of the thoracic segment with a pressure at the apical level without increasing the counter curvature. In GPR, this re-equilibration test aims to determine curve reducibility and the importance of body posture compensations to guide the clinician in the selection of active stretching postures and sensory integration exercises [9]. In the clinic, it is not possible to quantify the real correction. By having one hand on the thoracic region applying a corrective force while the other hand stabilizes the pelvis and overall posture, we can only limit upper trunk displacement by visual assessment. Radiographs could not be taken in this posture to verify the simulation results since the therapist stands behind the patient during this correction.

Self-correction

The self-correction resulted in a significant reduction of the main curve deformity indicating patient's motor control ability for an immediate and momentary spine correction [11]. The main thoracic curve was corrected without accentuating the lumbar counter curve in the coronal plane, but a slight reduction of sagittal curves was measured. Different correction strategies were observed that lead to posture compensations, such as decreasing of the sagittal curves or accentuating the coronal slit as seen on Fig. 3. These observations suggest that self-correction exercises must be progressively integrated in the treatment and only when patients have a better body posture control to avoid negative side-effects on the long term. GPR treatment aims to progressively reduce the posture compensations while maintaining the achieved curve correction as the treatment progresses [9].

Self-correction tended to decrease vertebral rotation, going from 11° to 7° on average. Initial rotation was small for most participants, except for participants 12 and 13 who had a rotation of 22°. For these patients, the correction percentage in self-correction was still 29 and 36% respectively, indicating that high vertebral rotation

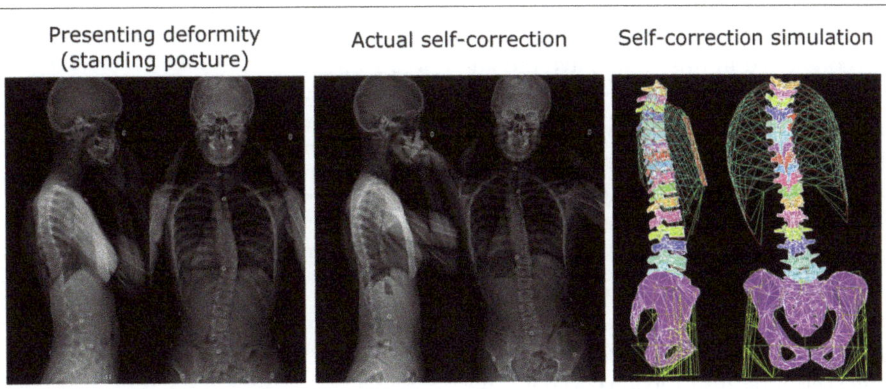

Fig. 3 Low dose biplanar radiographs in standing posture and during self-correction illustrate patient's potential to reduce the thoracic curvature immediately and momentarily. Self-correction numerical simulation agrees with self-correction radiographs

does not preclude self-correction. The simulation of the self-correction underestimated the actual correction in the coronal plane, despite the good correlation ($r = 0.9$), which could be attributed to other muscular recruitment correction mechanisms not included in the simulation.

Reaction forces computed at thoracic apical vertebra could be associated to the muscle recruitment needed to maintain the correction and balance. Since the reaction forces are concentrated on three vertebrae (T1 and apical vertebrae) their values are higher than the actual distributed muscle recruitment forces along the spine to maintain the self-correction, which could explain the high force values obtained (Table 2). Still, using this reaction force, the simulation allowed to compute a stiffness index for a relative patient ranking according to their effort to maintain posture. Patient P7 had the lowest simulated correction (1°), therefore obtained the highest stiffness index (21 N/°), suggesting a high spine stiffness.

Comparison between manual correction and self-correction

The absence of correlation between reductions obtained in the two postures suggests two different correction mechanisms. Manual correction is a passive correction, exclusively produced by the external forces from the therapist manipulation without active muscle recruitments. The obtained reduction hence is solely linked to the trunk inner resistance to the external force. On the contrary, self-correction is an active correction resulting exclusively from patient's inner ability to autocorrect.

Limitations

As for any computational model it is difficult to fully validate the FEM due to the limited data and standardized way to acquire it. For instance, for the manual correction, it was impossible to take radiographs while maintaining the posture. In the current study, simulations focussed on a specific subset of parameters such as the lateral force for the manual correction or apical vertebrae positions for the self-correction, which contributed to the complex mechanisms of correction exercises. While there are many unknowns in practice, numerical studies as the ones conducted in this study have the advantage of being able to evaluate the specific effects of the selected parameters. The various active muscle recruitment patterns, which may vary to assure a certain posture, were not tested. In this study, we only included the minimal forces needed to maintain a stable posture. Disk torsional rigidity was included in the FEM but not personalized to the patient-specific behavior, as it was not possible to measure using the available imaging data: this could affect the results for vertebrae with higher rotations, because intervertebral disc torsional rigidity increases with rotation [34]. Reproducibility of the inner forces needed for self-correction could not be assessed in this study due to the limited number of available radiographs, however self-correction reproducibility could eventually be measured by using a comparative non-irradiant method such as surface topography. Experimental limitations included different arm positions to comply with external topography and radiography protocols, which demanded additional attention from the patient to achieve self-correction and possibly altered their posture [35]. Hence even greater correction might be expected in self-correction during GPR treatment than during the current study.

Clinical implications

The current study featured a small patient sample with a large range of curves; some patients were treated with braces and other were not. The results should therefore not be interpreted as a clinical evaluation of PSSE efficacy. Rather, this study highlights the feasibility of using FEM to better understand the effect of GPR correction postures. The computed stiffness index through the use of FE modeling allowed to quantify the passive (manual correction) and active (self-correction) resistance of the trunk and may contribute to set personalized therapeutic objectives for postural correction. The next step to standardize the stiffness index would be to have a constant manual pressure applied and observe the correction obtained.

Conclusion

A FEM and experimental tools were developed to quantitatively assess two GPR curve reduction approaches and to better understand correction mechanisms. The forces exerted by the therapist during a manual correction approach, combined with the patient-specific FEM, allowed to simulate the scoliotic curve reduction. This would enable to quantify trunk stiffness without additional radiography. The self-correction simulation allowed to quantify the needed forces for the patient to reduce by him/her-self the main scoliotic spine curvature. Better understanding of correction mechanisms through GPR may help to support the contribution of this approach to scoliosis treatment.

Abbreviations

3D: Tridimensional; CSVL: Central sacral vertical line; FEM: Finite element model; GPR: Global Postural Re-education; IS: idiopathic scoliosis; PSSE: physiotherapy specific scoliosis exercises; SOSORT: Scoliosis Orthopaedic and Rehabilitation Treatment; T1: first thoracic vertebra; TLSO: thoraco-lombo-sacral orthosis

Acknowledgements

A big thank you to all participants for their participation in this study and to Soraya Barchi, Julie Joncas, Manivone Savann and Sylvain Deschênes for their precious collaboration.

Funding

Canada Research Chair

Project supported by the NSERC (Natural Sciences and Engineering Research Council of Canada).

C.Fortin is currently funded by a Junior 1 salary award from the Fonds de Recherche du Québec – Santé (FRQ-S).

Authors' contributions

CF, CEA, SD and CC designed the study. SD, CF and IL were responsible for data collection. SD, CF, CC and CEA were responsible for data analysis and interpretation. SD drafted the manuscript. CF, CC and CEA critically revised the manuscript. All authors revised and approved the final version of the manuscript.

Competing interests

The authors declare that they have no competing interests.

Author details

[1]Department of Mechanical Engineering, École Polytechnique de Montréal, P.O. Box 6097, Downtown Station, Station "Centre-ville", Montreal, Quebec H3C 3A7, Canada. [2]Research Centre, Sainte-Justine University Hospital Centre, 3175 chemin de la Côte-Sainte-Catherine, Montreal, Quebec H3T 1C5, Canada. [3]School of rehabilitation, Faculty of Medicine, University of Montreal, 2900 Edouard-Montpetit, Montreal, Quebec H3T 1J4, Canada.

References

1. Trobisch P, Suess O, Schwab F. Idiopathic scoliosis. Dtsch Arztebl Int. 2010; 107(49):875.
2. Negrini S, Aulisa AG, Aulisa L, Circo AB, de Mauroy JC, Durmala J, Grivas TB, Knott P, Kotwicki T, Maruyama T. 2011 SOSORT guidelines: orthopaedic and rehabilitation treatment of idiopathic scoliosis during growth. Scoliosis. 2012;7(1):3.
3. Negrini S, Donzelli S, Aulisa AG, Czaprowski D, Schreiber S, de Mauroy JC, Diers H, Grivas TB, Knott P, Kotwicki T, et al. 2016 SOSORT guidelines: orthopaedic and rehabilitation treatment of idiopathic scoliosis during growth. Scoliosis Spinal Disord. 2018;13(1):3.
4. Bonetti F, Curti S, Mattioli S, Mugnai R, Vanti C, Violante FS, Pillastrini P. Effectiveness of a 'Global postural Reeducation' program for persistent low back pain: a non-randomized controlled trial. BMC Musculoskelet Disord. 2010;11:285.
5. Fernández-de-las-Peñas C, Alonso-Blanco C, Morales-Cabezas M, Miangolarra-Page JC. Two exercise interventions for the management of patients with ankylosing spondylitis: a randomized controlled trial. Am J Phys Med Rehabil. 2005;84(6):407–19.
6. Fortin C, Ehrmann Feldman D, Tanaka C, Houde M, Labelle H. Inter-rater reliability of the evaluation of muscular chains associated with posture alterations in scoliosis. BMC Musculoskelet Disord. 2012;13(80):9.
7. Fortin C, Ehrmann Feldman D, Cheriet F, Labelle H. Differences in standing and sitting postures of youth with idiopathic scoliosis from quantitative analysis of digital photographs. Phys Occup Ther Pediatr. 2013;33(3):313–26.
8. Souchard P, Ollier M. Les scolioses; Traitement kinésithérapique et orthopédique, vol. 13, Masson Éditeur edn. Paris: Masson; 2002.
9. Souchard P. Déformations morphologiques de la colonne vertébrale : Traitement physiothérapique en Rééducation Posturale Globale-RPG. Issy-les-Moulineaux: Elsevier Masson; 2015.
10. Fusco C, Zaina F, Atanasio S, Romano M, Negrini A, Negrini S. Physical exercises in the treatment of adolescent idiopathic scoliosis: an updated systematic review. Physiother Theory Pract. 2011;27(1):80–114.
11. Monticone M, Ambrosini E, Cazzaniga D, Rocca B, Ferrante S. Active self-correction and task-oriented exercises reduce spinal deformity and improve quality of life in subjects with mild adolescent idiopathic scoliosis. Results of a randomised controlled trial. Eur Spine J. 2014;23(6):1204–14.
12. Kuru T, Yeldan İ, Dereli EE, Özdinçler AR, Dikici F, Çolak İ. The efficacy of three-dimensional Schroth exercises in adolescent idiopathic scoliosis: a randomised controlled clinical trial. Clin Rehabil. 2015;30(2):181-90.
13. Schreiber S, Parent EC, Moez EK, Hedden DM, Hill DL, Moreau M, Lou E, Watkins EM, Southon SC. Schroth physiotherapeutic scoliosis-specific exercises added to the standard of care lead to better cobb angle outcomes in adolescents with idiopathic scoliosis–an Assessor and statistician blinded randomized controlled trial. PLoS One. 2016;11(12): e0168746.
14. Płaszewski M, Bettany-Saltikov J. Non-surgical interventions for adolescents with idiopathic scoliosis: an overview of systematic reviews. PLoS One. 2014; 9(10):e110254.
15. Kalichman L, Kendelker L, Bezalel T. Bracing and exercise-based treatment for idiopathic scoliosis. J Bodyw Mov Ther. 2016;20(1):56–64.
16. Wang W, Baran GR, Betz RR, Samdani AF, Pahys JM, Cahill PJ. The use of finite element models to assist understanding and treatment for scoliosis: a review paper. Spine Deformity. 2014;2(1):10–27.
17. Clin J, Aubin CE, Sangole A, Labelle H, Parent S. Correlation between immediate in-brace correction and biomechanical effectiveness of brace treatment in adolescent idiopathic scoliosis. Spine. 2010;35(18):1706–13.
18. Périé D, Aubin C, Lacroix M, Lafon Y, Labelle H. Biomechanical modelling of orthotic treatment of the scoliotic spine including a detailed representation of the brace-torso interface. Med Biol Eng Comput. 2004;42(3):339–44.
19. Sattout A, Clin J, Cobetto N, Labelle H, Aubin C-E. Biomechanical assessment of providence nighttime brace for the treatment of adolescent idiopathic scoliosis. Spine Deformity. 2016;4(4):253–60.
20. Clin J, Aubin CE, Parent S, Labelle H. Biomechanical modeling of brace treatment of scoliosis: effects of gravitational loads. Med Biol Eng Comput. 2011;49(7):743–53.
21. Clin J, Aubin C-É, Parent S, Labelle H. A biomechanical study of the Charleston brace for the treatment of scoliosis. Spine. 2010;35(19):E940–7.
22. Cobetto N, Aubin C-E, Clin J, Le May S, Desbiens-Blais F, Labelle H, Parent S. Braces optimized with computer-assisted design and simulations are lighter, more comfortable, and more efficient than plaster-cast braces for the treatment of adolescent idiopathic scoliosis. Spine Deformity. 2014;2(4):276–84.
23. Desbiens-Blais F, Clin J, Parent S, Labelle H, Aubin CE. New brace design combining CAD/CAM and biomechanical simulation for the treatment of adolescent idiopathic scoliosis. Clin Biomech (Bristol, Avon). 2012;27(10):999–1005.
24. Cobetto N, Aubin C, Parent S, Clin J, Barchi S, Turgeon I, Labelle H. Effectiveness of braces designed using computer-aided design and manufacturing (CAD/CAM) and finite element simulation compared to CAD/CAM only for the conservative treatment of adolescent idiopathic scoliosis: a prospective randomized controlled trial. Eur Spine J. 2016;25(10):3056–64.
25. Cobetto N, Aubin C-É, Parent S, Barchi S, Turgeon I, Labelle H. 3D correction of AIS in braces designed using CAD/CAM and FEM: a randomized controlled trial. Scoliosis Spinal Disord. 2017; (in press)
26. Descrimes J, Aubin C, Skalli W, Zeller R, Dansereau J, Lavaste F. Introduction des facettes articulaires dans une modélisation par éléments finis de la colonne vertébrale et du thorax scoliotique: aspects mécaniques. Rachis. 1995;7(6):301–14.
27. Clin J, Aubin CE, Lalonde N, Parent S, Labelle H. A new method to include the gravitational forces in a finite element model of the scoliotic spine. Med Biol Eng Comput. 2011;49(8):967–77.
28. Périé D, Aubin CE, Petit Y, Beauséjour M, Dansereau J, Labelle H. Boston brace correction in idiopathic scoliosis: a biomechanical study. Spine. 2003; 28(15):1672–7.
29. Van den Hout J, Van Rhijn L, Van den Munckhof R, Van Ooy A. Interface corrective force measurements in Boston brace treatment. Eur Spine J. 2002; 11(4):332–5.
30. Romano M, Carabalona R, Petrilli S, Sibilla P, Negrini S. Forces exerted during exercises by patients with adolescent idiopathic scoliosis wearing fiberglass braces. Scoliosis. 2006;1:12.
31. Pham VM, Houilliez A, Schill A, Carpentier A, Herbaux B, Thevenon A. Study of the pressures applied by a Cheneau brace for correction of adolescent idiopathic scoliosis. Prosthetics Orthot Int. 2008;32(3):345–55.
32. Wong M, Mak A, Luk K, Evans J, Brown B. Effectiveness and biomechanics of spinal orthoses in the treatment of adolescent idiopathic scoliosis (AIS). Prosthetics Orthot Int. 2000;24(2):148–62.
33. Morrissy RT, Goldsmith G, Hall E, Kehl D, Cowie G. Measurement of the cobb angle on radiographs of patients who have scoliosis. Evaluation of intrinsic error. J Bone Joint Surg. 1990;72(3):320–7.
34. Aulisa L, Lupparelli S, Pola E, Aulisa AG, Mastantuoni G, Pitta L. Biomechanics of the conservative treatment in idiopathic scoliotic curves in surgical "grey-area". Stud Health Technol Inform. 2002;91:412–8.

Negative pressure pulmonary edema after percutaneous endoscopic interlaminar lumbar discectomy

Guo Chen[1,2†], Xian-di Wang[1†], Hong-fei Nie[1], Zhi-qiang Yang[1], Kang Chen[1], Zhu-hai Li[1], Yue-ming Song[1], Fu-xing Pei[1] and Jian-cheng Zeng[1*]

Abstract

Background: Negative pressure pulmonary edema (NPPE) is a rare complication that is more prevalent in young patients. NPPE usually results from acute upper airway obstruction, which is most commonly caused by laryngospasm during extubation. NPPE is characterized by the sudden onset of coughing, hemoptysis, tachycardia, tachypnea, and hypoxia, and is dramatically improved with supportive care, which prevents severe sequelae. To our knowledge, there is no report of a patient developing NPPE after percutaneous endoscopic interlaminar lumbar discectomy.

Case presentation: Herein, we report the case of a 22-year-old amateur basketball player with L5/S1 disc herniation who developed NPPE during extubation after general anesthesia for a minimally invasive spinal surgery (percutaneous endoscopic interlaminar lumbar discectomy). The NPPE was treated by maintaining the airway patency, applying positive-pressure ventilation, administering dexamethasone and antibiotics, and limiting the volume of fluid infused. The patient had an uneventful postoperative course, and was discharged to his home on postoperative day 3.

Conclusions: Although NPPE is an infrequent complication, especially in patients undergoing percutaneous endoscopic interlaminar lumbar discectomy, this case report highlights the importance of early diagnosis and prompt treatment of NPPE to prevent the development of potentially fatal complications.

Keywords: Percutaneous endoscopic lumbar discectomy, Negative pressure pulmonary edema, Complications

Background

Negative pressure pulmonary edema (NPPE) is an infrequent complication of acute upper airway obstruction, with an overall prevalence of 0.1% and no significant difference in the incidence between male versus female patients [1, 2]. The mechanism of NPPE is considered to involve the increased effort required to inspire against an obstructed upper airway; this exertion leads to a marked increase in negative intrathoracic pressure, an increase in normal inspiratory hemodynamic physiology, and an increase in the volume of blood that flows into the pulmonary vasculature from the systemic circulation. The increased hydrostatic pressure and lowered pericapillary interstitial pressure produce a large pressure difference between the alveoli and the capillaries, shearing the capillary membrane barrier and resulting in stress failure [1–3].

The most common causes of NPPE are near drowning, choanal stenosis, endotracheal tube obstruction, use of a laryngeal mask that causes airway obstruction or displacement, laryngeal tumor, and epistaxis. When NPPE occurs postoperatively, it is usually due to laryngospasm during extubation and postoperative vocal cord paralysis [4]. NPPE has reportedly occurred in patients undergoing many kinds of surgical procedures. In the field of orthopedics, NPPE is more likely to occur in patients undergoing spinal surgery, especially procedures involving the cervical spine [5–8]. However, there are no

* Correspondence: tomzeng5@126.com
[1]Department of Orthopaedic Surgery, West China Hospital, Sichuan University, N0.37 Guoxue Road, Chengdu, Sichuan Province 610041, China

reports of NPPE in patients undergoing percutaneous endoscopic interlaminar lumbar discectomy (PEID). The purpose of the present case report is to highlight the possibility of NPPE during PEID, and to highlight the importance of early diagnosis and prompt treatment of NPPE to prevent the development of potentially fatal complications.

Case presentation

A 22-year-old male amateur basketball player with no relevant medical history was admitted to our hospital due to continuous severe lower back pain with radiating nerve pain and numbness from the hip to the posterior part of the left leg. Physical examination revealed paravertebral muscle spasm, diminished sensation at the lateral aspect of the sole of the left foot, diminished strength in plantar flexion on the left side, a weakened Achilles tendon reflex on the left side, and a positive straight-leg raise test (30 degrees) on the left side. Magnetic resonance imaging of the lower spine showed a herniated nucleus pulposus at the left L5-S1 level, and so the patient was diagnosed with left lumbar disc herniation at L5-S1.

Preoperative evaluation was normal. The patient opted to undergo surgical treatment with PEID after failure of conservative treatment. Tracheal intubation was facilitated via the administration of atracurium and penehyclidine. General anesthesia was induced with propofol and fentanyl, and was maintained with sevoflurane, fentanyl, and atracurium. The PEID was successfully completed within 40 min, with complete removal of the herniated disc, annuloplasty of the annulus fibrosus, and thorough decompression of the S1 nerve root. Intraoperatively, the patient was infused with 1,100 mL of Ringer's lactate solution. Throughout the entire procedure, the urine volume was 400 mL, and the blood loss was less than 20 mL.

Extubation was performed when the patient was conscious, spontaneously breathing, and performing purposeful movements. The patient then suddenly began to respire forcefully. The heart rate was 130 beats/min, blood pressure was 155/90 mmHg, respiratory rate was 35 breaths/min, and SpO_2 had decreased from 98 to 65%, followed by the production of 5 ml of pink frothy sputum. Chest auscultation performed by the anesthetist revealed tachycardia and dispersed moist rales bilaterally. Arterial blood gas analysis showed that the pH was 7.34, PaO_2 was 71 mmHg, and $PaCO_2$ was 40 mmHg. Electrocardiography indicated sinus tachycardia. NPPE was diagnosed. The airway was kept unobstructed, and oxygen was delivered at 5 L/min via mask ventilation. The infusion volume was limited. Dexamethasone was administered to relieve spasm, and 20 mg of furosemide was administered intravenously to treat pulmonary edema. The SpO_2 improved and was maintained above 93%.

After stabilization with supportive treatment for about 60 min in the operating room, the patient was transferred to the orthopedic ward. Subsequent laboratory testing indicated an increased white cell count of 12.5×10^9/L, an elevated neutrophil percentage of 84%, and a hematocrit decrease from 45.3 to 40.7%. The D-dimer level was 1.0 ng/mL, while the other main laboratory parameters were within normal limits. Repeat arterial blood gas analysis indicated that the pH was 7.37, PaO_2 was 95 mmHg, and $PaCO_2$ was 48 mmHg with oxygenation via nasal catheterization. Compared with the normal chest radiograph preoperatively (Fig. 1a), the emergency chest radiograph showed bilateral infiltrates with opacities and nodules (Fig. 1b). Two hours later, chest computed tomography (CT) of a pulmonary window showed increased vascular diameter, a mosaic pattern of attenuation, and bilateral pleural effusion (Fig. 2a).

The patient was afebrile, and cefazolin was administered prophylactically. The oxygen requirement gradually decreased to room air, with the hematocrit remaining stable, and the vital signs remaining stable for the following 24 h. A chest radiograph obtained in the morning on postoperative day 1 still showed bilateral infiltrates with opacities and nodules; however, the severity of these was obviously decreased compared with the radiograph taken the previous evening (Fig. 1c). A chest radiograph taken in the afternoon on postoperative day 1 showed that the infiltrates had further decreased. In the evening on postoperative day 1, CT showed a marked decrease in bilateral pleural effusion (Fig. 2b). The vital signs were stable, without tachycardia, tachypnea, and/or hemoptysis. At 3 days postoperatively, radiography showed nearly complete resolution of the lung infiltrate (Fig. 1d, e) and CT (Fig. 2c). The patient was discharged 3 days after spinal surgery, at which time he reported that he was satisfied with the whole therapeutic process, and had marked improvement of the symptoms in the back and left leg.

At 6 weeks postoperatively, the patient was examined in the outpatient department. The pulse oxygenation was 100% on room air, and there were no abnormal findings on chest auscultation, radiography (Fig. 1f), and CT (Fig. 2d).

Conclusion

NPPE was first described in 1977 [1], and is an infrequent but recognized complication of upper airway obstruction. The overall prevalence of NPPE is less than 0.1% [2], with young, healthy males at greater risk compared with the general population [3]. NPPE can be caused by mechanical pressure due to hanging or strangulation [9], obstructive sleep apnea [10], aspiration of foreign material [11], endotracheal tube occlusion [12], complex intubation [13], epiglottitis and croup (especially in children) [14], and biting of the endotracheal tube [15]; one of the most common reasons for NPPE during the perioperative period is laryngospasm during extubation [2].

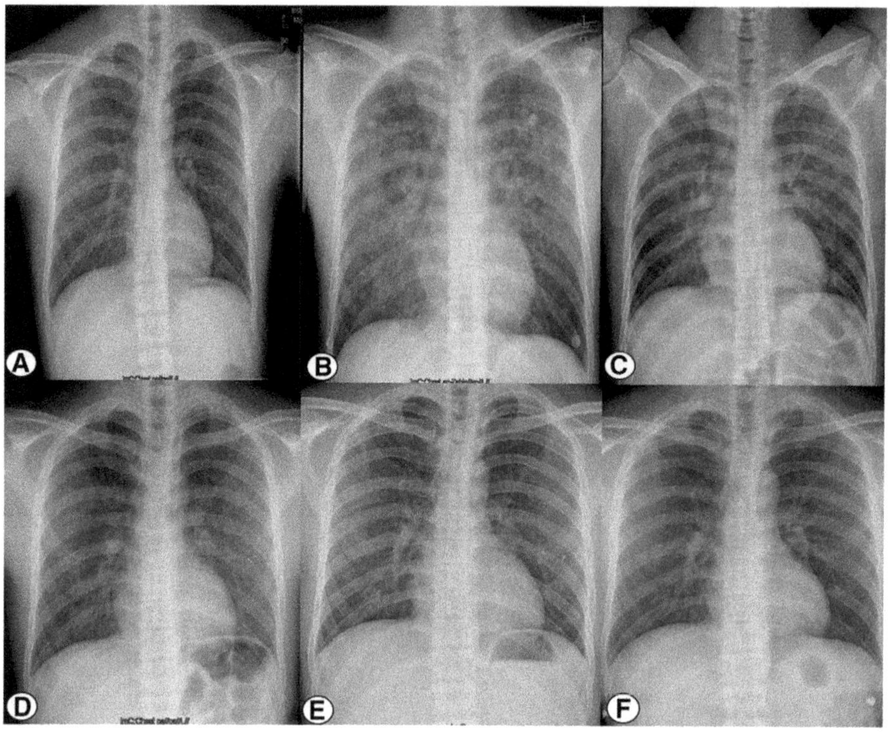

Fig. 1 a-f chest radiograph obtain preoperative, 2 h, 17 h, 23 h, 3 days and 6 weeks after the surgery. It was shown that bilateral infiltrates with opacities and nodules gradually decreased over time and completely disappeared on follow up

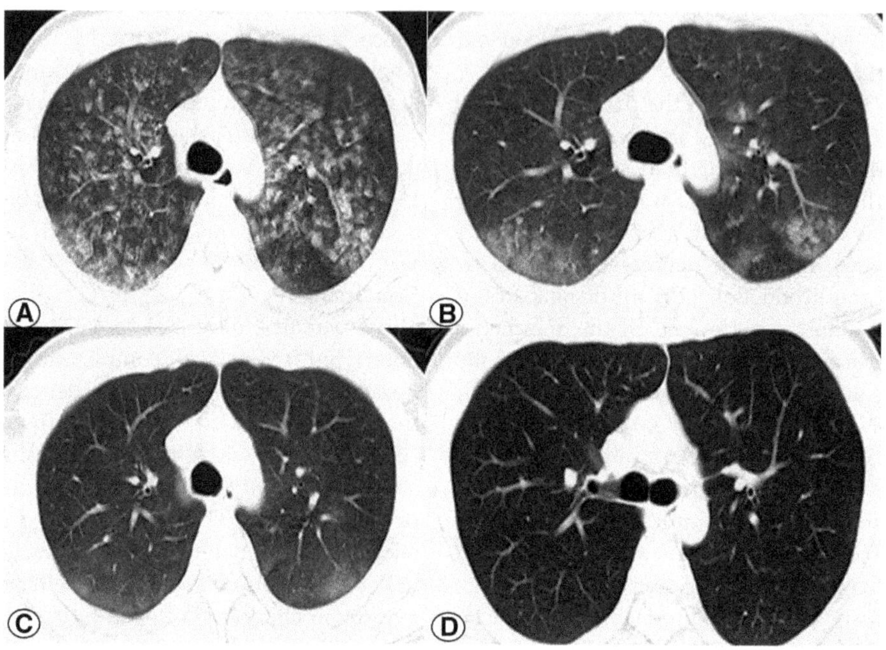

Fig. 2 a-d Chest computed tomographic scan obtained 2 h, 25 h, 3 days and weeks after the surgery. It was shown that bilateral pleural effusion gradually decreased over time and completely disappeared on follow up

The mechanism of NPPE is that the exertion of inspiring against an obstructed upper airway leads to a marked increase in negative intrathoracic pressure, an increase in normal inspiratory hemodynamic physiology, and an increased volume of blood flowing into the pulmonary vasculature from the systemic circulation [1–3]. The subsequent large pressure difference between the alveoli and the capillaries shears the capillary membrane barrier and results in stress failure [2, 16, 17]. Massive sympathetic discharge triggered by hypoxia [18] and changes in intrapleural pressure [19] were also reported.

The manifestations of NPPE are stridor, suprasternal and supraclavicular retractions, desperate use of accessory respiratory muscles, panic-stricken facial countenance, decreased SpO_2, pink frothy sputum, and crackles and wheezes on auscultation. Infiltrates in the lung with opacities and nodules may be seen on chest radiography and CT. Especially in high-risk patients, the diagnosis of NPPE can be made based on a history of a precipitating incident, typical symptoms and physical examination findings, and pulmonary edema on chest radiography. The differential diagnoses for NPPE include other causes of sudden respiratory distress, such as pneumonia, acute pulmonary edema, pulmonary embolism, and inhalation injury [17].

The treatment for NPPE should include assisted ventilation via a mask or endotracheal tube; mechanical ventilation via positive end expiratory pressure may be required if paralysis of the respiratory muscles eventuates and causes prolonged hypoxia and related complications. Patients with NPPE should have their fluid intake restricted, and dexamethasone should be administered to relieve spasm. Diuretic therapy should also be initiated to maintain a more beneficial hydrostatic balance in all capillary beds, especially in the pulmonary vasculature. In our experience, this treatment protocol results in marked improvement in most patients with NPPE, partly due to the intact of alveolar fluid clearance mechanisms.

Lumbar disc herniation is a type of spinal degeneration that generally occurs in those aged 39 to 70 years [20], with an increased incidence in those with obesity [21], a history of smoking [22], and those with specific occupations that involve sedentary behavior (such as civil servants, bank clerks, and drivers). In young patients, such as the present patient, the risk of NPPE may be increased due to genetic factors [23] and a history of trauma in daily life or during physical training [24]. Lumbar disc herniation is effectively treated by PEID, including in pediatric patients [25]. PEID is a minimally invasive procedure that has the advantages of minimal intraoperative fluoroscopy, clear exposure, complete decompression, and quick recovery with satisfactory long-term results [26–28]. We prefer to perform PEID under general anesthesia with nerve monitoring.

Young, healthy, athletic males are more susceptible to NPPE [2, 16], partly due to their relatively increased chest wall compliance and the enhanced capability to engender excessive negative intrathoracic pressure when upper airway obstruction occurs. This situation is similar to the present case in which NPPE developed in a 22-year-old amateur basketball player. Clinicians should be aware of the increased risk of NPPE in young, healthy, athletic males; caution is required when choosing anesthetic methods, and such patients should be monitored closely during extubation and the recovery period.

In our spine center, one surgical team performs more than 400 percutaneous endoscopic lumbar discectomy procedures every year (including PEID and percutaneous endoscopic transforaminal discectomy, PETD) or around six procedures every operation day. This high procedural volume involves rapid transition from one operation to the next. As PEID is minimally invasive and thus only takes a short amount of time, those undergoing PEID should be especially closely monitored to decrease the risk of NPPE; patients must be fully awake before extubation to decrease the possibility of laryngospasm, the anesthetist must provide adequate pharyngeal suctioning before extubation, and high-risk patients should be operated on early in the day to minimize the risk of anesthetist fatigue [29].

Although NPPE is an infrequent complication, especially in patients undergoing PEID, high-risk patients (young, healthy, athletic males) should be closely monitored and provided with appropriate treatment if NPPE does occur.

Abbreviations

NPPE: Negative pressure pulmonary edema; PEID: Percutaneous endoscopic interlaminar lumbar discectomy; PETD: Percutaneous endoscopic transforaminal discectomy

Acknowledgements

We are grateful to the staff of our department and anesthesiology department for their support and contribution in this study. We thank Dr. Kelly Zammit, BVSc, from Liwen Bianji, Edanz Editing China (www.liwenbianji.cn/ac), for editing the English text of a draft of this manuscript.

Funding

No commercial, public, or nonprofit organizations financially supported this research.

Authors' contributions

GC, XDW and JCZ designed this study. GC, HFN, ZQY and KC were responsible for gathering, analyzing and interpreting data, and writing the manuscript. ZHL, YMS, FXP and JCZ provided the valuable case, performed the operation and made contributions to revising the manuscript for crucial intellectual content. The final version of the text has been reviewed and approved by all authors.

Consent for publication
Written consent to publish this information was obtained from study participants. Proof of consent to publish from study participants can be requested at any time.

Competing interests
The authors declare that they have no competing interests.

Author details
[1]Department of Orthopaedic Surgery, West China Hospital, Sichuan University, N0.37 Guoxue Road, Chengdu, Sichuan Province 610041, China. [2]Department of Orthopaedic Surgery, the Affiliated Hospital of North Sichuan Medical College, No. 63 Wenhua Road, Nanchong, Sichuan Province 637000, China.

References
1. Oswalt CE, Gates GA, Holmstrom MG. Pulmonary edema as a complication of acute airway obstruction. JAMA. 1977;238(17):1833–5.
2. Bhattacharya M, Kallet RH, Ware LB, Matthay MA. Negative-pressure pulmonary edema. Chest. 2016;150(4):927–33.
3. Patton WC, Baker CL Jr. Prevalence of negative-pressure pulmonary edema at an orthopaedic hospital. J South Orthop Assoc. 2000;9(4):248–53.
4. Bhaskar B, Fraser JF. Negative pressure pulmonary edema revisited: pathophysiology and review of management. Saudi J Anaesth. 2011;5(3): 308–13.
5. Makan P. Neurologic compromise after an isolated laminar fracture of the cervical spine. Spine. 1999;24(11):1144–6.
6. Calvo Romero JM, Crespo Valades E. Acute dyspnea after lumbar spine surgery. Rev Clin Esp. 1999;199(2):103–4.
7. Gorospe L, Crespo-Aliseda PA, Garcia Gomez-Muriel I, Garcia-Latorre R, Campos-Ferrer C. Negative pressure pulmonary edema following cervical disc hernia surgery. Med Clin. 2017;149(6):280.
8. Shigematsu H, Yoneda M, Tanaka Y. Negative pressure pulmonary edema associated with anterior cervical spine surgery. Asian Spine J. 2014;8(6):827–30.
9. Koh MS, Hsu AA, Eng P. Negative pressure pulmonary oedema in the medical intensive care unit. Intensive Care Med. 2003;29(9):1601–4.
10. Chaudhary BA, Nadimi M, Chaudhary TK, Speir WA. Pulmonary edema due to obstructive sleep apnea. South Med J. 1984;77(4):499–501.
11. Zulueta JJ, Gerblich AA. Upper airway obstruction due to inhalation of a tracheal T-tube resulting in pulmonary edema. Chest. 1992;102(2):644–5.
12. Louis PJ, Fernandes R. Negative pressure pulmonary edema. Oral Surg Oral Med Oral Pathol Oral Radiol Endod. 2002;93(1):4–6.
13. Cascade PN, Alexander GD, Mackie DS. Negative-pressure pulmonary edema after endotracheal intubation. Radiology. 1993;186(3):671–5.
14. Travis KW, Todres ID, Shannon DC. Pulmonary edema associated with croup and epiglottitis. Pediatrics. 1977;59(5):695–8.
15. Devys JM, Balleau C, Jayr C, Bourgain JL. Biting the laryngeal mask: an unusual cause of negative pressure pulmonary edema. Can J Anaesth. 2000; 47(2):176–8.
16. Holmes JR, Hensinger RN, Wojtys EW. Postoperative pulmonary edema in young, athletic adults. Am J Sports Med. 1991;19(4):365–71.
17. Westreich R, Sampson I, Shaari CM, Lawson W. Negative-pressure pulmonary edema after routine septorhinoplasty: discussion of pathophysiology, treatment, and prevention. Arch Facial Plast Surg. 2006; 8(1):8–15.
18. Lorch DG, Sahn SA. Post-extubation pulmonary edema following anesthesia induced by upper airway obstruction. Are certain patients at increased risk? Chest. 1986;90(6):802–5.
19. Robotham JL, Lixfeld W, Holland L, MacGregor D, Bryan AC, Rabson J. Effects of respiration on cardiac performance. J Appl Physiol Respir Environ Exerc Physiol. 1978;44(5):703–9.
20. Miller JA, Schmatz C, Schultz AB. Lumbar disc degeneration: correlation with age, sex, and spine level in 600 autopsy specimens. Spine. 1988;13(2):173–8.
21. Flamme CH. Obesity and low back pain-biology, biomechanics and epidemiology. Orthopade. 2005;34(7):652–7.
22. Huang W, Han Z, Liu J, Yu L, Yu X. Risk factors for recurrent lumbar disc herniation: a systematic review and meta-analysis. Medicine. 2016;95(2):e2378.
23. Battie MC, Videman T, Parent E. Lumbar disc degeneration: epidemiology and genetic influences. Spine. 2004;29(23):2679–90.
24. Gray BL, Buchowski JM, Bumpass DB, Lehman RA Jr, Mall NA, Matava MJ. Disc herniations in the National Football League. Spine. 2013;38(22):1934–8.
25. Wang X, Zeng J, Nie H, Chen G, Li Z, Jiang H, Kong Q, Song Y, Liu H. Percutaneous endoscopic interlaminar discectomy for pediatric lumbar disc herniation. Childs Nerv Syst. 2014;30(5):897–902.
26. Nie H, Zeng J, Song Y, Chen G, Wang X, Li Z, Jiang H, Kong Q. Percutaneous endoscopic lumbar discectomy for L5-S1 disc herniation via an interlaminar approach versus a transforaminal approach: a prospective randomized controlled study with 2-year follow up. Spine. 2016;41:B30–7.
27. Nie HF, Zeng JC, Liu KX. A simple technique of accessing the L5-S1 disc space for transforaminal endoscopic spine surgery. Surg Technol Int. 2012;22:302–6.
28. Choi KC, Kim JS, Lee DC, Park CK. Percutaneous endoscopic lumbar discectomy: minimally invasive technique for multiple episodes of lumbar disc herniation. BMC Musculoskelet Disord. 2017;18(1):329.
29. Olsson GL, Hallen B. Laryngospasm during anaesthesia. A computer-aided incidence study in 136,929 patients. Acta Anaesthesiol Scand. 1984;28(5):567–75.

21

What do we know about managing Dupuytren's disease cost-effectively?

Melina Dritsaki[1*], Oliver Rivero-Arias[2], Alastair Gray[3], Catherine Ball[4] and Jagdeep Nanchahal[4]

Abstract

Background: Dupuytren's disease (DD) is a common and progressive, fibroproliferative disorder of the palmar and digital fascia of the hand. Various treatments have been recommended for advanced disease or to retard progression of early disease and to prevent deterioration of the finger contracture and quality of life. Recent studies have tried to evaluate the clinical and cost-effectiveness of therapies for DD, but there is currently no systematic assessment and appraisal of the economic evaluations.

Methods: A systematic literature review was conducted, following PRISMA guidelines, to identify studies reporting economic evaluations of interventions for managing DD. Databases searched included the Ovid MEDLINE/Embase (without time restriction), National Health Service (NHS) Economic Evaluation Database (all years) and the National Institute for Health Research (NIHR) Journals Library) Health Technology Assessment (HTA). Cost-effectiveness analyses of treating DD were identified and their quality was assessed using the CHEERS assessment tool for quality of reporting and Phillips checklist for model evaluation.

Results: A total of 103 studies were screened, of which 4 met the study inclusion criteria. Two studies were from the US, one from the UK and one from Canada. They all assessed the same interventions for advanced DD, namely collagenase Clostridium histolyticum injection, percutaneous needle fasciotomy and partial fasciectomy. All studies conducting a cost-utility analysis, two implemented a decision analytic model and two a Markov model approach. None of them were based on a single randomised controlled trial, but rather synthesised evidence from various sources. Studies varied in their time horizon, sources of utility estimates and perspective of analysis. The overall quality of study reporting was good based on the CHEERS checklist. The quality of the model reporting in terms of model structure, data synthesis and model consistency varied across the included studies.

Conclusion: Cost-effectiveness analyses for patients with advanced DD are limited and have applied different approaches with respect to modelling. Future studies should improve the way they are conducted and report their findings according to established guidance for conducting economic modelling of health care technologies.

Keywords: Dupuytren's disease, Systematic review, Economic evaluation, Economic modelling

* Correspondence: melina.dritsaki@ndorms.ox.ac.uk
[1]Oxford Clinical Trials Research Unit, Nuffield Department of Orthopaedics, Rheumatology and Musculoskeletal Sciences, University of Oxford, Oxford OX3 7LD, UK
Full list of author information is available at the end of the article

Background

Dupuytren's disease (DD) affects 4% of the general UK population and is a progressive, fibro-proliferative condition affecting the palmar and digital fascia of the hand, the 'bands' that anchor the skin of the palm [1–3]. Early manifestation of the disease is as a firm nodule. These nodules are the precursors to the development of fibrous collagenous cords which extend into the fingers. With further disease progression, cords thicken and contract, causing finger(s) to curl irreversibly into the palm. Approximately 40% of patients with early disease might eventually be expected to progress to develop cords [4, 5] and the flexion deformities that impair hand function, thereby greatly limiting activities of daily life, including self-care, usual activities and employment, and reducing health-related quality of life (HRQoL) [6].

The number of patients requiring treatment for DD in England increased by almost 50% between 1998 and 2011 (from 11,716 to 17,342 per annum). With the aging population it is predicted that there will be a further increase in the numbers of patients requiring treatment through to 2030 [7]. In an era of scarce health care resources, competing health care interventions must be subject to assessment of cost-effectiveness to identify those offering best value for money. Treatments for DD are no exception, and ensuring the condition is managed in a cost-effective way is especially important given the increasing demand on services placed by patients with the condition in the future.

Treatment for DD is recommended when the digital flexion contractures limit hand function and/or the proximal interphalangeal joint is flexed to 30^0 or more [3] and aims to correct the flexion deformities and restore hand function. Surgical interventions include fasciectomy whereby the diseased cords are surgically excised, usually under general or regional anaesthesia, or fasciotomy, where the cords are divided using a needle [8]. More recently there has been interest in using collagenase from Clostridium histolyticum, an enzyme which breaks down and weakens the collagen in the cords. Collagenase is injected directly into the affected tissue and manual straightening of the finger is performed 24 to 72 h later [9, 10]. Trade-offs are likely to exist when comparing the three treatments in terms of procedure-related morbidity and complications (likely to be higher with the more invasive fasciectomy), treatment failure and recurrence (potentially higher with fasciotomy and collagenase which both leave residual diseased tissue), time to return to work (likely to be longer with the more invasive fasciectomy), and cost [11, 12].

Treatments to retard the progression of early disease and to prevent both the deterioration in HRQoL associated with finger contracture and necessity for intervention and disease recurrence, have also been researched. A recent systematic review identified studies evaluating the clinical outcomes of radiotherapy, steroids, and physical therapy in patients with early DD [13]. A trial to evaluate the efficacy of a drug to inhibit tumour necrosis factor is ongoing (Repurposing Anti-TNF for Treating Dupuytren's Disease (RIDD) trial (ISRCTN27786905 DOI https://doi.org/10.1186/ISRCTN27786905) based on laboratory data showing the key role of this cytokine in the development and maintenance of the phenotype of myofibroblasts [14], the cells responsible for both the excessive matrix deposition and contraction [15].

The aim of this study is to conduct a systematic literature review to identify the extent and appraise the quality of the existing literature on the cost-effectiveness of treatments for DD.

Methods

The search included Ovid Medline/Embase (without time restriction), the NHS Economic Evaluation Database (NHS EED available at http://www.crd.york.ac.uk/CRDWeb/) (all years) and Health Technology Assessment (HTA) (available at http://www.crd.york.ac.uk/CRDWeb/). Following extraction of eligible papers, forward and back-citation searches were conducted using Google Scholar. When potentially eligible abstracts were identified, the authors were contacted to ascertain whether further details of the study were available. The search strategy for Ovid Medline is shown in Additional file 1 and contains a combination of MeSH headings and free text words relating to both the clinical condition and health economic evaluation. We used the search strategy originally developed by Brazzelli et al. [2] on the cost-effectiveness of interventions for DD, which has proven to be sensitive and specific, with the inclusion of an additional clinical term (see line 4 in Additional file 1).

The search aimed to identify any study reporting on the cost-effectiveness of one or more interventions for managing DD in adult patients aged 18 years and over. Invasive and non-invasive interventions for both early and advanced disease were sought, as were all types of full economic evaluation, including cost-consequence analysis (CCA), cost-effectiveness analysis (CEA), cost-utility analysis (CUA), and cost-benefit analysis (CBA). Any study design was permitted, including economic evaluations conducted as part of patient-based studies such as randomised controlled trials, non-randomised studies and decision analytical models. To identify current practices, only studies published between January 1996 and November 2016 were eligible for inclusion. No restrictions were placed on language or on publication type. Studies reporting on the management of DD prior to 1996, or in adolescents, were excluded, as were cost minimisation analyses and cost analyses whereby interventions are compared on the basis of cost only. The review was registered on the PROSPERO register of systematic reviews (registration number CRD42016032989).

All records returned by searching were imported into EndNote bibliographic software (EndNote 2016 Thomson Reuters) and duplicate publications removed. A first screen of titles and abstracts was conducted by one reviewer (OR-A) and full text versions of potentially eligible publications were obtained. Two reviewers (MD and OR-A) then independently read and classified each full text publication as eligible or not based upon the criteria outlined above. The resulting classifications were compared and disagreements resolved through discussion.

The Consolidated Health Economic Evaluation Reporting Standards (CHEERS) statement [16] was used to extract data and also assess the quality of data reporting (see Additional file 2). CHEERS was developed using CONSORT methodology [17] to improve the quality of the reporting of economic evaluations and includes a checklist of 24 items. The items include study title, background and objectives, target population, setting and location, treatment alternatives being compared, methodological issues such as study time horizon, use of discount rates for both costs and outcomes, choice of models applied, assumptions made, and ways of accounting for model uncertainty and heterogeneity. Economic evaluations based on a single study and those based on evidence synthesis from a variety of sources were also distinguished. Two authors (MD and OR-A) independently extracted data from the included studies, and any disagreements were again resolved through discussion. We contacted the authors of three published abstracts for further information. All three responded and two were able to provide further information in the form of conference poster presentations.

A literature review reported existing reporting guidelines for economic evaluations that were relevant to population modelling studies [18]. The authors identified a total of 69 quality criteria among seven economic evaluation studies, including one which provided a detailed framework for model quality assessment [19] (see Additional file 3). The overarching themes of the checklist published by these authors relate to 1) structure of the model (20 items), 2) data issues (31 items), 3) consistency (& validity) of the model (5 items). Two authors (MD and OR-A) independently assessed the models from the included studies against the Philips checklist [19]. The purpose of this exercise was to identify, in a systematic approach, the strengths and any particular issues or weakness of the models identified so as to inform any future modelling applications.

Results

Summary of studies included in the review

The searches of Ovid Medline, Embase and NHS EED identified 102 studies, and one additional publication was included from cross-references. Thirty-eight duplicate articles were identified and removed, leaving the titles and abstracts of 65 publications to be screened (by OR-A and MD) (see Additional file 4 for details). Fifty-one of these publications were not eligible for inclusion in the review: 32 did not include an economic evaluation, 14 reported a cost-analysis only, 3 conducted a quality of life analysis only, and 2 manuscripts were a letter to the editor and an erratum. The remaining 14 publications were obtained in full, and following independent review and discussion, four were considered eligible for inclusion [2, 20–22], two of which overlap with the findings reported by Brazzelli et al. [2]. Figure 1 (PRISMA flowchart) reports a breakdown of the reasons for exclusion of the remaining 10 manuscripts at this stage.

A search of the HTA database returned ten potentially eligible records that were studied for additional missing references. Five records and their associated publications were reviewed but revealed no further eligible studies. The remaining five were for commercially conducted HTAs covering two interventions for advanced DD. The reports could be purchased but no summary information was available about the content with regards to cost-effectiveness analysis and therefore they were excluded.

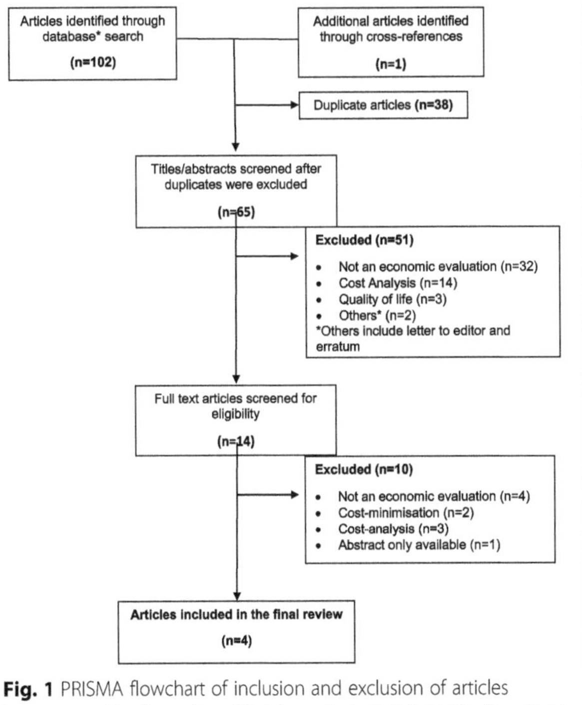

Fig. 1 PRISMA flowchart of inclusion and exclusion of articles incorporated in the review. *Databases included Ovid Medline, Ovid Embase and NHS EED

Details on the CHEERS assessment of the four included studies are described in Additional file 5. None of the studies evaluated the cost-effectiveness of interventions for early DD. Published from 2011 onwards, all four (two from the US, one from Canada, and one from the UK) assessed the same three interventions for patients with advanced disease manifest as contractures of one or more digits, namely collagenase Clostridium histolyticum, percutaneous needle fasciotomy (aponeurotomy) and partial (limited) fasciotomy. Two were full journal articles, one a chapter in a Health Technology Assessment (HTA) report, and one was a conference poster presentation. All four utilised modelling as the framework for estimating costs and effects.

Summary conclusions differed across the four studies (see Additional file 5). Two concluded that fasciectomy was not cost-effective, and that collagenase was unlikely to offer value for money unless the injection cost was significantly lower than the current market price [20, 22]. In contrast, the third report found fasciectomy to be the most cost-effective treatment, dominating both collagenase and percutaneous needle fasciotomy [21]. The fourth study also concluded that fasciectomy offered the best value for money, dominating collagenase and offering a favourable cost per QALY when compared with percutaneous fasciotomy [2].

Table 1 Reporting standards in the included studies

		Yes	No	Not Applicable
CHEERS reporting item				
1	Title	4		
2	Abstract	4		
3	Background and objectives	4		
4	Target population and subgroups	4		
5	Setting and location	4		
6	Study perspective	4		
7	Comparators	4		
8	Time horizon	4		
9	Discount rate	3	1	
10	Choice of health outcomes	4		
11a	Measurement of effectiveness (single study-based estimates)			4
11b	Measurement of effectiveness (synthesis-based estimates)	4		
12	Measurement and valuation of preference-based outcomes	4		
13a	Estimating resources and costs (single study-based economic evaluation)			4
13b	Estimating resources and costs (model-based economic evaluation)	4		
14	Currency, price date and conversion	4		
15	Choice of model	4		
16	Assumptions	4		
17	Analytic method	4		
18	Study parameters	4		
19	Incremental costs and outcomes	3	1	
20a	Characterising uncertainty (single study-based economic evaluation)			4
20b	Characterising uncertainty (model-based economic evaluation)	3	1	
21	Characterising heterogeneity	1	3	
22	Study findings, limitations, generalisability and current knowledge	4		
23	Source of funding		3	1
24	Conflicts of interest		3	1

Quality of reporting

Table 1 summarises the CHEERS assessment results of the four studies included in the current systematic literature review. The overall quality of the papers was good. All the studies conducted a cost-utility analysis. Two [20, 22] implemented an expected value decision analytic model whereas the others [2, 21] employed a Markov model. None of the studies was based on a single RCT, but rather used evidence synthesised from various sources. The time horizon varied between the studies, ranging from 10 to 37 years, with a starting age of 63 years assumed in all studies apart from one [21] which assumed a starting age of 50. All the studies discounted costs and effects at 3%, 3.5% or 5% except one [20], which did not report discounting for future cost and outcomes, although the time horizon of the analysis was more than 1 year. Uncertainty was addressed in 3 out of 4 studies, but only one group [2] conducted a probabilistic sensitivity analysis to test the robustness of results to simultaneous changes in model parameters. Characterisation of both deterministic and probabilistic sensitivity analysis is particularly important in decision analytical model and therefore should be included [23].

Sources of utility estimates varied across the four included studies: two studies [20, 22] conducted a utility survey using standard gamble techniques (SG) specific to their study in a US setting and surveyed participants living with Dupuytren's contracture. One study [21] used utility valuations from patients with carpal tunnel syndrome, and another one [2] used a discrete choice experiment (DCE) based on the general UK population [24]. For the latter, the values were scaled to be approximately relative to an EQ-5D-3 L health state. QALYs derived from the US survey-SG questionnaire ranged from 0.971 for successful treatment with complications to 0.994 for successful treatment without any complications. When no treatment was provided, the utility was

0.987. The DCE approach provided results that were significantly different to the SG-based results, with utilities for affected dominant hands, non-dominant hands or ambidextrous hands being respectively 0.49, 0.57 and 0.63 [24].

The framework described by Phillips et al. [19] for quality assessment was applied to evaluate the models of the four included studies (see Additional file 6). Table 2 summarises the evidence in terms of model structure, data synthesis and model consistency. All authors provided a clear statement about the decision problem, prompting the analysis which in all cases defined the population as Duyputren's contracture and the available treatment options. The perspective of the analyses, although defined clearly, was not always consistent with the scope of the models. For example, although one study considered a societal perspective, the authors did not include any cost bourne by patients, out of pocket expenses or productivity loss due to treatment for Dupuytren's contracture [20]. All treatment comparators evaluated within the models were feasible and practical within the reference healthcare systems. All studies compared up to three treatment options and none of them provided justification of the exclusions of any other feasible options. Vehicle to calculate the decision analysis were decision trees and Markov models. Although all models took a long term or life time horizon, only two publications [2, 22] provided justification of the time frame used.

Methods used to identify data were transparent in all studies and consistent with the objectives of the models. The quality and reliability of the retrieved data and data input parameters were not described in any of the studies, although trial data or prospective naturalistic studies are recommended as the highest quality sources of data [25]. An example of a parameter that may have a significant impact on the modelling process for treatments Dupuytren's disease is the definition of risk of recurrence. Further treatment option following a treatment failure should be based on clinical opinion and expertise. Also, decisions should be made on whether patients failing after a specific treatment should proceed for further treatment or instead enter a semi-absorbing state with no accumulated cost and lower health related quality of life.

Data parameters were incorporated in the studies either as point estimates (deterministic) or as distributions (probabilistic), or both [2]. In the first case, parameter uncertainty was explored through univariate sensitivity analysis on recurrence rate, complication rate and various cost items [20–22]. In the case of probabilistic parameter distributions the functional form of the distributions was described but not justified clearly. Only one study [2] made a distinction and addressed different forms of uncertainty, namely parameter, structural and methodological. Only two studies [2, 22] examined the external consistency of their models by comparing their results with available evidence and other models that addressed similar research questions. The internal consistency (mathematical logic) of the model was partly assessed in the two aforementioned studies as well.

Discussion

In this study we searched for and systematically reviewed cost-effectiveness analyses of potential interventions for DD. We identified only four studies (3 peer-review manuscripts and one poster conference presentation), suggesting that the country-specific economic evidence to date is sparse. All four studies used an economic model and focused on late rather than early stage DD. The quality of reporting varied, but overall was good. Studies used different time horizons and had different analytical perspectives and different pricing systems. These differences had a major impact on the cost effectiveness results, with two studies [20, 22] suggesting that fasciectomy was not cost-effective whereas the remaining two studies [2, 21] concluded that fasciectomy was the most cost-effective treatment. None of the studies used a common guideline to report the results of their modelling exercise. Therefore, it is difficult to assess how the results of a study in a particular country are relevant to other jurisdictions.

The quality-adjusted life year (QALY) was the main health outcome measure in all models. Two main approaches were taken to derive utility estimates: the standard gamble (SG) approach, and discrete choice experiments (DCEs). The standard gamble approach is associated with a number of limitations [2, 24]. In particular, participants offered a choice between two extreme alternative outcomes, such as taking a pill (which would lead to an immediate state of full health or immediate death), or living in a particular chronic state for the rest of their life, were often strongly death-averse, with the result that very high utilities (0.971 to 0.994) were estimated for some health states. The resulting implication is that for an intervention to be cost-effective it should be both highly successful and very inexpensive [20], which suggests that the utility elicitation method is unrealistic and lacks face validity [20].

The authors of the included studies primarily used decision modelling to estimate costs and outcomes of alternative treatments for DD. The versatility of health economic modelling was likely to be well suited to the assessment of cost-effectiveness in the field of DD for a number of reasons. Firstly, treatments span both early and advanced disease, and modelling can facilitate a comparison of early versus late intervention in the absence of trial-based head to head comparisons. Secondly, progression and recurrence of DD following initial treatment is common, and modelling can be used to

Table 2 Reporting standards for modelling studies [19]

Quality criteria	Question(s) for critical appraisal	Yes	No	YES/NO	?	Not applicable
Structure (S)						
S1	Is there a clear statement of the decision problem?	4				
	Is the objective of the evaluation and model specified and consistent with the stated decision problem?	4				
	Is the primary decision maker specified?		4			
S2	Is the perspective of the model stated clearly?	4				
	Are the model inputs consistent with the stated perspective?	2	1		1	
	Has the scope of the model been stated and justified?	2		2		
	Are the outcomes of the model consistent with the perspective, scope and overall objective of the model?	3	1			
S3	Has the evidence regarding the model structure been described? Is the structure of the model consistent with a coherent theory of the health condition under evaluation?	4				
	Are the sources of data used to develop the structure of the model specified?	4				
	Are the causal relationships described by the model structure justified appropriately?		4			
S4	Are the structural assumptions transparent and justified?	3		1		
	Are the structural assumptions reasonable given the overall objective, perspective and scope of the model?	4				
S5	Is there a clear definition of the options under evaluation?	4				
	Have all feasible and practical options been evaluated?		4			
	Is there justification for the exclusion of feasible options?		4			
S6	Is the chosen model type appropriate given the decision problem and specified causal relationships within the model?	3		1		
S7	Is the time horizon of the model sufficient to reflect all important differences between options?	3			1	
	Is the time horizon of the model, the duration of treatment and the duration of treatment effect described and justified?	2	1	1		
S8	Do the disease states (state transition model) or the pathways (decision tree model) reflect the underlying biological process of the disease in question and the impact of interventions?	4				
S9	Is the cycle length defined and justified in terms of the natural history of disease?	1		1		2
DATA (D)						
D1	Are the data identification methods transparent and appropriate given the objectives of the model?	4				
	Where choices have been made between data sources, are these justified appropriately?	3				1
	Has particular attention been paid to identifying data for the important parameters in the model?	4				
	Has the process of selecting key parameters been justified and systematic methods used to identify the most appropriate data?	3	1			
	Has the quality of the data been assessed appropriately?		4			
	Where expert opinion has been used, are the methods described and justified?	1				3
D2	Is the pre-model data analysis methodology based on justifiable statistical and epidemiological techniques?		3		1	
D2a	Is the choice of baseline data described and justified?	2	2			
	Are transition probabilities calculated appropriately?	2				2
	Has a half cycle correction been applied to both cost and outcome?	1		1		2
	If not, has this omission been justified?		1			3

Table 2 Reporting standards for modelling studies [19] *(Continued)*

Quality criteria	Question(s) for critical appraisal	Yes	No	YES/NO	?	Not applicable
D2b	If relative treatment effects have been derived from trial data, have they been synthesised using appropriate techniques?		1			3
	Have the methods and assumptions used to extrapolate short-term results to final outcomes been documented and justified?	2	1	1		
	Have alternative extrapolation assumptions been explored through sensitivity analysis?	2	2			
	Have assumptions regarding the continuing effect of treatment once treatment is complete been documented and justified?	3	1			
	Have alternative assumptions regarding the continuing effect of treatment been explored through sensitivity analysis?	1	3			
D2c	Are the utilities incorporated into the model appropriate?			1	3	
	Is the source for the utility weights referenced?	3	1			
	Are the methods of derivation for the utility weights justified?	2	2			
D3	Have all data incorporated into the model been described and referenced in sufficient detail?	3		1		
	Has the use of mutually inconsistent data been justified (i.e. are assumptions and choices unclear appropriate)?					4
	Is the process of data incorporation transparent?	3		1		
	If data have been incorporated as distributions, has the choice of distribution for each parameter been described and justified?			2		2
	If data have been incorporated as distributions, is It clear that second order uncertainty is reflected?		2			2
D4	Have the four principal types of uncertainty been addressed?	1	3			
	If not, has the omission of particular forms of uncertainty been justified?		3			1
D4a	Have methodological uncertainties been addressed by running alternative versions of the model with different methodological assumptions?	1	3			
D4b	Is there evidence that structural uncertainties have been addressed via sensitivity analysis?	1	3			
D4c	Has heterogeneity been dealt with by running model separately for different sub-groups?	1	3			
D4d	Are the methods of assessment of parameter uncertainty appropriate?	4				
	If data are incorporated as point estimates, the ranges used for sensitivity analysis stated clearly and justified?	2		1		1
Consistency (C)						
C1	Is there evidence that the mathematical logic of the model has been tested thoroughly before use?	2	2			
C2	Are the conclusions valid given the data presented?	4				
	Are any counterintuitive results from the model explained and justified?	2				2
	If the model has been calibrated against independent data, have any differences been explained and justified?	1				3
	Have the results of the model been compared with those of previous models and any differences in results explained?	2	2			

extrapolate and capture the costs and consequences of these repeated events into the future. Thirdly, modelling can be used to identify future research priorities in the field.

A potential limitation of the paper is that it cannot be considered as a meta-analysis of the cost-effectiveness of treatment of Dupuytren's disease, and does not use statistical techniques to combine the results from retrieved studies to obtain a quantitative estimate of the effect of a particular intervention or outcome. The aim of this study was to conduct a systematic literature review to identify any existing literature on the cost-effectiveness of treatments for DD and assess the quality of such studies. We are not using any primary data because this literature review will ultimately inform the economic evaluation and modelling alongside a pragmatic randomised clinical trial (RIDD). Another limitation arises from the potential underestimation of the quality of the model applied to the publication by Sau et al. [21] based on the Phillips checklist. The nature of evidence (provided in a conference abstract format) makes it difficult to fully critically appraise it since available information is restricted to a page. Regardless of this limitation, the inclusion of this publication in this literature review was considered essential.

Recommendations for the design of a model- based economic evaluation of Dupuytren's disease:

- We recommend that an improved and systematic reporting following CHEERS standards to facilitate interpretation and comparison between studies and help to clearly identify study methods, quality and limitations. If possible, both a healthcare and broader societal perspective should be adopted. DD affects daily function as well as capacity to work (productivity loss), and these wider effects should also be captured. Employment-related information should be collected using a custom-made questionnaire specific for this patient population.
- DD is a musculoskeletal disease which, although not life-threatening, has a chronic element. Therefore, a lifetime perspective should be taken when modelling costs and outcomes beyond a trial's time horizon. Costs and outcomes should be discounted at the customary 3.5% discount rate.
- Quality-adjusted life years (QALYs) should be used as the main health outcome measure in the model.
- The structure of the model and the identification of the Dupuytren's disease health state history should be developed using previous published epidemiological and economic models and in discussion with clinicians treating patients with the disorder. Transition probabilities associated with each health state should be taken from patient-level data and/or from the literature. When the disease recurs or is predicted to recur, the impact of any associated surgical treatment on costs and quality of life should be evaluated. Information on rates of recurrence and their impact on costs and quality of life should be taken from the literature.
- The model structure, the uncertainty around data parameters, and the internal and external validation of the model should receive particular attention during the preparation of the model. Uncertainty around cost-effectiveness results should be handled using probabilistic sensitivity analysis and cost-effectiveness acceptability curves. Areas of methodological uncertainty, such as discount rates for costs and outcomes, should be explored using sensitivity analysis. Heterogeneity should be explored using pre-specified sub-groups. Current value judgements from the National Institute for Health and Clinical Excellence should be used to guide willingness to pay for health benefits and hence calculate likelihood of being cost-effective [26].

We anticipate the above recommendation to contribute to the planned economic analysis alongside the Repurposing Anti-TNF for Treating Dupuytren's Disease (RIDD) trial (ISRCTN27786905 DOI https://doi.org/10.1186/ISRCTN27786905), which began recruiting patients in 2016. Identification of previous cost-effectiveness analyses will help identify likely cost drivers, key model parameters and variables most likely to require sensitivity analyses, and provide context for new evidence. The economic analysis alongside the RIDD study is expected to synthesise information from the trial with literature searches to populate a model evaluating alternative treatments to delay the progression to advanced DD. The model will capture progression and recurrence of DD following initial treatment and will extrapolate and capture the future costs and consequences of these repeated events. It will also help identify and prioritise future research priorities in this field.

Conclusion

Our results suggest that the current cost-effectiveness evidence on potential treatments for patients with DD is limited. We have identified areas for improvement in the reporting and conduct of these studies, in particular with respect to modelling. The conduct and reporting of future studies evaluating the cost-effectiveness of alternative treatments for DD should be improved. This can be achieved using established guidance on good research practice for the conduct of economic modelling of health care technologies [27].

Additional files

Additional file 1: Search strategy used in the systematic review.

Additional file 2: CHEERS checklist-item to include when reporting economic evaluations of health interventions [16].

Additional file 3: Checklist items for reporting modelling studies [19].

Additional file 4: List of 65 publications identified in the first stage after removing duplicates.

Additional file 5: Cheers Assessments of included studies.

Additional file 6: Quality assessments framework to the modelling studies [19].

Abbreviations

CBA: Cost-benefit analysis; CCA: Cost-consequence analysis; CEA: Cost-effectiveness analysis; CHEERS: Consolidated health economics evaluation reporting standards; CUA: Cost-utility analysis; DCE: Discrete choice experiment; DD: Dupuytren's Disease; HRQoL: Health- Related Quality of Life;

HTA: Health technology assessment; NHS: National Healthcare System; QALY: Quality adjusted life years; RCT: Randomised controlled trial; SG: Standard and gamble

Acknowledgements
We would like to thank Helen Campbell, National Perinatal Epidemiology Unit (NPEU), Nuffield Department of Population Health, University of Oxford for her assistance with the literature search.
We would like to acknowledge funding from the Health Innovation Challenge Fund (HICF), a parallel funding partnership between the Wellcome Trust and the Department of Health, and the National Institute for Health Research (NIHR) Oxford Biomedical Research Centre (BRC). The views expressed are those of the authors and not necessarily those of the NHS, the NIHR or the Department of Health

Funding
The article processing charge is funded by a Health Innovation Challenge Fund (HICF), a parallel funding partnership between the Wellcome Trust and the Department of Health UK.

Authors' contributions
The concept of the manuscript was conceived by OR-A and JN. MD and OR-A gathered and reviewed the literature and data and drafted the initial manuscript. CB assisted with the literature search. OR-A, JN, MD, AG and CB participated in the interpretation of data and preparation of the final manuscript. All authors read and approved the final manuscript.

Consent for publication
Not applicable

Competing interests
All named authors declare that they have no competing interest with respect to the research, authorship, and/or publication of this article.

Author details
[1]Oxford Clinical Trials Research Unit, Nuffield Department of Orthopaedics, Rheumatology and Musculoskeletal Sciences, University of Oxford, Oxford OX3 7LD, UK. [2]National Perinatal Epidemiology Unit (NPEU), Nuffield Department of Population Health, University of Oxford, Oxford OX3 7LF, UK. [3]Health Economics Research Centre, Nuffield Department of Population Health, University of Oxford, Oxford OX3 7LF, UK. [4]Kennedy Institute of Rheumatology, Nuffield Department of Orthopaedics, Rheumatology and Musculoskeletal Sciences, University of Oxford, Oxford OX3 7FY, UK.

References

1. Hindocha S, McGrouther DA, Bayat A. Epidemiological evaluation of Dupuytren's disease incidence and prevalence rates in relation to etiology. Hand (NY). 2009;4(3):256–69.
2. Brazzelli M, Cruickshank M, Tassie E, McNamee P, Robertson C, Elders A, Fraser C, Hernandez R, Lawrie D, Ramsay C. Collagenase clostridium histolyticum for the treatment of Dupuytren's contracture: systematic review and economic evaluation. Health Technol Assess. 2015;19(90):1–202.
3. Townley WA, Baker R, Sheppard N, Grobbelaar AO. Dupuytren's contracture unfolded. BMJ. 2006;332(7538):397–400.
4. Gudmundsson KG, Arngrimsson R, Jonsson T. Eighteen years follow-up study of the clinical manifestations and progression of Dupuytren's disease. Scand J Rheumatol. 2001;30(1):31–4.
5. Reilly RM, Stern PJ, Goldfarb CA. A retrospective review of the management of Dupuytren's nodules. J Hand Surg Am. 2005;30(5):1014–8.
6. Wilburn J, McKenna SP, Perry-Hinsley D, Bayat A. The impact of dupuytren disease on patient activity and quality of life. J Hand Surg Am. 2013;38(6): 1209–14.
7. Bebbington E, Furniss D. Linear regression analysis of hospital episode statistics predicts a large increase in demand for elective hand surgery in England. J Plast Reconstr Aesthet Surg. 2015;68(2):243–51.
8. MD BA. Management of Dupuytren's disease – clear advice for an elusive solution. Ann R Coll Surg. 2006;38(1):3–8.
9. Hurst LC, Badalamente MA, Hentz VR, Hotchkiss RN, Kaplan FTD, Meals RA, et al. Injectable collagenase clostridium histolyticum for Dupuytren's contracture. N Engl J Med. 2009;361:968–79.
10. Gilpin D, Coleman S, Hall S, Houston A, Karrasch J, Jones N. Injectable collagenase clostridium histolyticum: a new nonsurgical treatment for Dupuytren's disease. J Hand Surg Am. 2010;35(12):2027–38. e1
11. van Rijssen AL, ter Linden H, Werker PM. 5-year results of randomized clinical trial on treatment in Dupuytren's disease: percutaneous needle fasciotomy versus limited fasciectomy. Plast Reconstr Surg. 2012;129:469–77.
12. Peimer CA, Blazar P, Coleman S, et al. Dupuytren contracture recurrence following treatment with Collagenase clostridium Histolyticum (CORDLESS study): 3-year data. J Hand Surg. 2013;38:12–22.
13. Ball C, Izadi D, Verjee LV, Chan J, Nanchahal J. Systematic review of non-surgical treatments for early Dupuytren's disease. BMC Musculoskelet Disord. 2016;17:345.
14. Verjee LS, Verhoekx JS, Chan JKK, et al. Unraveling the signaling pathways promoting fibrosis in Dupuytren's disease reveals TNF as a therapeutic target. PNAS. 2013;110(10):E928–E37.
15. Nanchahal J, Hinz B. Strategies to overcome the hurdles to treat fibrosis, a major unmet clinical need. PNAS. 2016;5(113):7291–3.
16. Husereau D, Drummond M, Petrou S, Carswell C, Moher D, Greenberg D, Augustovski F, Briggs AH, Mauskopf J, Loder E, Force I. Consolidated health economic evaluation reporting standards (CHEERS)–explanation and elaboration: a report of the ISPOR health economic evaluation publication guidelines good reporting practices task force. Value Health. 2013;16(2):231–50.
17. Moher D, Hopewell S, Schulz K, et al. CONSORT 2010 explanation and elaboration: updated guidelines for reporting parallel group randomised trials. BMJ. 2010;340:c869.
18. Bennett C, Manuel DG. Reporting guidelines for modelling studies. BMC Med Res Methodol. 2012;12:168.
19. Philips Z, Bojke L, Sculpher M, Claxton K, Golder S. Good practice guidelines for decision-analytic modelling in health technology assessment. A review and consolidation of quality assessment. PharmacoEconomics. 2006;24(4):355–71.
20. Chen NC, Shauver MJ, Chung KC. Cost-effectiveness of open partial fasciectomy, needle aponeurotomy, and collagenase injection for dupuytren contracture. J Hand Surg Am. 2011;36(11):1826–34. e32
21. Sau C, Bounthavong M, Tran JN, Wilson RL. Cost-utility analysis of collagenase clostridium histolyticum, limited fasciectomy, and percutaneous needle fasciotomy in dupuytren's contracture. Value Health. 2011;14(3):A128.
22. Baltzer H, Binhammer PA. Cost-effectiveness in the management of Dupuytren's contracture. A Canadian cost-utility analysis of current and future management strategies. Bone Joint J. 2013;95-B(8):1094–100.
23. (NICE) NIfHaCE. Guide to the Methods of Technolog Appraisal. London: NICE. 2013;URL: http://publications.nice.org.uk/guide-to-the-methods-oftechnology-appraisal-2013-pmg9.
24. Gu NY, Botteman MF, Gerber RA, Ji X, Postema R, Wan Y, et al. Eliciting health state utilities for Dupuytren's contracture using a discrete choice experiment. Acta Orthop. 2013;84:571–8.
25. Halpern MT, Luce BR, Brown RE, et al. Health and economic outcomes modeling practices: a suggested framework. Value Health. 1998;1(2):131–47.
26. Excellence NIfHaC. Social Value Judgments. Principles for the development of NICE guidance. London: National Institute for Health and Clinical Excellence; 2008.
27. Caro JJ, Briggs AH, Siebert U, Kuntz KM. Modeling good research practices—overview: a report of the ISPOR-SMDM modeling good research practices task Force-1. Value Health. 2012;15(6):796–803.

22

Effectiveness of ultrasonography and nerve conduction studies in the diagnosing of carpal tunnel syndrome

Benedito Felipe Rabay Pimentel[1*], Flávio Faloppa[2], Marcel Jun Sugawara Tamaoki[2] and João Carlos Belloti[2]

Abstract

Background: The aim of this study was to evaluate the effectiveness of two diagnostic tests routinely used for diagnosing carpal tunnel syndrome (CTS)—ultrasonography (US) and nerve conduction studies (NCS)—by comparing their accuracy based on surgical results, with the remission of paresthesia as the reference standard.

Methods: We enrolled 115 patients, all of the female gender with a high probability of a clinical diagnosis of CTS. All patients underwent US and NCS for a diagnosis and subsequent surgical treatment. As a primary outcome, the accuracy of the US and NCS diagnoses was measured by comparing their diagnoses compared with those determined by the surgical outcomes. Their accuracy was secondarily evaluated based on before and after scores of the Boston Carpal Tunnel Questionnaire (BCTQ).

Results: Overall, 104 patients (90.4%) were diagnosed with CTS by the surgical reference standard, 97 (84.3%) by NCS, and 90 (78.3%) by US. The concordance of NCS and surgical treatment ($p < 0.001$; kappa = 0.648) was superior to that of US and surgical treatment ($p < 0.001$; kappa = 0.423). The sensitivity and specificity of US and NCS were similar ($p = 1.000$ and $p = 0.152$, respectively: McNemar's test). The BCTQ scores were lower after surgery in patients diagnosed by both US and NCS ($p < 0.001$and $p < 0.001$, respectively: analysis of variance).

Conclusions: US and NCS effectively diagnosed CTS with good sensitivity but were not effective enough to rule out a suspicion of CTS.

Keywords: Carpal tunnel syndrome, Diagnostic accuracy, Diagnostic practices, Clinical diagnosis, Surgical treatment, Ultrasonography, Ultrasound, Nerve conduction studies, Electrodiagnostic testing, Electromyograph

Background

Carpal tunnel syndrome (CTS), characterized by compression of the median nerve at the wrist level, is the most common compressive neuropathy of the upper limb [1, 2]. Ultrasonography (US) and nerve conduction studies (NCS) are diagnostic tests routinely used to confirm the diagnosis of CTS [3, 4]. As the parameters of US and NCS have not been standardization for this diagnosis, and the cutoff point for a CTS diagnosis has not been established, the diagnostic accuracy values for both tests vary widely in the literature. These variations could be related to different study designs, sample sizes, and reference standards that do not reflect routine clinical practice [1, 2]. Thus, the diagnosis of CTS is inconsistent and controversial, with no universally accepted reference standard [5, 6].

Well-designed primary CTS studies of methodological quality sufficient to guide diagnostic practices are uncommon and challenging [7–10]. Hence, we propose a strategy for diagnosing CTS in routine clinical practice.

* Correspondence: befecil@gmail.com
[1]Division of Hand Surgery and Upper Limb, Discipline of Orthopaedics and Traumatology, Paraiba Valley Regional Hospital and Taubaté University Hospital, University of Taubaté, 239 Francisco de Barros, Taubaté, São Paulo zip code 12020-230, Brazil

It includes a methodological resource, based on an algorithm, that could help obtain answers to the question of what is the best pathway to an accurate diagnosis of CTS. This study aimed to evaluate the effectiveness of two diagnostic tests routinely used for diagnosing CTS by comparing the accuracy of US and NCS with the results of the surgical treatment for the CTS. Remission of paresthesia following surgery was the reference standard.

Methods

Ethical approval, registration, guidelines and study design

The ethics and research committees of Federal University of São Paulo/Paulista School of Medicine, São Paulo, Brazil (approval No. 244468) and Paraiba Valley Regional Hospital and Taubaté University Hospital, University of Taubaté, Taubaté, Brazil (No. 009/13) approved this study. It was registered in "ClinicalTrials.gov" (No. NCT02553811) and followed the recommendations of the STARD [11]. It is a primary, longitudinal, prospective clinical trial to determine accuracy performed at a single center.

Participants and eligibility criteria

Initially were evaluated 173 participants with a clinical suspicion of CTS. All participants who agreed to participate in this study signed the informed consent form and underwent an initial clinical evaluation by the same specialist in hand surgery. According to the sample calculation, it was necessary to include a total of 115 eligible patients.

Probability of the clinical diagnosis: CTS-6 model

The CTS-6 [5], represents a logistic regression model that estimates the diagnostic probability of CTS. "See Additional file 1: Table S6". A total score ≥ 12 was considered to indicate a high probability of a clinical diagnosis of CTS. There are six criteria for the probability of a clinical diagnosis (CTS-6), with their respective scores evaluated based clinical history and physical examination on the patient's initial clinical evaluation.

1. *Paresthesia*: in the territory of distribution of the median nerve of the affected hand during any period of the day and when performing manual tasks (3.5 points)
2. *Night paresthesia*: in the territory of distribution of the median nerve of the affected hand during sleep or in the morning upon awakening (4.0 points)
3. *Weakness and hypotrophy or atrophy of the tenar musculature*: loss of strength needed to grasp objects, dropping them; evaluated by testing the tenar musculature with the thumb in opposition (5.0 points)
4. *Tinel test*: performed by applying digital percussion in the anatomical path of the median nerve at wrist level; test is positive when the patient reports a sensation of "shock" at the percussion site that irradiates to the territory of distribution of the median nerve in the affected hand (4.0 points)
5. *Phalen test*: performed by the positioning the wrist and elbow at 90° of flexion for 30–60 s; test is positive when the patient reports the onset or exacerbation of paresthesia in the territory of distribution of the median nerve of the affected hand (5.0 points)
6. *Discrimination of sensory stimuli applied between two points*: performed by applying at least 10 cutaneous sensorial stimuli using a discriminator instrument positioned longitudinally in the digital pulp of the indicators, not in direct view of the patient; test is positive when the patient does not identify at least 7 of the 10 discriminator stimuli placed at intervals of ≤6 mm (4.5 points)

Inclusion and exclusion criteria

Inclusion criteria were a CTS-6 score of ≥12 points, female gender, aged 40–80 years, unilateral or bilateral

Table 1 Distribution of patients by US and NCS results in relation to results of surgical treatment

Parameter	Surgical treatment				Total	
	No remission of paresthesia (CTS absent)		Remission of paresthesia (CTS present)			
	N	%	n	%	N	%
US	11	9.6	104	90.4	115	100.0
CSA < 10 mm^2 (CTS absent)	9	7.8	16	13.9	25	21.7
CSA ≥10 mm^2 (CTS present)	2	1.7	88	76.5	90	78.3
NCS	11	9.6	104	90.4	115	100.0
SCV ≥50 m/s and DML < 4.2 ms (CTS absent)	10	8.7	8	7.0	18	15.7
SCV < 50 m/s and DML ≥4.2 ms (CTS present)	1	0.9	96	83.5	97	84.3

n = 115 patients
Results are given as the total percent
CSA cross sectional area, *CTS* carpal tunnel syndrome, *NCS* nerve conduction studies, *DML* distal motor latency, *US* ultrasonography, *SCV* sensory conduction velocity

Table 2 Observed and expected concordances and Kappa coefficient for the comparisons between US, NCS and surgery

Comparison	Observed concordance	Expected concordance	Kappa coefficient	Standard error	z	*p*
US vs. surgery	84.4%	72.9%	0.423	0.083	5.08	< 0.001
NCS vs. surgery	92.2%	77.8%	0.648	0.090	7.22	< 0.001
US vs. NCS	76.5%	69.4%	0.232	0.091	2.54	0.006

NCS nerve conduction studies, *US* ultrasonography
There were 115 subjects in each comparison group

involvement (only a more symptomatic hand was considered for inclusion), previous conservative treatment for CTS without clinical improvement. Exclusion criteria were the presence of cervical radiculopathy, thoracic outlet syndrome, pronator syndrome; a history of previous surgical release of the carpal tunnel, with sequelae of fracture of the wrist; a CTS-6 score of ≤12 points; lack of compliance at any stage of the study.

Diagnostic interventions

After the initial physical examination, eligible patients underwent both US and NCS. These diagnostic interventions were performed in our institution, consecutively and randomly on different days by the same professional experts who were specialized and experienced with US and NCS. They were unaware of the clinical situation of the patients at the time of the examination.

US

All US evaluations were performed on the same equipment (model M2540A; Philips Healthcare, Bothell, WA USA) with high resolution and broadband linear transducers, 4–6 MHz and 9–13 MHz. The US examination technique consisted of positioning the patient comfortably: sitting with the affected forearm in a supine position in slight flexion and supported on the examination table. The wrist is in neutral position and the fingers in extension [12]. The objective of US was to determine the cross-sectional area (CSA) of the median nerve at the proximal limit ("in let") of the carpal tunnel by direct measurement. To evaluate the diagnostic accuracy of US, an CSA value ≥10.0 mm^2 was the cutoff point to confirm a diagnosis of CTS [3, 12–15].

NCS

All NCS was performed on the same equipment (model MEB 9400 K, two channels; Nihon Kohden, Tokyo, Japan). The NCS technique consisted of positioning the patient comfortably in a horizontal dorsal decubitus position with the upper limbs positioned at rest along the body and prepared for a comparative assessment of the muscular groups and the median, ulnar and radial nerves, to exclude other conditions and differential diagnoses [16–20]. The temperature of the upper limb to be examined was acclimatized at 32 °C. The age and temperature of the patients were considered in the diagnostic parameters of CTS by NCS evaluation [16]. The objective of the NCS was to determine the sensory conduction velocity (SCV) of the median nerve in the third finger–wrist segment for a length of 13 cm and the distal motor latency (DML) of the median nerve from the wrist to the tenar eminence. To evaluate the diagnostic accuracy of NCS, the cutoff values to confirm a

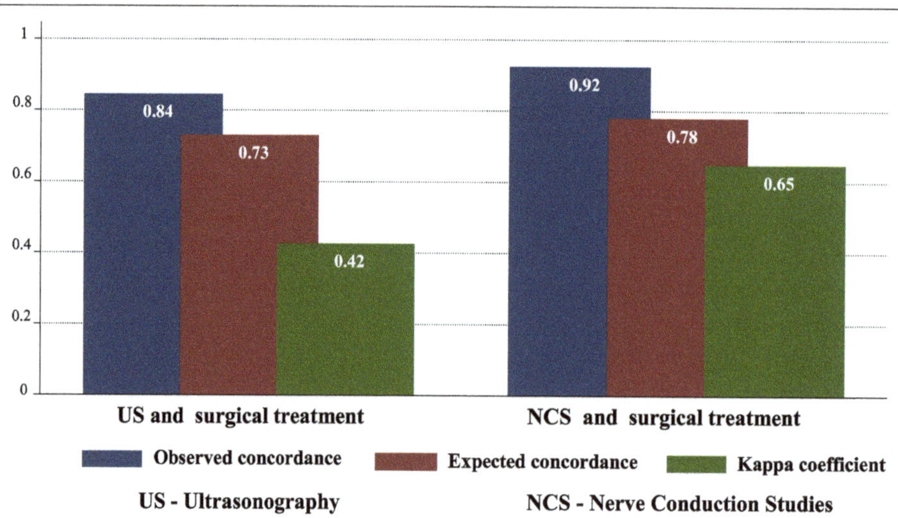

Fig. 1 Comparison between observed, expected concordances and Kappa coefficient of the US and NCS

diagnosis of CTS were < 50 m/s for SCV and ≥ 4.2 ms for DML [3, 16–20].

Evaluation of the performance of diagnostic tests

Surgical treatment

After US and NCS had been performed, the patients were forwarded and underwent to surgical treatment in our institution, by one and the same surgeon. All patients underwent intravenous regional Bier block anesthesia [21]. The surgical technique used was classic open release through a palmar longitudinal incision about 2 cm in length that did not extend proximally beyond the distal flexion fold of the wrist or distally beyond the Kaplan line [22]. The patients were sent home on the same day and were followed through the fourth postoperative month [23].

Primary outcome

Paresthesia remission after surgical treatment was considered the reference standard for diagnosing CTS. Patients with CTS who achieved paresthesia remission postoperatively were considered truly affected by CTS, and patients who did not experience remission were considered not to have CTS [8]. The accuracy of the two preoperative diagnostics methods was measured the evaluating the US and NCS results (positive or negative) relative to the results of the surgery (remission/no remission of paresthesia) [9, 10].

Secondary outcome

The Boston Carpal Tunnel Questionnaire (BCTQ) is a disease-specific (CTS) questionnaire that is self-

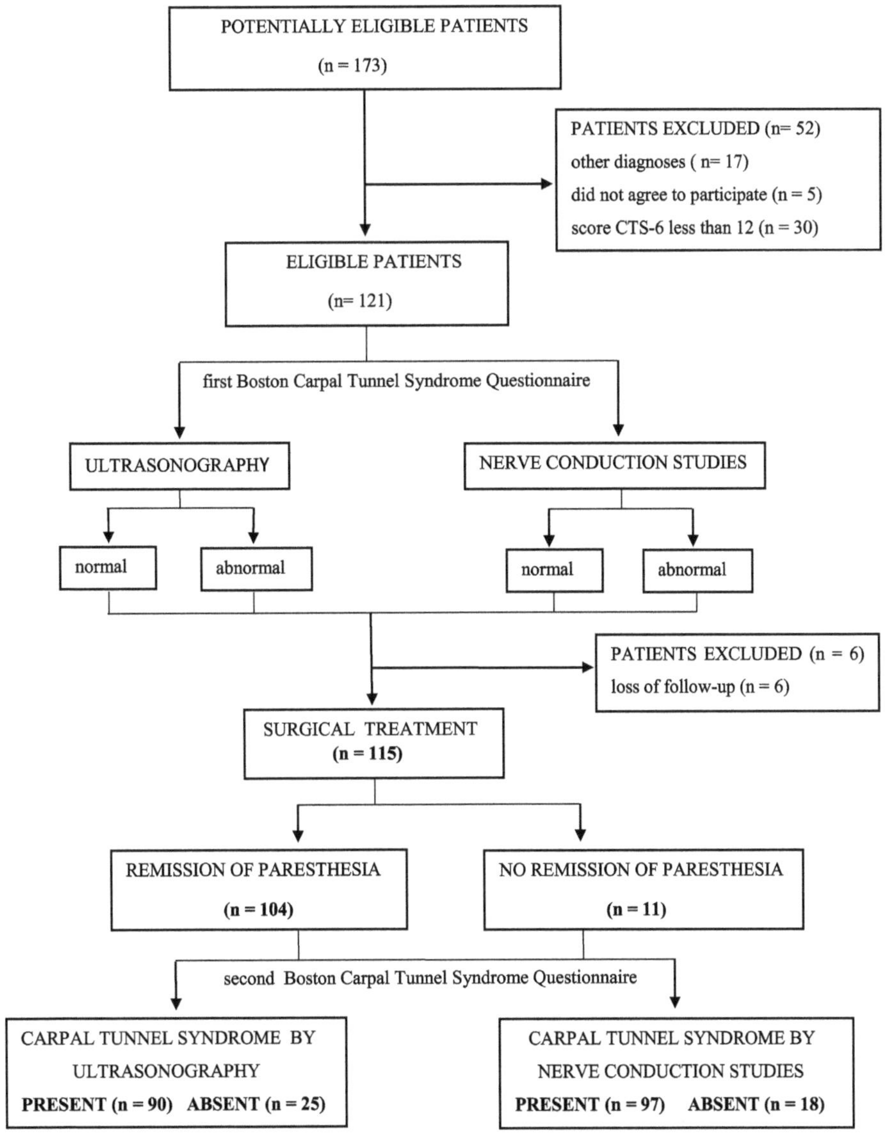

Fig. 2 Flowchart of the diagnostic intervention results

administered and has been translated into the portuguese language and validated, which evaluates two components: a scale of severity of symptoms and a scale of functional status [24, 25]. All patients in this study responded to two BCTQs: the first after the initial clinical evaluation and the second at the end of the fourth month of postoperative follow-up.

Statistical analysis

The categorical variables were presented as relative and absolute frequencies, and numerical variables were presented as a measures summary. The evaluation of the observed and expected concordance between US and NCS and the surgical treatment were performed using the kappa coefficient. The accuracy of the US and NCS relative to the paresthesia remission after surgical treatment (reference standard) was evaluated using the McNemar. Sensitivity, specificity, positive and negative predictive values, and positive and negative likelihood ratios were analyzed by statistical calculations of expected values and obtained in a 2×2 contingency table. The evolution of the BCTQ score by moments of evaluation and diagnostic results was evaluated using analysis of variance with repeated measures. For all statistical tests, a significance level of 5% was adopted [26]. The statistical package SPSS 20.0 (IBM Corp., Armonk, NY, USA) and Stata12 (Stata Corp., College Station, TX, USA) software was used for the analyses.

The statistical sampling was performed considering a 20% difference between the sensitivity of the NCS and US diagnostic tests using the McNemar test, with a statistical power of 84.0% and a significance level of 5%. For this calculation, we assumed as percentage of total concordance the value of 60% and a prevalence of 80% for STC, requiring a total sample of 115 patients [26]. Statistical software PASS 14 (Power Analysis and Sample Size System; NCSS, https://www.ncss.com) was used.

Results

Study population

A total of 115 women were evaluated (average age ± SD 52.9 ± 9.1 years, range 40–79 years, median 52 years). The average ± SD disease duration was 4.0 ± 3.2 years, range 1–20 years, median 3 years. "See Additional file 2: Table S7".

Concordance between the diagnoses

Table 1 shows the total percentages of diagnoses of CTS by the US and NCS relative to the total percentage of diagnoses according to the surgical results (based on remission, or not, of paresthesia). "See Additional file 3: Table S8".

As seen in Table 2, there was moderate concordance between US and the surgical outcomes ($p < 0.001$, kappa = 0.423), good concordance between NCS and the surgical outcomes ($p < 0.001$, kappa = 0.648), and reasonable concordance between US and NCS ($p = 0.006$, kappa = 0. 232) (Fig. 1).

Accuracy of diagnostic tests

The results of the diagnostic interventions are summarized in Fig. 2.

The sensitivity, specificity, and positive predictive values for US ($p = 1.000$, McNemar test) and NCS ($p = 0.$ 152, McNemar test) were similar, with no statistical differences between the two diagnostic methods (Fig. 3). The negative predictive values, however, were lower than expected for both US and NCS. "Additional file 4: Table

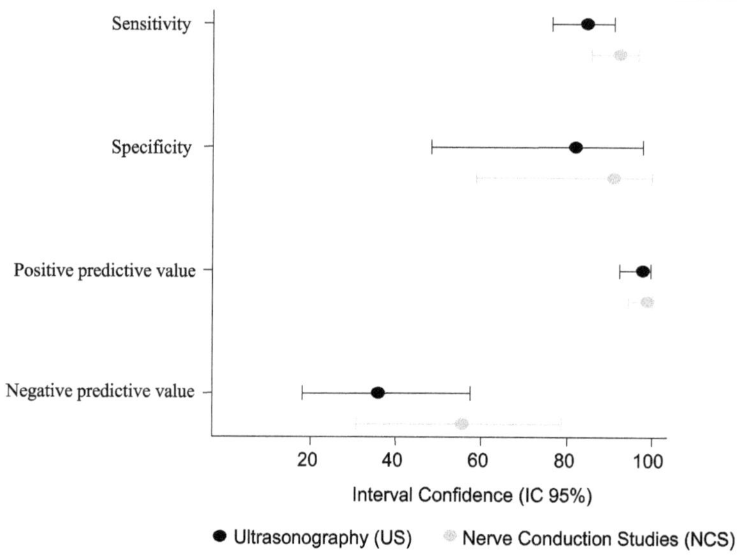

Fig. 3 Interval confidence for sensitivity, specificity, positive and negative predictive value of the US and NCS

S9, Additional file 5: Table S10, Additional file 6: Table S11, Additional file 7: Table S12". The positive and negative likelihood values were accurate and associated with few false-positive and false-negative results for the cutoff point considered and according to the reference standard used (Figs. 4 and 5). "Additional file 8: Table S13 and Additional file 9: Table S14 respectively, shows this with more details". The diagnostic accuracies for US and NCS, according to the statistical parameters of this study, are summarized in Table 3.

Assessment of severity of symptoms and functional status

According to Tables 4 and 5, the mean symptom severity score was reduced by 1.8 points and the functional status score by 1.6 points on the second BCTQ, applied 4 months after surgery in patients with a CTS diagnosis (Figs. 6, 7, 8 and 9).

Discussion

Well-designed studies that have focused on the diagnosis of CTS are uncommon. The deficiencies in the design of studies involving clinical and complementary tests for CTS are associated with a super-estimation of the performance of these diagnostic tests and the lack of a universally accepted reference standard for diagnosing CTS [6, 8–10]. Most CTS diagnostic accuracy studies were unlikely to report results that are applicable in clinical practice [1, 27]. The current study design followed an algorithm based on evaluating an actual clinical practice routine for diagnosing CTS: from the consecutive and random eligibility of patients based on a high probability of a clinical diagnosis of CTS, confirmed (or not) by US and NCS—performed such that the examiners were unaware of the clinical condition of the patients and the results of the concurrent complementary examination treatment follow-up and its clinical outcomes. To ensure good diagnostic accuracy it is important that the estimates provided by a diagnostic test reflect its good performance in clinical practice [1]. The remission of paresthesia (reference standard) after surgical treatment was used in this study to evaluate the effectiveness and performance of the diagnosis of CTS by the US and NCS [3]. The classical open approach is considered a definitive surgical treatment for CTS with good results in 75 to 90% of patients [23]. In this study, 90.4% of the 115 operated patients obtained remission of paresthesia with four months pos operative, while in another study 78.9% of the 113 operated patients obtained remission of paresthesia with ten years pos operative by same surgical technique. [28]. As for the 9.6% of operated patients who did not obtain remission of paresthesia with surgical treatment in our study, it can be attributed to proximal compressions of the median nerve, double cervical

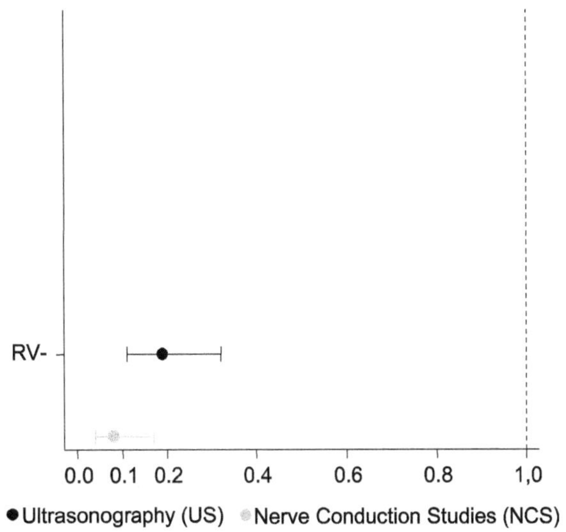

Fig. 5 Confidence Interval for negative likelihood ratios (RV-) of the US and NCS

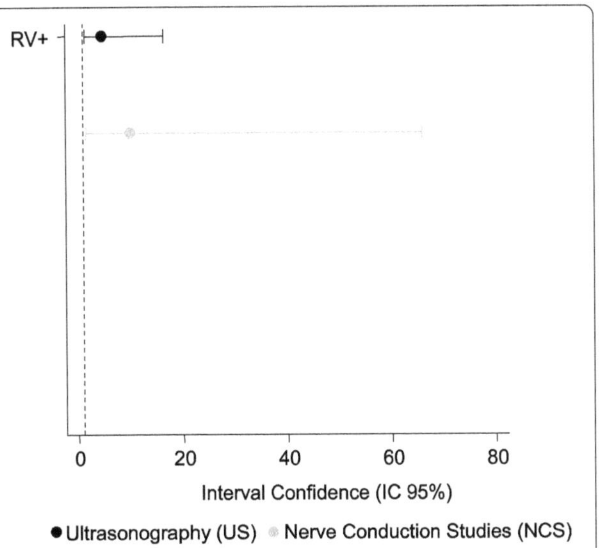

Fig. 4 Confidence Interval for positive likelihood ratios (RV+) of the US and NCS

Table 3 Comparison of US and NCS: statistical values

Statistical parameter	US	NCS
Sensitivity(%)	84.6 (76.2–90.9)	92.3 (85.4–96.6)
Specificity(%)	81.8 (48.2–97.7)	90.9 (58.7–99.8)
Positive predictive value(%)	97.8 (92.2–99.7)	99.0 (94.4–100.0)
Negative predictive value(%)	36.0 (18.0–57.5)	55.6 (30.8–78.5)
Positive likelihood ratio(%)	4.7 (1.3–16.4)	10.2 (1.6–65.9)
Negative likelihoodratio(%)	0.2 (0.1–1.3)	0.1 (0–0.2)

NCS nerve conduction studies, *US* ultrasonography

Table 4 BCTQ scores for severity scale of symptoms relative to CTS diagnosis by US and NCS

Parameter	After treatment	Before treatment	Difference between after and before treatment
US			
CSA ≥10 mm^2 (presence)	1.7 (0.7)	3.5 (0.7)	−1.8 (0.9)
CSA < 10 mm^2 (absence)	1.9 (0.8)	3.7 (0.8)	−1.8 (1.0)
NCS			
SCV < 50 m/s and DML ≥4.2 ms (presence)	1.7 (0.7)	3.5 (0.7)	− 1.8 (0.9)
SCV ≥50 m/s and DML < 4.2 ms (absence)	2.1 (0.9)	3.7 (0.8)	−1.6 (1.0)

$n = 115$ patients
Results are given as the mean (SD)
CSA cross sectional area, *ANOVA* analysis of variance, *BCTQ* Boston Carpal Tunnel Questionnaire, *NCS* nerve conduction studies, *DML* distal motor latency, *US* ultrasonography, *SCV* sensory conduction velocity
ANOVA for repeated measurements—diagnostic effect: US ($p = 0.135$), NCS ($p = 0.059$)
ANOVA for repeated measures—effect of surgical treatment: US ($p < 0.001$), NCS ($p < 0.001$)
ANOVA for repeated measurements—effect of interaction between diagnosis and surgical treatment: US ($p = 0.990$), NCS ($p = 0.246$)

compression syndrome, cervical radiculopathy or even to an advanced degree of CTS [22]. The evaluation of the patients who did not obtain remission of paresthesia after 4 months of the surgical treatment was based on clinical criteria, using the parameters to the CTS-6 and secondly BCTQ [1, 5, 24]. Though the false-negative patients had normal (absent) results for STC by US and NCS in this study, they were submitted to surgical treatment, supported by the results obtained by the clinical diagnosis for CTS in the initial clinical evaluation. Patients with normal results (absent) for CTS by the US showed better performance in the remission of paresthesia after surgical treatment, as shown in the Table 1. To obtain good quality of evidence in this accuracy study, the degree of CTS impairment provided by US and NCS was discarded and reduced to a simple dichotomous (present / absent, abnormal / normal) diagnosis to make these tests useful in clinical practice of routine [8, 9, 11]. The parameters and cut-off points considered in this study for the diagnosis of CTS by the US and NCS had a direct impact on the primary and secondary outcomes, producing the four possible types of results of a diagnostic test, showing balanced results for the values of accuracy, especially between sensitivity and specificity. The positive results obtained by the kappa index in the evaluation of NCS and US concordance in relation to the reference standard in this study expressed the reliability of these tests for the diagnosis of CTS, with NCS showing a better performance. Mondelli et al. evaluated the diagnostic usefulness of US and NCS in patients with a clinical diagnosis of CTS and obtained positive kappa values with good concordance [19]. The confirmation of the clinical diagnosis of CTS in 90.4% of patients, with a total of 84.3% for NCS and 78.3% for the US—using remission of paresthesia as the reference standard—validated the CTS-6 clinical diagnostic probability instrument used during the initial clinical evaluation. Fowler et al. compared US and NCS using CTS-6 as a reference standard and obtained results relative to confirmation of the clinical diagnosis of CTS in 65% of patients, relative to US diagnosis in 61%, and relative to NCS diagnosis in 65% [29].

The sensitivity, specificity, and positive predictive value of the US and NCS obtained in the current study were similar, showing that both diagnostic methods were effective for diagnosing CTS, with good sensitivity. Well-designed diagnostic accuracy studies with STARD-

Table 5 BCTQ scores for functional status scale relative to CTS diagnosis by US and NCS

Parameter	After treatment	Before treatment	Difference between after and before treatment
US			
CSA ≥ 10 mm^2 (presence)	2.0 (0.9)	3.6 (0.9)	−1.6 (1.1)
CSA < 10 mm^2 (absence)	2.1 (0.9)	3.6 (1.0)	−1.5 (1.1)
NCS			
SCV < 50 m/s and DML ≥4.2 ms (presence)	2.0 (0.9)	3.6 (0.9)	−1.6 (1.1)
SCV ≥ 50 m/s and DML < 4.2 ms (absence)	2.3 (0.9)	3.7 (0.8)	−1.5 (1.1)

$n = 115$ patients
Results are given as the mean (SD)
CSA cross sectional area, *ANOVA* analysis of variance, *BCTQ* Boston Carpal Tunnel Questionnaire, *NCS* nerve conduction studies, *DML* distal motor latency, *US* ultrasonography, *SCV* sensory conduction velocity
ANOVA for repeated measurements—diagnostic effect: US ($p = 0.634$), NCS ($p = 0.821$)
ANOVA for repeated measures—effect of surgical treatment: US ($p < 0.001$), NCS ($p < 0.001$)
ANOVA for repeated measures—effect of interaction between diagnosis and surgical treatment: US ($p = 0.629$), NCS ($p = 0.622$)

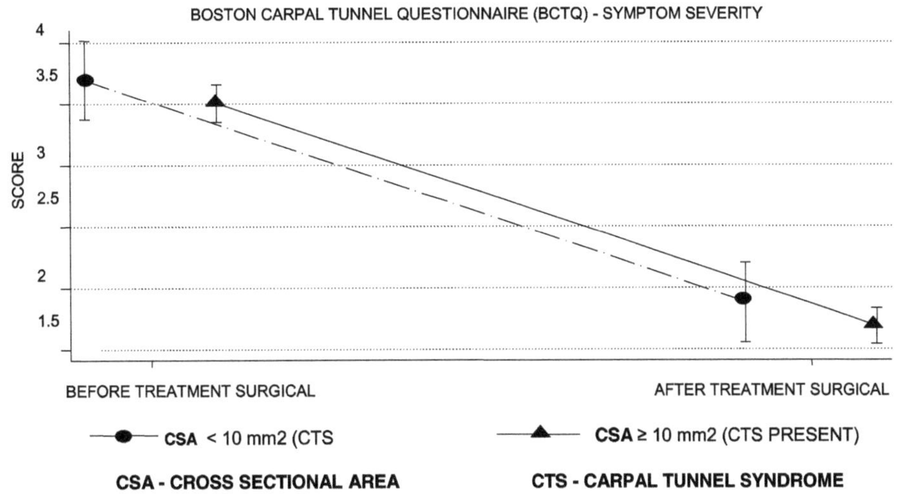

Fig. 6 Evolution of the BCTQ score averages for symptom severity scale by the ultrasonography

compliant methodology obtained similar results when comparing US and NCS [15, 29, 30]. Because of the low negative predictive values, however, neither US nor NCS could adequately rule out the clinical suspicion of CTS in this study when compared with other studies with different reference standards [3, 29–32].

The reduced average of the two scores obtained with the second BCTQ were statistically significant in the current study, indicating improvement of the paresthesia. Thus, the results of the surgical treatment in this study were effective, according to the minimal clinical difference proposed by Ozer et al. [33].

The main limitation of this study was that we did not consider the degree of severity of the initial clinical and complementary diagnosis of CTS. The two-point discrimination test and atrophy of the thenar musculature used in the CTS-6 model are directly linked to the severity of CTS [34]. A value of > 13 mm2 for the median nerve area found during US would correspond to a moderate degree of impairment [35, 36]. Absence of a

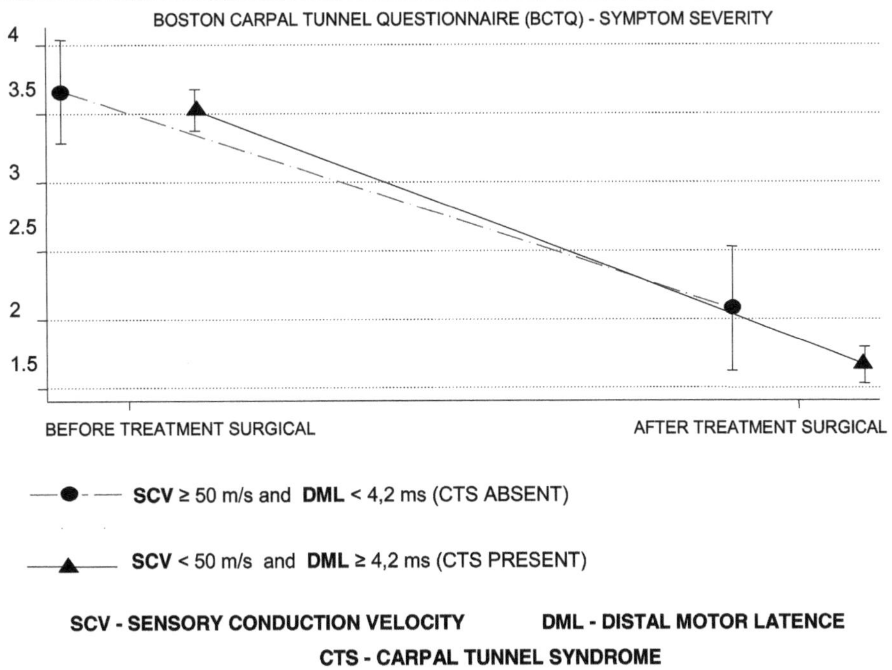

Fig. 7 Evolution of the BCTQ score averages for symptom severity by nerve conduction studies

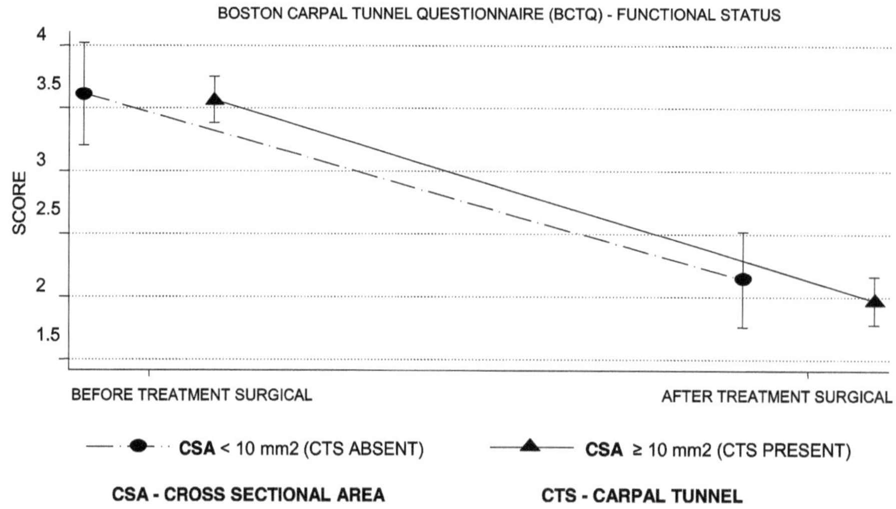

Fig. 8 Evolution of the mean BCTQ scores for functional status by the ultrasonograph

sensory response and abnormal distal motor latency during NCS would correspond to a severe degree of impairment [3, 19].

Another limitation of this study was the inclusion of only female patients, having the disadvantage of limiting the generalization capacity of available information [10].

Conclusions

US and NCS were effective in the diagnosis of CTS, showing a good sensitivity for the detection of patients with CTS. The US and NCS did not show adequate complementary exams to avoid the clinical suspicion of CTS. The NCS presented better concordance regarding the reference standard (remission of paresthesia) than the US. The CTS-6 clinical diagnostic probability instrument was effective and validated for the suspected cases of CTS, through the results obtained by the reduction of the means of the scores at the postoperative in relation to the preoperative evaluated by the BCTQ. The conclusions obtained by study will be useful for areas that routinely handle the diagnosis-treatment algorithm of CTS such as rheumatology, neurology, neurosurgery and orthopedics. This accuracy clinical trial provided further data regarding clinical diagnosis and surgical treatment that may be useful in future research.

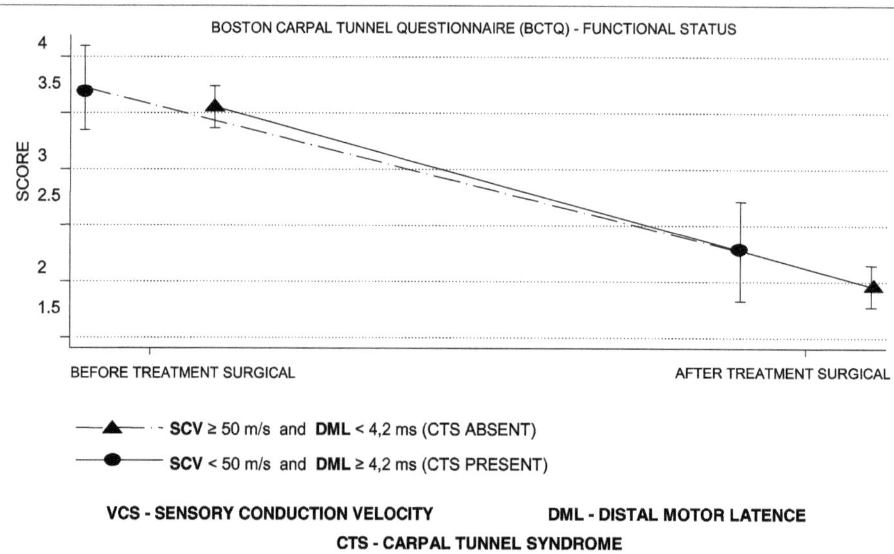

Fig. 9 Evolution of the mean BCTQ scores for functional status by nerve conduction studies

Additional files

Additional file 1: Table S6. Clinical diagnostic probability instrument CTS-6.

Additional file 2: Table S7. Distribution of patients by clinical characteristics.

Additional file 3: Table S8. Distribution of patients in percentages of CTS diagnosis for US, NCS and reference standard.

Additional file 4: Table S9. Sensitivity and specificity of the US in relation to the reference standard.

Additional file 5: Table S10. Sensitivity and Specificity of the NCS in relation to the reference standard.

Additional file 6: Table S11. Positive and negative predictive value of the US in relation to the reference standard.

Additional file 7: Table S12. Positive and negative predictive value of the NCS in relation to the reference standard.

Additional file 8: Table S13. Positive and negative likelihood ratios of US in relation to the reference standard.

Additional file 9: Table S14. Positive and negative likelihood ratios of the NCS in relation to the reference standard.

Abbreviations

BCTQ: Boston carpal tunnel questionnaire; CSA: Cross sectional area; CTS: Carpal tunnel syndrome; CTS-6: Instrument of probability diagnostic for carpal tunnel syndrome; DML: Distal motor latency; NCS: Nerve conduction studies; SCV: Sensory conduction velocity; STARD: Standards for reporting of diagnostic accuracy studies; US: Ultrasonography

Acknowledgements

The authors thank Drs Marcel Saiji Takeshita and Ruschansky Vilela de Azevedo for their friendship, confidence and valuable time spent on the US and NCS examinations, respectively, of the patients who participated in this study. The authors thank all colleagues, residents, and staff of the Department of Orthopedics and Traumatology, Federal University of São Paulo/Paulista School of Medicine and Discipline of Orthopedics and Traumatology, Paraiba Valley Regional Hospital and Taubaté University Hospital, University of Taubaté for their collaboration, care, and support. We thanks Nancy Schatken, BS, MT (ASCP), from Edanz Group (global@edanzediting.com) for editing a draft of this manuscript.

Funding

The authors declare that they have no funding for this study.

Authors' contributions

BFRP: developed the study protocol and contributed to put into practice the design of the study and its methodology, being the main investigator of this clinical trial. FF: participated in the design of the study and actively collaborated in the review and orientation of this clinical trial; MJST collaborated in the correction and revision of this clinical trial; JCB: was the founder of the study design and the main coordinator of this clinical trial, was responsible given final approval of the version to be published. All authors contributed to the improvement of this study and approved the final manuscript.

Competing interests

The authors declare that they have no competing interests.

Author details

[1]Division of Hand Surgery and Upper Limb, Discipline of Orthopaedics and Traumatology, Paraiba Valley Regional Hospital and Taubaté University Hospital, University of Taubaté, 239 Francisco de Barros, Taubaté, São Paulo zip code 12020-230, Brazil. [2]Division of Hand Surgery and Upper Limb, Department of Orthopedics and Traumatology, Federal University of São Paulo, Paulista School of Medicine, 786 Borges Lagoa, São Paulo, São Paulo zip code 04038-030, Brazil.

References

1. Kwon BC, Jung KI, Baek GH. Comparison of sonography and electrodiagnostic testing in the diagnosis of carpal tunnel syndrome. J Hand Surg Am. 2008;33:65–71.
2. Bickel KD. Carpal tunnel syndrome. J Hand SurgAm. 2010;35:147–52.
3. El Miedany YM, Aty SA, Ashour S. Ultrasonography versus nerve conduction study in patients with carpal tunnel syndrome: substantive or complementary tests? Rheumatology (Oxford). 2004;43:887–95.
4. Pimentel BF, Abicalaf CA, Braga L, et al. Cross-sectional area of the median nerve characterized by ultrasound in patients with carpal tunnel syndrome before and after release of the transverse carpal ligament. J Diagn Med Sonography. 2013;29:116–21.
5. Graham B, Regehr G, Naglie G, et al. Development and validation of diagnostic criteria for carpal tunnel syndrome. J Hand Surg Am. 2006;31: 919–24.
6. Prime SM, Palmer J, Khan WS, et al. Is there light at the end of the tunnel? Controversies in the diagnosis and management of carpal tunnel syndrome. Hand (NY). 2010;5:354–60.
7. Scott IA, Glasziou PP. Improving effectiveness of clinical medicine: the need for better translation of science into practice. Med J Aust. 2012;197:374–8.
8. Rutjes AW, Reitsma JB, Coomarasamy A, et al. Evaluation of diagnostic tests when there is no gold standard: a review of methods. Health Technol Assess 2007;11:iii, ix–51.
9. McCabe SJ. Diagnosis of carpal tunnel syndrome. J Hand Surg Am. 2010;35: 646–8.
10. Boyer K, Wies J, Turkelson CM. Effects of bias on the results of diagnostic studies of carpal tunnel syndrome. J Hand Surg Am. 2009;34:1006–13.
11. Bossuyt PM, Reistma JB, Bruns DE, et al. STARD 2015: an updated list of essential items for reporting diagnostic accuracy studies. BMJ. 2015;351: h5527.
12. Sernik RA, Abicalaf CA, Pimentel BF, et al. Ultrasound features of carpal tunnel syndrome: a prospective case-control study. Skelet Radiol. 2008;37: 49–53.
13. Duncan I, Sullivan P, Lomas F. Sonography in the diagnosis of carpal tunnel syndrome. AJR Am J Roentgenol. 1999;173:681–4.
14. Martinoli C, Bianchi S, Gandolfo N, et al. US of nerve entrapments in osteofibrous tunnels of the upper and lower limbs. Radiographics 2000; 20(Spec No):S199–S213; discussion S213–7.
15. Visser LH, Smidt MH, Lee ML. High-resolution sonography versus EMG in the diagnosis of carpal tunnel syndrome. J Neurol Neurosurg Psychiatry. 2008; 79:63–7.
16. Werner RA, Andary M. Electrodiagnostic evaluation of carpal tunnel syndrome. Muscle Nerve. 2011;44:597–607.
17. Padua L, Lo Monaco M, Padua R, et al. Neurophysiological classification of carpal tunnel syndrome: assessment of 600 symptomatic hands. Ital J Neurol Sci. 1997;18:145–50.
18. Jablecki CK, Andary MT, Floeter MK, et al. Practice parameter: electrodiagnostic studies in carpal tunnel syndrome. Report of the American Association of Electrodiagnostic Medicine, American Academy of Neurology, and American Academy of physical medicine and rehabilitation. Neurology. 2002;58:589–92.
19. Mondelli M, Filippou G, Gallo A, et al. Diagnostic utility of ultrasonography versus nerve conduction studies in mild carpal tunnel syndrome. Arthritis Rheum. 2008;59:357–66.
20. Ntani G, Palmer KT, Linaker C, et al. Symptoms, signs and nerve conduction velocities in patients with suspected carpal tunnel syndrome. BMC Musculoskelet Disord. 2013;14:242.
21. Brill S, Middleton W, Brill G, et al. Bier's block: 100 years old and still going strong! Acta Anaesthesiol Scand. 2004;48:117–22.
22. Rodner CM, Katarincic J. Open carpal tunnel release. Tech Orthopaedics. 2006;21:3–11.
23. Louie D, Earp B, Blazar P. Long-term outcomes of carpal tunnel release: a critical review of the literature. Hand (NY). 2012;7:242–6.
24. Levine DW, Simmons BP, Koris MJ, et al. A self-administered questionnaire for the assessment of severity of symptoms and functional status in carpal tunnel syndrome. J Bone Joint Surg Am. 1993;75:1585–92.

25. De Campos CC, Manzano GM, De Andrade LB, Castelo FILHOA, Nóbrega JA. Translation and validation of an instrument for evaluation of severity of symptoms and the functional status in carpal tunnel syndrome. Arq Neuropsiquiatr. 2003;61:51–5. (in Portuguese)
26. Machin D, Campbell MJ, Tan SB, et al. Sample size tables for clinical trials. 3rd ed. Wiley-Blackwell: Chichester, UK; 2009.
27. Alfonso C, Jann S, Massa R, et al. Diagnosis, treatment and follow-up of the carpal tunnel syndrome: a review. Neurol Sci. 2010;31:243–52.
28. Louie DL, Earp BE, Collins JE, Losina E, Katz JN, Black EM, Simmons BP, Blazar PE. Outcomes of carpal tunnel release at a minimum of ten years. J Bone Joint Surg Am. 2013;95(12):1067–73.
29. Fowler JR, Munsch M, Tosti R, et al. Comparison of ultrasound and electrodiagnostic testing for diagnosis of carpal tunnel syndrome: study using a validated clinical tool as the reference standard. J Bone Joint Surg Am. 2014;96:e148.
30. Fowler JR, Cipolli W, Hanson T. A comparison of three diagnostic tests for carpal tunnel syndrome using latent class analysis. J Bone Joint Surg Am. 2015;97:1958–61.
31. Taylor-Gjevre RM, Gjevre JA, Nair B. Suspect carpal tunnel syndrome: do nerve conduction study results and symptoms match? Can Fam Physician. 2010;56:e250–4.
32. Pastare D, Therimadasamy AK, Lee E, et al. Sonography versus nerve conduction studies in patients referred with a clinical diagnosis of carpal tunnel syndrome. J Clin Ultrasound. 2009;37:389–93.
33. Ozer K, Malay S, Toker S, et al. Minimal clinically important difference of carpal tunnel release in diabetic and nondiabetic patients. Plast Reconstr Surg. 2013;131:1279–85.
34. D'Arcy CA, McGee S. The rational clinical examination: does this patient have carpal tunnel syndrome? JAMA. 2000;283:3110–7.
35. Karadağ YS, Karadağ O, Çiçekli E, et al. Severity of carpal tunnel syndrome assessed with high frequency ultrasonography. Rheumatol Int. 2010;30:761–5.
36. Ghasemi M, Abrishamchi F, Basiri K, et al. Can we define severity of carpal tunnel syndrome by ultrasound. Adv Biomed Res. 2015;4:138.

23

Reliability and validity of a novel quality of life questionnaire for female patients with adolescent idiopathic scoliosis: scoliosis Japanese Questionnaire-27

Toru Doi[1*], Hirokazu Inoue[2], Yasuhisa Arai[3], Osamu Shirado[4], Tokuhide Doi[5], Ken Yamazaki[6], Koki Uno[7], Haruhisa Yanagida[8] and Katsushi Takeshita[2]

Abstract

Background: A progressive deformity associated with adolescent idiopathic scoliosis (AIS) negatively affects a patient's health-related quality of life (HRQOL). Although the Scoliosis Research Society-22 (SRS-22) is the standard measurement tool for assessing HRQOL in patients with AIS, it is partially suboptimal for evaluating HRQOL in Japanese patients with AIS because of cultural differences. The purpose of this study was to develop a novel patient-reported outcome measure for Japanese female patients with AIS and to evaluate the reliability and validity of this questionnaire in comparison with the SRS-22 tool.

Methods: We developed 27 questions based on the psychosocial problems in the daily life of young female patients with AIS in Japan, the Scoliosis Japanese Questionnaire-27 (SJ-27). To evaluate its reliability, the internal consistency was assessed using Cronbach's alpha coefficient. Concurrent validity was evaluated using Spearman's correlation coefficient between the SJ-27 and the SRS-22. To investigate the construct validity of the SJ-27, the correlation between the SJ-27 questions was assessed using Akaike's information criterion (AIC).

Results: We analyzed 384 female patients with AIS. Cronbach's alpha coefficients were 0.914 and 0.829 for the SJ-27 and the SRS-22, respectively. Spearman's correlation coefficient between the SJ-27 and the SRS-22 was 0.692 ($p < 0.001$). The AIC analysis indicated that the SJ-27 items are divided into five domains, indicating that the SJ-27 covered a wide range of health-related problems among female patients with AIS.

Conclusions: The results suggest that the SJ-27 is a reliable and valid patient-reported outcome measure for evaluating HRQOL in female patients with AIS in Japan.

Keywords: Adolescent idiopathic scoliosis, Questionnaires, Patient-reported outcome measure, Validation study, Reliability study, Scoliosis Japanese Questionnaire-27, Scoliosis Research Society-22, Health-related quality of life, AIC network

* Correspondence: tooru.doi@gmail.com
[1]Department of Orthopaedic Surgery, University of Tokyo, 7-3-1 Hongo, Bunkyo-ku, Tokyo, Japan
Full list of author information is available at the end of the article

Background

Adolescent idiopathic scoliosis (AIS) is the most common childhood-onset spinal deformity and is present in 2–3% of adolescents worldwide [1]. A curve progression of >30° is more commonly observed in female patients than in male patients [2]. A recent study of AIS prevalence in Japan showed that the overall prevalence in school-age children (11–14 years) is 0.87% [3].

The progressive spinal deformity associated with AIS has been reported to negatively affect a patient's health-related quality of life (HRQOL) [4–6], with increased back pain, reduced physical activity, and psychosocial problems being associated with a disfigured appearance [7–10].

Patient-reported outcome measures are useful instruments for assessing patients' HRQOL [11] and are widely used for patients with orthopedic diseases [12–14], including spinal disorders [15]. The Scoliosis Research Society (SRS) patient-reported outcome measure has been established as a practical and disease-specific measure for assessing HRQOL in patients with AIS [16–19]. An earlier version of the SRS Questionnaire, SRS-24, was developed by Haher et al. [20]. The latest version, SRS-22, which was developed by Asher in 2003 [18], is a practical questionnaire for facilitating the assessment of HRQOL in patients with AIS and has been reported to have a high reliability and validity [16–19, 21]. The SRS-22 questionnaire was revised in 2006 (SRS-22r) [22] in order to improve the internal consistency in the Function domain and this revised version of the SRS-22 questionnaire is commonly used worldwide for the assessment of HRQOL in patients with AIS. The SRS-22 questionnaire covers four domains (Function, Pain, Self image, Mental health) consisting five questions each and one domain (Satisfaction/Dissatisfaction with management) consisting two questions. Each question has five verbal response alternatives ranging from 1 (worst) to 5 (best). The results of the SRS-22 questionnaire are expressed as the mean (total sum of the domain divided by the number of items answered) for each domain and for the total score (minimum: 1 point, maximum: 5 points). To apply the SRS-22 questionnaire in non-English speaking countries, translated and adapted versions of the SRS-22 questionnaire have been developed, and their reliability and validity have been reported [23–34]. For Japanese patients with AIS, the SRS-24 was translated into Japanese; however, previous studies demonstrated that its internal consistency and discriminative validity are not optimal [35, 36], showing definite differences between American and Japanese patients in all the domain scores. These differences may reflect the cultural differences between the assessed populations [37]. The Japanese version of the SRS-22 questionnaire was established in 2007, and its reliability and validity were approved [38]. However, in comparison to its corresponding scale in the original English version, the self-image subscale showed a different pattern of correlation with other variables. This resulted in the study authors suggesting further psychometric assessments to better understand clinical HRQOL. Basically, the self-image subscale questions in the SRS-22 (e.g., Q19 "Do you feel attractive with your current back condition?") are thought to be suboptimal for the modest or reserved personality types observed in a majority of Japanese people. Moreover, the question related to economic burden (Q15 "Are you and/or your family experiencing financial difficulties because of your back?") is also suboptimal for Japanese patients due to the different types of medical insurance systems in Japan, relative to the USA. A previous study on the Turkish version of the SRS-22 reported that Q15 had poor internal consistency, resulting in this item being omitted from this version of the questionnaire [23]. Thus, we sought to develop a novel, patient-reported outcome measure for patients with AIS that is adapted to the Japanese population. The purpose of this study was to develop and introduce a new and unique patient-reported outcome measure for assessing HRQOL in Japanese female patients with AIS and to evaluate its validity and reliability.

Methods

Development of the Scoliosis Japanese Questionnaire-27 (SJ-27)

An original patient-reported outcome measure for Japanese female patients with AIS, the SJ-27, was developed and refined over 17 sessions by an expert committee of the Japanese Scoliosis Society consisting 10 specialists in spinal surgery, rehabilitation, pediatric psychiatrics, and biostatistics. A group of three Japanese Scoliosis Society board-certified experts with extensive spinal disorder treatment experience repeatedly discussed and selected items based on their relevance to the aims of the questionnaire. These experts also sought the advice of a professional pediatric psychiatrist regarding items related to psychosocial problems among adolescent patients with AIS. During the development of the questionnaire, the focus was directed to young female patients because the curve progression and prevalence are greater in females than in males. Additionally, a progressive spinal deformity can result in greater appearance-related psychological problems in females than in males [7, 39]. Furthermore, we also focused on the discomfort when wearing clothes or underwear caused by the spinal deformity because this is an important problem in the daily life of young female patients. To develop the items related to such problems, we interviewed a few young Japanese female patients with AIS and took their opinions into consideration for the development of the SJ-27. Ultimately, each

SJ-27 question essentially reflects the lifestyle of young female patients in Japan.

SJ-27 contents

SJ-27 is a self-administered, disease-specific outcome measure that consists of 27 items (Table 1), summarized as follows:

1. Four questions regarding back pain while lying down and after sitting or standing, or neck/shoulder stiffness or soreness (Q1–4)
2. Seven questions regarding discomfort while wearing clothes or holding bags (Q5–10 and 27)
3. Four questions regarding difficulties associated with participating in physical activities (Q11, 15, 16, and 19)
4. Six questions regarding being self-conscious about one's appearance while in public (Q12–14, 22, 25, and 26)
5. Six questions related to feelings of anxiety or depression due to the spinal deformity (Q17, 18, 20, 21, 23, and 24)

The SJ-27 is intended to cover a wide range of HRQOL issues among female patients with AIS. The 27 items are scored on a 5-point scale from no impairment (0 point) to severe impairment (4 points) and then added to yield a total score (minimum: 0 point, maximum: 108 points). We adopted the scoring method whereby a higher score indicates a much worse HRQOL, which is opposite to the scoring method of the SRS-22. The reason why we adopted the opposite scoring method to the SRS-22 is because we hope to adopt the same scoring method as the visual analog scale (VAS) or Oswestry disability index (ODI), which are broadly utilized patient-reported outcome instruments in spine disease.

Study design and patient recruitment

This study is a multicenter cross-sectional analysis designed to assess the reliability and validity of the SJ-27. Female participants with AIS were recruited from outpatient clinics at 24 institutions located throughout Japan between July 2009 and June 2011. These patients were invited to participate in this study regardless of severity and variation in treatment methods. The inclusion criteria were as follows:

1. Young women 10 to 18 years of age.
2. Radiographic findings of a main curve Cobb angle >10°.
3. Diagnosis of AIS confirmed by experienced specialists.

Table 1 Contents of the Scoliosis Japanese Questionnaire-27

Please fill out the following questions about your upper and lower back from the past month. Tick the most appropriate answer for each question. If you wear a brace, answer the questions for the times when you were not wearing the brace.

1. To what extent do you feel pain in your upper or lower back while lying down?
□Not at all □Mild □Moderate □Considerable □Severe

2. To what extent do you feel pain in your upper or lower back after sitting for an hour?
□Not at all □Mild □Moderate □Considerable □Severe

3. To what extent do you feel pain in your upper or lower back after standing for long periods?
□Not at all □Mild □Moderate □Considerable □Severe

4. To what extent do you feel stiffness or soreness in your shoulders or neck?
□Not at all □Mild □Moderate □Considerable □Severe

5. To what extent do you feel uncomfortable when wearing a jacket or coat?
□Not at all □Mild □Moderate □Considerable □Severe

6. To what extent are you concerned about the waistline of a skirt?
□Not at all □Mild □Moderate □Considerable □Severe

7. To what extent do you have difficulty putting on socks or stockings?
□Not at all □Mild □Moderate □Considerable □Severe

8. To what extent are you concerned about the fit of T-shirts?
□Not at all □Mild □Moderate □Considerable □Severe

9. To what extent are you bothered by the slipping of bra or camisole straps from your shoulders?
□Not at all □Mild □Moderate □Considerable □Severe

10. To what extent are you self-conscious about the curve of your back when wearing lighter clothing in warmer weather?
□Not at all □Slightly □Moderately □Strongly □Extremely

11. Do you find yourself wanting to avoid exercise?
□Not at all □Slightly □Moderately □Strongly □Extremely

12. Have parents, friends, or teachers told you that you have a back problem?
□Never □Rarely □Sometimes □Often □Very often

13. Do you feel embarrassed to bathe with your mother or sisters because of the curve of your back?
□Not at all □Slightly □Somewhat □Quite □Very much

14. How self-conscious are you about classmates or colleagues noticing your appearance?
□Not at all □Slightly □Somewhat □Quite □Very much

15. Do you become anxious when standing in front of a group of people?
□Not at all □Slightly □Somewhat □Quite □Very much

16. To what extent are you reluctant to participate in sporting events or performances?
□Not at all □Slightly □Somewhat □Quite □Very much

17. To what extent does your appearance in the mirror make you self-conscious?
□Not at all □Slightly □Somewhat □Quite □Very much

18. To what extent are you self-conscious about the x-ray images on your back?
□Not at all □Slightly □Somewhat □Quite □Very much

19. Do you feel sports or exercise will have a negative effect on your spine?
□Not at all □Slightly □Somewhat □Quite □Very much

20. Do you worry about your future regarding marriage, childbirth, and your children inheriting your condition?

Table 1 Contents of the Scoliosis Japanese Questionnaire-27 *(Continued)*

Please fill out the following questions about your upper and lower back from the past month. Tick the most appropriate answer for each question. If you wear a brace, answer the questions for the times when you were not wearing the brace.
□Not at all □Slightly □Somewhat □Quite □Very much
21. To what extent do you wish you could change the current condition of your spine? □Not at all □Slightly □Somewhat □Quite □Very much
22. To what extent do you feel shy or reclusive because of the shape of your spine? □Not at all □Slightly □Somewhat □Quite □Very much
23. To what extent do you feel depressed due to the condition of your spine? □Not at all □Slightly □Somewhat □Quite □Very much
24. To what extent do you feel an inferiority complex due to the shape of your spine? □Not at all □Slightly □Somewhat □Quite □Very much
25. To what extent do you feel overly self-conscious about your appearance due to the shape of your spine? □Not at all □Slightly □Somewhat □Quite □Very much
26. To what extent do you think of yourself as less capable than others because of your spine? □Not at all □Slightly □Somewhat □Quite □Very much
27. To what extent do you feel self-conscious about how you hold bags? □Not at all □Slightly □Somewhat □Quite □Very much

Patients who were unable to respond to the Japanese questionnaire were excluded. The adequate sample size was calculated using the following simple formula [40]: $n = Z^2 P(1\text{-}P)/d^2$ where n is the sample size, Z is the statistic corresponding to the level of confidence (for the 95% level of confidence, which is conventional, the Z value is 1.96), P is the expected response rate (a P value of 50% was applied because it would result in a larger sample size), and d is the precision (a precision of 5% was applied if a P value is between 10% and 90%). Accordingly, the sample size computed using the given formula resulted in 384 participants. We thus aimed to enroll approximately 400 participants in this study.

Testing the questionnaire

Patients invited to participate in this study were given SJ-27 questionnaire booklets and copies of the Japanese version of the SRS-22. It takes approximately 5 min to complete both questionnaires. In the questionnaire instructions, we specified that patients must complete both questionnaires by themselves, but provided that if there were a need for help in filling out the questionnaire, their parents or attendants may help them fill out the questionnaire, but the answer must be patient's own. The attending physicians recorded the patient's AIS treatment history, including observation, therapeutic exercise, brace, surgery, and other treatments (multiple choices allowed).

Spinal radiographic examination

Standing anteroposterior radiographs of the whole spine were taken to confirm the AIS diagnosis. The Cobb method was used to measure curve angles at the time the questionnaire was administered.

Statistical analysis

Floor and ceiling effects for the total SJ-27 score and mean total SRS-22 score were examined by calculating the percentage of patients who achieved the lowest (SJ-27: 0 point, SRS-22: 1 point) or the highest (SJ-27: 108 points, SRS-22: 5 points) score, respectively. We adopted the commonly used 15% threshold for the percentage of patients achieving the lowest or the highest score to define floor and ceiling effects [41, 42]. Cronbach's alpha coefficients were calculated for both scales to indicate internal consistency. A Cronbach's alpha coefficient of 0.7 or higher was considered acceptable for internal consistency, while a score above 0.8 was good and above 0.9 was excellent [43]. Cronbach's alpha coefficients were also used to assess how each item contributed to internal consistency by recalculating the Cronbach's alpha coefficient upon deletion of each item in the SJ-27 respectively and then comparing this to the Cronbach's alpha coefficient for all items. Furthermore, we evaluated Cronbach's alpha coefficients for the top three treatment groups in both questionnaires to examine whether each treatment method for AIS affects the internal consistency.

To evaluate the concurrent validity, the correlation between the SJ-27 and the SRS-22 was assessed using Spearman's correlation coefficient. The correlation coefficient was interpreted as follows: ±0.1 was considered weak, ±0.3 moderate, and ± 0.5 a strong correlation [43].

To evaluate the construct validity of the SJ-27, the correlation between SJ-27 questions was evaluated using categorical principal component analysis (CATPCA) and Akaike's information criterion (AIC) [44, 45]. The AIC values were calculated for all combinations of questions and sorted in ascending order using a categorical data analysis program (CATDAP)-02 developed by the Institute of Statistical Mathematics in Japan [46]. CATDAP-02, running with R language software, simultaneously searched for the best subset and categorization of explanatory variables and automatically indicated matching combinations using AIC. SJ-27 construct structures, identified using CATPCA, and AIC factor plotting were performed using IBM SPSS Statistics, version 23 (IBM Corp, Armonk, NY, USA) and an open-source graph visualization software (Graphviz, http://www.graphviz.org), respectively.

Results

Patient characteristics

A total of 405 female patients diagnosed with AIS were recruited, and 21 patients over 18 years of age were excluded. Thus, 384 participants were enrolled in this study. Table 2 shows the demographic characteristics of the 384 participants and the number of participants in each institution. The mean patient age was 14.3 (standard deviation (SD), 1.9) years, and the mean Cobb angle was 31.0° (SD, 12.6). The AIS treatment history survey showed that 161 patients were treated using braces, 120 were observed, and 78 underwent surgery, respectively.

Floor and ceiling effects

The floor and ceiling effects for the total SJ-27 score and mean total SRS-22 score were evaluated in this patient group. A total of 370 out of 384 participants (96.4%) completed the SJ-27, while a total of 367 out of 384 participants (95.6%) completed the SRS-22. The mean score in the SJ-27 and the SRS-22 were 23.2 (SD, 16.7) and 4.1 (SD, 0.4), respectively. The minimum and maximum points of both scales were 0.0 and 86.0 points, respectively, for the SJ-27 and 2.9 and 5.0 points, respectively, for the SRS-22. The percentages of patients who achieved the lowest score were 0.5% for the SJ-27 and 0. 0% for the SRS-22, respectively. The percentages of patients who achieved the highest score were 0.0% for the SJ-27 and 0.3% for the SRS-22, respectively.

Internal consistency

The response completion rates were 99.9% for the SJ-27 and 99.8% for the SRS-22, respectively. Cronbach's alpha coefficients were 0.914 for the SJ-27 (14 of the 384 participants were excluded due to missing or incomplete answers) and 0.829 for the SRS-22 (17 of the 384 participants were excluded due to missing or incomplete answers), respectively. Table 3 shows the Cronbach's alpha coefficient upon deletion of each item in the SJ-27. Only when Q16 was experimentally deleted, Cronbach's alpha coefficient increased slightly to 0.915 (Table 3). Cronbach's alpha coefficient showed a minimum value of 0.907 when Q10 or Q17 was deleted from the SJ-27 (Table 3). Cronbach's alpha coefficients in each of the top three treatment groups (brace, observation, and surgery) were 0.909, 0.

Table 2 Demographic characteristics of the participants and the number of participants in each institution

		Patients with AIS ($n = 384$)	
Mean age (SD), years		14.3 (1.9)	
Mean body mass (SD), kg		45.0 (7.2)	
Mean body height (SD), cm		155.7 (7.1)	
Mean body mass index (SD), kg / m2		18.5 (2.3)	
Treatment, n (multiple choices allowed)		31.0 (12.6)	
Mean Cobb angle (SD), degrees		14.3 (1.9)	
Mean age (SD), years		45.0 (7.2)	
Treatment, n (multiple choices allowed)			
Observation		120	
Exercise		28	
Brace		161	
Surgery		78	
Other		23	
Institution, n			
Okayama Medical Center	10	Shiba Clinic	14
Aizu Medical Center	2	Jikei University Hospital	20
Iwate Medical University Hospital	16	Akita University Hospital	8
Gifu University Hospital	17	Juntendo University Hospital	26
Kurume University Hospital	3	Niigata Spine Surgery Center	19
University of Miyazaki Hospital	20	Niigata University Medical and Dental Hospital	9
Kanazawa Medical University Hospital	5	Gunma Spine Center of Harunaso Hospital	20
Keio University Hospital	23	Sendai Nishitaga Hospital	20
Hirosaki University Hospital	14	Tokai University Hospital	18
Hirosaki Memorial Hospital	5	University of Tokyo Hospital	26
Saitama Medical University Hospital	30	Hamamatsu University Hospital	20
Saitama Medical Center	19	Fukuoka Children's Hospital	20

Table 3 Cronbach's alpha coefficient upon deletion of each item in the Scoliosis Japanese Questionnaire-27

	Scale mean if item is deleted	Scale variance if item is deleted	Corrected item - total correlation	Cronbach's alpha if item is deleted
Q01	48.76	269.209	.409	.912
Q02	48.20	260.097	.525	.911
Q03	48.23	261.917	.473	.911
Q04	47.82	262.736	.349	.914
Q05	48.57	257.850	.644	.909
Q06	48.43	256.343	.588	.909
Q07	48.78	270.137	.317	.914
Q08	48.54	258.222	.600	.909
Q09	48.30	256.656	.611	.909
Q10	48.35	251.967	.729	.907
Q11	48.34	265.733	.335	.914
Q12	48.12	261.379	.430	.912
Q13	49.03	273.229	.325	.913
Q14	48.68	258.542	.663	.909
Q15	47.99	261.827	.382	.914
Q16	48.59	271.398	.234	.915
Q17	48.23	252.714	.694	.907
Q18	47.10	254.560	.560	.910
Q19	48.56	265.082	.445	.912
Q20	48.30	257.582	.575	.910
Q21	46.70	260.103	.396	.914
Q22	48.90	267.523	.552	.911
Q23	48.28	253.539	.653	.908
Q24	48.34	253.855	.659	.908
Q25	48.50	254.570	.689	.908
Q26	48.63	262.212	.545	.910
Q27	48.11	259.620	.486	.911

903, and 0.916, respectively, for the SJ-27 and 0.506, 0.395, and 0.606, respectively, for the SRS-22.

Concurrent and construct validity

A total of 357 out of 384 participants (93.0%) completed both the SJ-27 and the SRS-22 questionnaires. Spearman's correlation coefficient between the SJ-27 and the SRS-22 was 0.692 ($p < 0.001$). Four domains were identified using the three-dimensional components plotted with CATPCA (Fig. 1), but these domains were not as clearly categorized as expected; thus, further analysis was required for spatial relationships between these domains, according to the calculated SJ-27 groupings. The AIC calculation of SJ-27 produced 351 (= ${}_{27}C_2$) "minimal distance" assortments (degree of independence) for the two-item groupings. Among all the 351 AIC pairs, Q2 and Q3 produced the minimum AIC value (– 252.49), indicating this as the best matched pair. The AIC analysis enabled the division of SJ-27 items into five distinct domains: (1) Pain, (2) Discomfort when wearing clothes, (3) Appearance, (4) Cognition, and (5) Participation, with the five domains being interlinked (Fig. 2). Q17 ("To what extent does your appearance in the mirror make you self-conscious?") was centered between domains (2) and (4).

Discussion

A progressive spinal deformity associated with AIS negatively influences a patient's HRQOL by limiting physical ability and causing back pain, mental disorders, and a negative perception of one's body [4–6]. A patient's HRQOL can be determined using patient-reported outcome measures [11] and the SRS scale is currently the gold standard for assessing HRQOL in patients with AIS [16–19, 21]. A Japanese version of the SRS scale has been established, and its reliability and validity were proven [35–38]. However, this scale is thought to be at least partially suboptimal for Japanese patients with AIS

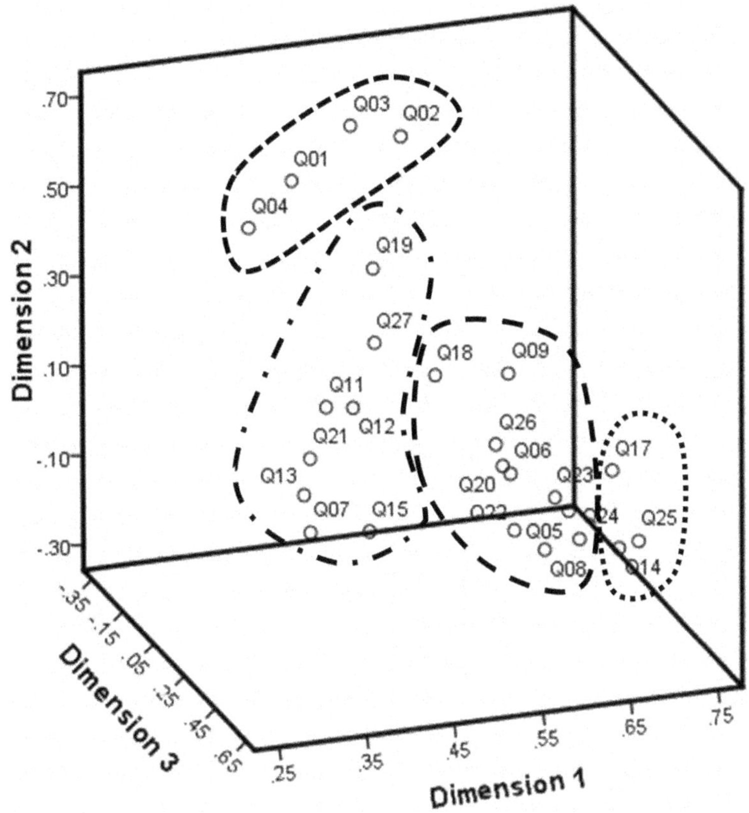

Fig. 1 Three-dimensional graph showing the four question subgroups in the Scoliosis Japanese Questionnaire-27

because of cultural differences. The need for an original, patient-reported outcome measure for Japanese patients resulted in the development of a new instrument by us, the SJ-27.

The percentage of patients who achieved the lowest score in the SJ-27 and the SRS-22 were 0.5% and 0.0%, respectively. The percentage of patients who achieved the highest score in the SJ-27 and the SRS-22 were 0.0% and 0.3%, respectively. These results indicated that there were no floor and ceiling effects associated with the SJ-27 and the SRS-22 according to the widely used definition of this phenomenon. Based on the results of the current assessment, the SJ-27 showed an excellent internal consistency (Cronbach's alpha coefficient, 0.914) and a strong correlation with the SRS-22 (Spearman's correlation efficient, 0.692). With regard to construct validity, the AIC analysis revealed that five distinct domains (Pain, Discomfort when wearing clothes, Appearance, Cognition, and Participation) were identified in the SJ-27 (Fig. 2) and these domains are comparable to the theoretically designed domains originally developed for the SJ-27 questionnaire. These results suggest that the SJ-27 questionnaire covers a wide range of health-related issues, from pain to psychosocial problems. Consequently, our study demonstrates that the SJ-27 questionnaire is a reliable and valid patient-reported outcome measure for female patients with AIS in Japan.

In the formulation of the questions for the SJ-27, we utilized modest and mild expressions, such as that in Q22 ("To what extent do you feel shy or reclusive because of the shape of your spine?"), which reflect the typical modest and reserved characteristics associated with Japanese individuals. These characteristics may also be common in other Eastern countries. Furthermore, we excluded the question on economic burden because of the nature of the Japanese medical insurance system. Accordingly, these considerations may lead to the improved reliability and validity of the SJ-27.

During the development of the SJ-27, we created seven questions regarding scoliosis-related discomfort when wearing clothes or holding bags (Q5–10 and Q27). These items were independently categorized into a distinct domain ("Discomfort when wearing clothes") using AIC analysis (Fig. 2). Furthermore, Cronbach's alpha coefficient upon deletion of each item in the SJ-27 (Table 3) revealed that Q10 ("To what extent are you self-conscious about the curve of your back when wearing lighter clothing in warmer weather?") was a one of the major contributors to its excellent internal consistency. These findings suggest that problems associated with wearing clothes may be

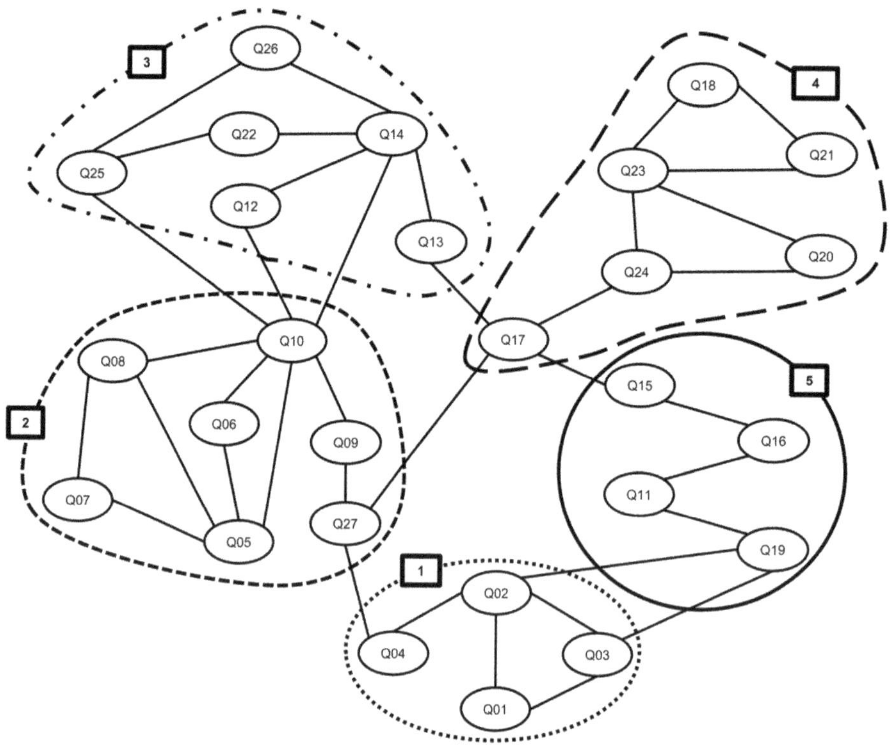

Fig. 2 Akaike's information criterion network for the Scoliosis Japanese Questionnaire-27. Five domains were identified: (1) Pain, (2) Discomfort when wearing clothes, (3) Appearance, (4) Cognition, and (5) Participation

closely associated with the HRQOL in patients with AIS and may be important for young female patients who are likely to have a strong interest in fashion. Moreover, the problems associated with wearing clothes in female patients with AIS may arise from changing their dressing habits to conceal their body deformity. Further studies are warranted to determine whether these problems are crucial for female patients with AIS, relative to controls.

An analysis of the relationships between items in the SJ-27 using the AIC method revealed that Q17 ("To what extent does your appearance in the mirror make you self-conscious?") was centered between domains (2) and (4), indicating that Q17 is a key item for assessing HRQOL in female patients with AIS. These patients usually realize and accept their deformity by observing their body shape in a mirror after being diagnosed with scoliosis or when pointed out by family members or colleagues. We speculate that viewing themselves in mirrors may result in self-image problems among adolescent girls and that these constant visible reminders may negatively influence various aspects of the patient's HRQOL.

The main purpose of using outcome measures is to examine disease clinical severity, determine the proper timing of therapeutic interventions, and choose the most suitable management method for a patient's condition. The SRS scale has often been utilized for making decisions regarding the initiation of treatment and evaluating the effects of therapeutic interventions. In the future, we wish to evaluate the relationship between the total SJ-27 score and scoliosis severity (e.g., a Cobb angle >30°) and determine the SJ-27 threshold influencing the decision to initiate therapeutic interventions, especially surgery.

This study has several limitations. First, the participants included untreated patients and patients treated with various approaches. However, given that each of the top three treatment methods (brace, observation, and surgery) has little influence on the internal consistency of the SJ-27 (Cronbach's alpha coefficient of each treatment group: brace, 0.909; observation, 0.903; surgery, 0. 916), this instrument may be useful for the assessment of HRQOL in patients with AIS regardless of variation in treatment methods. Second, a healthy control group was not included. Hence, further study is required to validate the SJ-27 by comparing the results of the study group with the results of a control group. Third, some institutions had a small number of female patients with AIS (Table 2), which leads to the possibility of selection bias in this study. Fourth, we did not assess for any physical comorbidities among the participants, which may affect the SJ-27 results. Fifth, we did not specify the timing of the questionnaire administration, whether it should be done prior to or after clinical examination. If patients were given questionnaires after clinical examination, the examination results may have a positive or negative impact on the responses. Finally, test-retest reliability, age effect, and severity effect were not evaluated due to the lack of opportunity to repeatedly administer the SJ-27 to the same participants. In future work, we hope to examine the test-retest reliability, age effect, and severity effect of the SJ-27 by employing longitudinal assessment.

Conclusions

Our study demonstrated that the SJ-27, which is a novel patient-reported outcome measure for Japanese female patients with AIS, showed good reliability and validity. Therefore, the SJ-27 could assist clinicians in assessing their female patients and help individuals with spinal deformities understand their health status.

Abbreviations

AIC: Akaike's information criterion; AIS: Adolescent idiopathic scoliosis; CATDAP: Categorical data analysis program; CATPCA: Categorical principal component analysis; HRQOL: Health-related quality of life; SJ-27: Scoliosis Japanese Questionnaire-27; SRS: Scoliosis Research Society

Acknowledgements

The authors thank all the orthopedic surgeons, their staff, and the patients who willingly participated in this study. We especially thank M. Akai (International University of Health and Welfare Graduate School), T. Iwaya (Nagano University of Health and Medicine), and K. Denda (Department of Health Science, School of Medicine, Hokkaido University). This work was supported by the Japanese Society for Musculoskeletal Medicine. The following hospitals and clinics are also greatly appreciated: Okayama Medical Center, Aizu Medical Center, Iwate Medical University Hospital, Gifu University Hospital, Kurume University Hospital, University of Miyazaki Hospital, Kanazawa Medical University Hospital, Keio University Hospital, Hirosaki University Hospital, Hirosaki Memorial Hospital, Saitama Medical University Hospital, Saitama Medical Center, Shiba Clinic, Jikei University Hospital, Akita University Hospital, Juntendo University Hospital, Niigata Spine Surgery Center, Niigata University Medical and Dental Hospital, Gunma Spine Center of Harunaso Hospital, Sendai Nishitaga Hospital, Tokai University Hospital, University of Tokyo Hospital, Hamamatsu University Hospital, and Fukuoka Children's Hospital.

Funding

No funds were received in support of this work.

Authors' contributions

TD 1, HI, and KT designed the research, analyzed data, and wrote the manuscript. YA, OS, and TD 2 designed the research, developed the questionnaire, and supervised the study. KY, KU, and HY designed the research and supervised the study. All authors have read and approved the final manuscript.

Consent for publication

Not applicable.

Competing interests

The authors declare that they no competing interests.

Author details

[1]Department of Orthopaedic Surgery, University of Tokyo, 7-3-1 Hongo, Bunkyo-ku, Tokyo, Japan. [2]Department of Orthopaedic Surgery, Jichi Medical University, 3311-1 Yakushiji, Shimotsuke, Tochigi 329-0498, Japan. [3]Tokyo Metropolitan Rehabilitation Hospital, 2-14-1 Tsutsumidori, Sumida-ku, Tokyo, Japan. [4]Department of Orthopaedic and Spinal Surgery, Aizu Medical Center, Fukushima Medical University, 21-2 Kawahigashimachitanisawa, Aizuwakamatsu, Fukushima, Japan. [5]Shizu Clinic, 1669 Kamishizu, Sakura, Chiba, Japan. [6]Iwate Spinal Scoliosis Center, 103-1 Ogamayoshimizu, Takizawa, Iwate, Japan. [7]Department of Orthopaedic Surgery, National Hospital Organization Kobe Medical Center, 3-1-1 Nishiochiai, Suma-ku, Kobe, Hyogo, Japan. [8]Fukuoka Children's Hospital, 5-1-1 Kashiiteriha, Higashi-ku, Fukuoka, Japan.

References

1. Weinstein SL. Natural history. Spine (Phila Pa 1976). 1999;24(24):2592–600.
2. Roach JW. Adolescent idiopathic scoliosis. Orthop Clin North Am. 1999;30(3): 353–65. vii-viii
3. Ueno M, Takaso M, Nakazawa T, Imura T, Saito W, Shintani R, Uchida K, Fukuda M, Takahashi K, Ohtori S, et al. A 5-year epidemiological study on the prevalence rate of idiopathic scoliosis in Tokyo: school screening of more than 250,000 children. J Orthop Sci. 2011;16(1):1–6.
4. Danielsson AJ, Wiklund I, Pehrsson K, Nachemson AL. Health-related quality of life in patients with adolescent idiopathic scoliosis: a matched follow-up at least 20 years after treatment with brace or surgery. Eur Spine J. 2001; 10(4):278–88.
5. Freidel K, Petermann F, Reichel D, Steiner A, Warschburger P, Weiss HR. Quality of life in women with idiopathic scoliosis. Spine (Phila Pa 1976). 2002;27(4):E87–91.
6. Tones M, Moss N, Polly DW Jr. A review of quality of life and psychosocial issues in scoliosis. Spine (Phila Pa 1976). 2006;31(26):3027–38.
7. Clayson D, Luz-Alterman S, Cataletto MM, Levine DB. Long-term psychological sequelae of surgically versus nonsurgically treated scoliosis. Spine (Phila Pa 1976). 1987;12(10):983–6.
8. Danielsson AJ. What impact does spinal deformity correction for adolescent idiopathic scoliosis make on quality of life? Spine (Phila Pa 1976). 2007;32(19 Suppl):S101–8.
9. Payne WK 3rd, Ogilvie JW, Resnick MD, Kane RL, Transfeldt EE, Blum RW. Does scoliosis have a psychological impact and does gender make a difference? Spine (Phila Pa 1976). 1997;22(12):1380–4.
10. White SF, Asher MA, Lai SM, Burton DC. Patients' perceptions of overall function, pain, and appearance after primary posterior instrumentation and fusion for idiopathic scoliosis. Spine (Phila Pa 1976). 1999;24(16):1693–9. discussion 1699-1700
11. Greenhalgh J. The applications of PROs in clinical practice: what are they, do they work, and why? Qual Life Res. 2009;18(1):115–23.
12. Gagnier JJ, Mullins M, Huang H, Marinac-Dabic D, Ghambaryan A, Eloff B, Mirza F, Bayona M. A systematic review of measurement properties of patient-reported outcome measures used in patients undergoing Total knee arthroplasty. J Arthroplast. 2017;32(5):1688–97.
13. Hunt KJ, Hurwit D. Use of patient-reported outcome measures in foot and ankle research. J Bone Joint Surg Am. 2013;95(16):e118. (111–119)
14. Phillips L, Carsen S, Vasireddi A, Mulpuri K. Use of patient-reported outcome measures in pediatric Orthopaedic literature. J Pediatr Orthop. 2016. https://doi.org/10.1097/BPO.0000000000000847
15. Guzman JZ, Cutler HS, Connolly J, Skovrlj B, Mroz TE, Riew KD, Cho SK. Patient-reported outcome instruments in spine surgery. Spine (Phila Pa 1976). 2016;41(5):429–37.
16. Asher M, Min Lai S, Burton D, Manna B. Discrimination validity of the scoliosis research society-22 patient questionnaire: relationship to idiopathic scoliosis curve pattern and curve size. Spine (Phila Pa 1976). 2003;28(1):74–8.
17. Asher M, Min Lai S, Burton D, Manna B. Scoliosis research society-22 patient questionnaire: responsiveness to change associated with surgical treatment. Spine (Phila Pa 1976). 2003;28(1):70–3.

18. Asher M, Min Lai S, Burton D, Manna B. The reliability and concurrent validity of the scoliosis research society-22 patient questionnaire for idiopathic scoliosis. Spine (Phila Pa 1976). 2003;28(1):63–9.
19. Bridwell KH, Cats-Baril W, Harrast J, Berven S, Glassman S, Farcy JP, Horton WC, Lenke LG, Baldus C, Radake T. The validity of the SRS-22 instrument in an adult spinal deformity population compared with the Oswestry and SF-12: a study of response distribution, concurrent validity, internal consistency, and reliability. Spine (Phila Pa 1976). 2005;30(4):455–61.
20. Haher TR, Gorup JM, Shin TM, Homel P, Merola AA, Grogan DP, Pugh L, Lowe TG, Murray M. Results of the Scoliosis Research Society instrument for evaluation of surgical outcome in adolescent idiopathic scoliosis. A multicenter study of 244 patients. Spine (Phila Pa 1976). 1999;24(14):1435–40.
21. Berven S, Deviren V, Demir-Deviren S, Hu SS, Bradford DS. Studies in the modified Scoliosis Research Society outcomes instrument in adults: validation, reliability, and discriminatory capacity. Spine (Phila Pa 1976). 2003;28(18):2164–9. discussion 2169
22. Asher M, Min Lai S, Glattes C, Burton D, Alanay A, Bago J. Refinement of the SRS-22 health-related quality of life questionnaire function domain. Spine (Phila Pa 1976). 2006;31(5):593–7.
23. Alanay A, Cil A, Berk H, Acaroglu RE, Yazici M, Akcali O, Kosay C, Genc Y, Surat A. Reliability and validity of adapted Turkish version of Scoliosis Research Society-22 (SRS-22) questionnaire. Spine (Phila Pa 1976). 2005; 30(21):2464–8.
24. Antonarakos PD, Katranitsa L, Angelis L, Paganas A, Koen EM, Christodoulou EA, Christodoulou AG. Reliability and validity of the adapted Greek version of scoliosis research society - 22 (SRS-22) questionnaire. Scoliosis. 2009;4:14.
25. Beauséjour M, Joncas J, Goulet L, Roy-Beaudry M, Parent S, Grimard G, Forcier M, Lauriault S, Labelle H. Reliability and validity of adapted French Canadian version of scoliosis research society outcomes questionnaire (SRS-22) in Quebec. Spine (Phila Pa 1976). 2009;34(6):623–8.
26. Cheung KM, Senkoylu A, Alanay A, Genc Y, Lau S, Luk KD. Reliability and concurrent validity of the adapted Chinese version of scoliosis research society-22 (SRS-22) questionnaire. Spine (Phila Pa 1976). 2007;32(10):1141–5.
27. Climent JM, Bago J, Ey A, Perez-Grueso FJ, Izquierdo E. Validity of the Spanish version of the scoliosis research society-22 (SRS-22) patient questionnaire. Spine (Phila Pa 1976). 2005;30(6):705–9.
28. Danielsson AJ, Romberg K. Reliability and validity of the Swedish version of the scoliosis research society-22 (SRS-22r) patient questionnaire for idiopathic scoliosis. Spine (Phila Pa 1976). 2013;38(21):1875–84.
29. Lee JS, Lee DH, Suh KT, Kim JI, Lim JM, Goh TS. Validation of the Korean version of the scoliosis research society-22 questionnaire. Eur Spine J. 2011; 20(10):1751–6.
30. Lonjon G, Ilharreborde B, Odent T, Moreau S, Glorion C, Mazda K. Reliability and validity of the French-Canadian version of the scoliosis research society 22 questionnaire in France. Spine (Phila Pa 1976). 2014;39(1):E26–34.
31. Monticone M, Carabalona R, Negrini S. Reliability of the scoliosis research society-22 patient questionnaire (Italian version) in mild adolescent vertebral deformities. Eura Medicophys. 2004;40(3):191–7.
32. Mousavi SJ, Mobini B, Mehdian H, Akbarnia B, Bouzari B, Askary-Ashtiani A, Montazeri A, Parnianpour M. Reliability and validity of the persian version of the scoliosis research society-22r questionnaire. Spine (Phila Pa 1976). 2010; 35(7):784–9.
33. Niemeyer T, Schubert C, Halm HF, Herberts T, Leichtle C, Gesicki M. Validity and reliability of an adapted german version of scoliosis research society-22 questionnaire. Spine (Phila Pa 1976). 2009;34(8):818–21.
34. Sathira-Angkura V, Pithankuakul K, Sakulpipatana S, Piyaskulkaew C, Kunakornsawat S. Validity and reliability of an adapted Thai version of scoliosis research society-22 questionnaire for adolescent idiopathic scoliosis. Spine (Phila Pa 1976). 2012;37(9):783–7.
35. Watanabe K, Hasegawa K, Hirano T, Uchiyama S, Endo N. Use of the scoliosis research society outcomes instrument to evaluate patient outcome in untreated idiopathic scoliosis patients in Japan: part II: relation between spinal deformity and patient outcomes. Spine (Phila Pa 1976). 2005;30(10):1202–5.
36. Watanabe K, Hasegawa K, Hirano T, Uchiyama S, Endo N. Use of the scoliosis research society outcomes instrument to evaluate patient outcome in untreated idiopathic scoliosis patients in Japan: part I: comparison with nonscoliosis group: preliminary/limited review in a Japanese population. Spine (Phila Pa 1976). 2005;30(10):1197–201.
37. Watanabe K, Lenke LG, Bridwell KH, Hasegawa K, Hirano T, Endo N, Cheh G, Kim YJ, Hensley M, Stobbs G, et al. Cross-cultural comparison of the scoliosis research society outcomes instrument between American and Japanese idiopathic scoliosis patients: are there differences? Spine (Phila Pa 1976). 2007;32(24):2711–4.
38. Hashimoto H, Sase T, Arai Y, Maruyama T, Isobe K, Shouno Y. Validation of a Japanese version of the scoliosis research society-22 patient questionnaire among idiopathic scoliosis patients in Japan. Spine (Phila Pa 1976). 2007; 32(4):E141–6.
39. Clayson D, Levine DB. Adolescent scoliosis patients. Personality patterns and effects of corrective surgery. Clin Orthop Relat Res. 1976;116:99–102.
40. Daniel WW. Biostatistics: a foundation for analysis in the health sciences. 7th ed. New York: John Wiley & Sons; 1999.
41. McHorney CA, Tarlov AR. Individual-patient monitoring in clinical practice: are available health status surveys adequate? Qual Life Res. 1995;4(4):293–307.
42. Terwee CB, Bot SD, de Boer MR, van der Windt DA, Knol DL, Dekker J, Bouter LM, de Vet HC. Quality criteria were proposed for measurement properties of health status questionnaires. J Clin Epidemiol. 2007;60(1):34–42.
43. Streiner DL, Norman GR. Health measurement scales: a practical guide to their development and use. 4th ed. Oxford: Oxford University Press; 2008.
44. Akaike H. Information theory and an extension of the maximum likelihood principle. In: Petrov B, Caski F, editors. The Second International Symposium on Information Theory 1973. Budapest: Akadémiai Kiadó; 1976. p. 267–81.
45. Wagenmakers EJ, Farrell S. AIC model selection using Akaike weights. Psychon Bull Rev. 2004;11(1):192–6.
46. Sakamoto Y. Appendix: FORTRAN program CATDAP-02. In: Sakamoto Y, editor. Categorical data analysis by AIC. Tokyo: KTK Scientific Publishers and Kluwer Academic Publishers; 1991. p. 163–206.

Permissions

All chapters in this book were first published in MD, by BioMed Central; hereby published with permission under the Creative Commons Attribution License or equivalent. Every chapter published in this book has been scrutinized by our experts. Their significance has been extensively debated. The topics covered herein carry significant findings which will fuel the growth of the discipline. They may even be implemented as practical applications or may be referred to as a beginning point for another development.

The contributors of this book come from diverse backgrounds, making this book a truly international effort. This book will bring forth new frontiers with its revolutionizing research information and detailed analysis of the nascent developments around the world.

We would like to thank all the contributing authors for lending their expertise to make the book truly unique. They have played a crucial role in the development of this book. Without their invaluable contributions this book wouldn't have been possible. They have made vital efforts to compile up to date information on the varied aspects of this subject to make this book a valuable addition to the collection of many professionals and students.

This book was conceptualized with the vision of imparting up-to-date information and advanced data in this field. To ensure the same, a matchless editorial board was set up. Every individual on the board went through rigorous rounds of assessment to prove their worth. After which they invested a large part of their time researching and compiling the most relevant data for our readers.

The editorial board has been involved in producing this book since its inception. They have spent rigorous hours researching and exploring the diverse topics which have resulted in the successful publishing of this book. They have passed on their knowledge of decades through this book. To expedite this challenging task, the publisher supported the team at every step. A small team of assistant editors was also appointed to further simplify the editing procedure and attain best results for the readers.

Apart from the editorial board, the designing team has also invested a significant amount of their time in understanding the subject and creating the most relevant covers. They scrutinized every image to scout for the most suitable representation of the subject and create an appropriate cover for the book.

The publishing team has been an ardent support to the editorial, designing and production team. Their endless efforts to recruit the best for this project, has resulted in the accomplishment of this book. They are a veteran in the field of academics and their pool of knowledge is as vast as their experience in printing. Their expertise and guidance has proved useful at every step. Their uncompromising quality standards have made this book an exceptional effort. Their encouragement from time to time has been an inspiration for everyone.

The publisher and the editorial board hope that this book will prove to be a valuable piece of knowledge for researchers, students, practitioners and scholars across the globe.

List of Contributors

U. Flodin, B. Krapi and F. Nyqvist
Occupational and Environmental Medicine, and Department of Clinical and Experimental Medicine, Linköping University, Östergötland, 581 85 Linköping, Sweden

B. Rolander
Department of Behavioral Science and Social Work, School of Health Sciences, Jönköping University, Jönköping, Sweden
Futurum, Academy for Health and Care, Region Jönköping County, Jönköping, Sweden

H. Löfgren
Neuro-Orthopedic Center, Ryhov Hospital, Jönköping, Sweden

C. Wåhlin
Occupational and Environmental Medicine, and Department of Clinical and Experimental Medicine, Linköping University, Östergötland, 581 85 Linköping, Sweden
Unit of Intervention and Implementation Research, Institute for Environmental Medicine, Karolinska Institutet, Stockholm, Sweden

Carole Fortin and Isabelle Leclair
Research Centre, Sainte-Justine University Hospital Centre, 3175 chemin de la Côte-Sainte-Catherine, Montreal, Quebec H3T 1C5, Canada
School of rehabilitation, Faculty of Medicine, University of Montreal, 2900 Edouard-Montpetit, Montreal, Quebec H3T 1J4, Canada

Benedito Felipe Rabay Pimentel
Division of Hand Surgery and Upper Limb, Discipline of Orthopaedics and Traumatology, Paraiba Valley Regional Hospital and Taubaté University Hospital, University of Taubaté, 239 Francisco de Barros, Taubaté, São Paulo, Brazil

Flávio Faloppa, Marcel Jun Sugawara Tamaoki and João Carlos Belloti
Division of Hand Surgery and Upper Limb, Department of Orthopedics and Traumatology, Federal University of São Paulo, Paulista School of Medicine, 786 Borges Lagoa, São Paulo, São Paulo Brazil

Melina Dritsaki
Oxford Clinical Trials Research Unit, Nuffield Department of Orthopaedics, Rheumatology and Musculoskeletal Sciences, University of Oxford, Oxford OX3 7LD, UK

Oliver Rivero-Arias
National Perinatal Epidemiology Unit (NPEU), Nuffield Department of Population Health, University of Oxford, Oxford OX3 7LF, UK

Alastair Gray
Health Economics Research Centre, Nuffield Department of Population Health, University of Oxford, Oxford OX3 7LF, UK

Catherine Ball and Jagdeep Nanchahal
Kennedy Institute of Rheumatology, Nuffield Department of Orthopaedics, Rheumatology and Musculoskeletal Sciences, University of Oxford, Oxford OX3 7FY, UK

Carl-Éric Aubin
Department of Mechanical Engineering, École Polytechnique de Montréal, Downtown Station, Station "Centre-ville", Montreal, Quebec H3C 3A7, Canada
Research Centre, Sainte-Justine University Hospital Centre, 3175 chemin de la Côte-Sainte-Catherine, Montreal, Quebec H3T 1C5, Canada
School of rehabilitation, Faculty of Medicine, University of Montreal, 2900 Edouard-Montpetit, Montreal, Quebec H3T 1J4, Canada

Guo Chen
Department of Orthopaedic Surgery, West China Hospital, Sichuan University, N0.37 Guoxue Road, Chengdu, Sichuan Province 610041, China
Department of Orthopaedic Surgery, the Affiliated Hospital of North Sichuan Medical College, No. 63 Wenhua Road, Nanchong, Sichuan Province 637000, China

Xian-di Wang, Hong-fei Nie, Zhi-qiang Yang, Kang Chen, Zhu-hai Li, Yue-ming Song, Fu-xing Pei and Jian-cheng Zeng
Department of Orthopaedic Surgery, West China Hospital, Sichuan University, N0.37 Guoxue Road, Chengdu, Sichuan Province 610041, China

Irena Kovačević
University of Applied Health Sciences, Mlinarska 38, 10 000 Zagreb, Croatia

Višnja Majerić Kogler
School of Medicine, University of Zagreb, Šalata 3, Zagreb, Croatia

Tihana Magdić Turković, Lidija Fumić Dunkić and Željko Ivanec
Sisters of Charity University Hospital Centre, Vinogradska cesta 29, Zagreb, Croatia

Davorina Petek
Department of Family Medicine, Faculty of Medicine, University of Ljubljana, Poljanski nasip 58, 1000 Ljubljana, Slovenia

Maciej J. K. Simon
Department of Orthopedics, University Medical Center Hamburg-Eppendorf, Martinistrasse 52, 20246 Hamburg, Germany
Department of Osteology and Biomechanics, University Medical Center Hamburg-Eppendorf, Martinistrasse 52, 20246 Hamburg, Germany
Spinal Surgery Center, Schön Klink Neustadt, Am Kiebitzberg 10, 23730 Neustadt in Holstein, Germany

Henry F. H. Halm and Markus Quante
Spinal Surgery Center, Schön Klink Neustadt, Am Kiebitzberg 10, 23730 Neustadt in Holstein, Germany

Sang Ho Kwak, Seung-Jun Lee, Min Uk Do and Kuen Tak Suh
Department of Orthopaedic Surgery, Pusan National University Yangsan Hospital, Pusan National University School of Medicine, 20, Geumo-ro, Mulgeum-eup, Yangsan-si, Gyeongsangnam-do, Republic of Korea

Hee Seok Jeong
Department of Radiology, Pusan National University Yangsan Hospital, Pusan National University School of Medicine, 20, Geumo-ro, Mulgeum-eup, Yangsan-si, Gyeongsangnam-do, Republic of Korea

Hao Wang and Weitao Jin
Department of Orthopaedics, Beijing Tiantan Hospital, Capital Medical University, 6 TiantanXili, Dongcheng District, Beijing 100050, China

Haibin Li
Department of Epidemiology and Biostatistics, School of Public Health, Capital Medical University, Beijing 100069, China

Qi Lai, Tian Gao, Xin Lv, Xuqiang Liu, Zongmiao Wan, Min Dai, Bin Zhang and Tao Nie
Department of Orthopedics, The First Affiliated Hospital of Nanchang University, Artificial Joints Engineering and Technology Research Center of Jiangxi Province, Nanchang, Jiangxi 330006, People's Republic of China

Rong Xing, Wangmi Liu, Xilei Li, Libo Jiang, Mumingjiang Yishakea and Jian Dong
Department of Orthopaedic Surgery, Zhongshan Hospital, Fudan University, 180 Fenglin Road, Shanghai 200032, China

Heidi Arponen
Department of Oral and Maxillofacial Diseases, University of Helsinki, FI-00014 Helsinki, Finland

Janna Waltimo-Sirén
Department of Oral and Maxillofacial Diseases, University of Helsinki, FI-00014 Helsinki, Finland
Department of Oral and Maxillofacial Diseases, Helsinki University Hospital, Helsinki, Finland

Helena Valta
Children's Hospital, University of Helsinki and Helsinki University Hospital, Helsinki, Finland

Outi Mäkitie
Children's Hospital, University of Helsinki and Helsinki University Hospital, Helsinki, Finland
Folkhälsan Research Center, Helsinki, Finland
Center for Molecular Medicine, Karolinska Institutet, and Department of Clinical Genetics, Karolinska University Hospital, Stockholm, Sweden

Daniela Converso, Sara Viotti, Ilaria Sottimano and Gloria Guidetti
Department of Psychology, University of Turin, Via Giuseppe Verdi 8, 10124 Turin, Italy

Vincenza Cascio
ASL TO1, Turin, Italy

Giuseppe Salvatore, Alessandra Berton, Mauro Ciuffreda, Pino Florio, Umile Giuseppe Longo and Vincenzo Denaro
Department of Orthopaedic and Trauma Surgery, Campus Bio-Medico University, Via Alvaro del Portillo, 200, 00128 Trigoria, Rome, Italy

Hugo Giambini, Andrew Thoreson and Kai-Nan An
Biomechanics Laboratory, Division of Orthopaedic Research, Mayo Clinic, Rochester, MN, USA

Xinjie Wu and Mingsheng Tan
Department of Spinal Surgery, China-Japan Friendship Hospital, Beijing 100029, People's Republic of China
Graduate School of Peking Union Medical College, Beijing 100730, People's Republic of China

Yingna Qi
Department of Spinal Surgery, China-Japan Friendship Hospital, Beijing 100029, People's Republic of China
Graduate School of Beijing University of Chinese Medicine, Beijing 100029, People's Republic of China

Ping Yi, Feng Yang, Xiangsheng Tang and Qingying Hao
Department of Spinal Surgery, China-Japan Friendship Hospital, Beijing 100029, People's Republic of China

Qiuliang Zhu, Bin Xu, Jinzhu Lv and Maohua Yan
Department of Orthopedics, People's Hospital of Anji, Zhejiang 313000, China

Wenhao Hu, Xuesong Zhang, Fanqi Hu, Hao Zhang and Yan Wang
The Department of Orthopedics, Chinese PLA General Hospital, Fuxing Rd. 28, Haidian District, Beijing, China

Jiayi Yu
Department of Renal cancer and Melanoma, Peking University Cancer Hospital, Fucheng Rd. 28, Haidian District, Beijing, China

Akinobu Nishimura
Departments of Orthopaedic Surgery, Mie University Graduate School of Medicine, 2-174 Edobashi, Tsu City, Mie 514-8507, Japan
Departments of Orthopaedic and Sports Medicine, Mie University Graduate School of Medicine, Tsu City 514-8507, Mie, Japan

Naoya Ito and Akihiro Sudo
Departments of Orthopaedic Surgery, Mie University Graduate School of Medicine, 2-174 Edobashi, Tsu City, Mie 514-8507, Japan

Shigeto Nakazora and Ko Kato
Department of Orthopaedic Surgery, Suzuka Kaisei Hospital, Suzuka City 513-8505, Mie, Japan

Toru Ogura
Clinical Research Support Center, Mie University Hospital, 2-174 Edobashi, Tsu City, Mie 514-8507, Japan

Jeffrey R. Cooley, Bruce F. Walker and Emad M. Ardakani
School of Health Professions, Murdoch University, 90 South Street, Murdoch, Western Australia 6150, Australia

Per Kjaer
Department of Sports Science and Clinical Biomechanics, University of Southern Denmark, Campusvej 55, 5230, Odense M, DK, Denmark

Tue S. Jensen
Spine Centre of Southern Denmark, Ostre Hougvej 55, 5500 Middelfart, DK, Denmark
Nordic Institute of Chiropractic and Clinical Biomechanics, Campusvej 55, 5230 Odense M, DK, Denmark

Jeffrey J. Hebert
Faculty of Kinesiology, University of New Brunswick, 3 Bailey Drive, Fredericton, New Brunswick E3B 5A3, Canada
School of Psychology and Exercise Science, Murdoch University, 90 South Street, Murdoch, Western Australia 6150, Australia

Yen-Ting Cho and Wen-Yen Hsu
Department of Physical Medicine and Rehabilitation, Wan Fang Hospital, Taipei Medical University, No.111, Hsing-Long Road, Section 3, Taipei 116, Taiwan

Li-Fong Lin
Department of Physical Medicine and Rehabilitation, Shuang-Ho Hospital, Taipei Medical University, New Taipei City, Taiwan

Yen-Nung Lin
Department of Physical Medicine and Rehabilitation, Wan Fang Hospital, Taipei Medical University, No.111, Hsing-Long Road, Section 3, Taipei 116, Taiwan
Graduate Institute of Injury Prevention and Control, Taipei Medical University, Taipei, Taiwan

Hailey C. Cunningham
Biomedical Engineering Graduate Group, University of California Davis, Davis, CA, USA

Daniel W. D. West and Leslie M. Baehr
Department of Physiology & Membrane Biology, University of California Davis, Davis, CA, USA

Franklin D. Tarke
Department of Orthopaedic Surgery, University of California Davis Medical Center, Lawrence J. Ellison Musculoskeletal Research Center, 4635 2nd Avenue, Suite 2000, Sacramento, CA 95817, USA

Keith Baar
Biomedical Engineering Graduate Group, University of California Davis, Davis, CA, USA
Department of Physiology & Membrane Biology, University of California Davis, Davis, CA, USA
Department of Neurobiology, Physiology, and Behavior, University of California Davis, Davis, CA, USA

Sue C. Bodine
Department of Physiology & Membrane Biology, University of California Davis, Davis, CA, USA
Department of Neurobiology, Physiology, and Behavior, University of California Davis, Davis, CA, USA

Blaine A. Christiansen
Biomedical Engineering Graduate Group, University of California Davis, Davis, CA, USA
Department of Orthopaedic Surgery, University of California Davis Medical Center, Lawrence J. Ellison Musculoskeletal Research Center, 4635 2nd Avenue, Suite 2000, Sacramento, CA 95817, USA

Tai-Hua Yang, Anne Gingery, Andrew R. Thoreson and Chunfeng Zhao
Biomechanics & Tendon and Soft Tissue Biology Laboratory, Division of Orthopedic Research, Rochester, USA

Dirk R. Larson
Division of Biomedical Statistics and Informatics, Department of Health Science Research, Mayo Clinic, Rochester, MN 55905, USA

Peter C. Amadio
Biomechanics & Tendon and Soft Tissue Biology Laboratory, Division of Orthopedic Research, Rochester, USA
Tendon and Soft Tissue Biology Laboratory, Division of Orthopedic Research, Mayo Clinic, 200 First Street SW, Rochester, MN 55905, USA

Sarah Dupuis and Christiane Caouette
Department of Mechanical Engineering, École Polytechnique de Montréal, Downtown Station, Station "Centre-ville", Montreal, Quebec H3C 3A7, Canada
Research Centre, Sainte-Justine University Hospital Centre, 3175 chemin de la Côte-Sainte-Catherine, Montreal, Quebec H3T 1C5, Canada

Toru Doi
Department of Orthopaedic Surgery, University of Tokyo, 7-3-1 Hongo, Bunkyo-ku, Tokyo, Japan

Hirokazu Inoue and Katsushi Takeshita
Department of Orthopaedic Surgery, Jichi Medical University, 3311-1 Yakushiji, Shimotsuke, Tochigi 329-0498, Japan

Yasuhisa Arai
Tokyo Metropolitan Rehabilitation Hospital, 2-14-1 Tsutsumidori, Sumida-ku, Tokyo, Japan

Osamu Shirado
Department of Orthopaedic and Spinal Surgery, Aizu Medical Center, Fukushima Medical University, 21-2 Kawahigashimachitanisawa, Aizuwakamatsu, Fukushima, Japan

Tokuhide Doi
Shizu Clinic, 1669 Kamishizu, Sakura, Chiba, Japan

Ken Yamazaki
Iwate Spinal Scoliosis Center, 103-1 Ogamayoshimizu, Takizawa, Iwate, Japan

Koki Uno
Department of Orthopaedic Surgery, National Hospital Organization Kobe Medical Center, 3-1-1 Nishiochiai, Suma-ku, Kobe, Hyogo, Japan

Haruhisa Yanagida
Fukuoka Children's Hospital, 5-1-1 Kashiiteriha, Higashi-ku, Fukuoka, Japan

Index

CPSIA information can be obtained
at www.ICGtesting.com
Printed in the USA
LVHW060901030122
707669LV00002B/286

9 781639 273928